Midwives, Research and Childbirth

VOLUME 3

Midwives, Research and Childbirth

VOLUME 3

Edited by

Sarah Robinson

Senior Research Fellow, Nursing Research Unit
King's College, London

and

Ann M. Thomson

Senior Lecturer in Midwifery, School of Nursing Studies,
University of Manchester/Director, Health Care Research Unit,
Stockport, Tameside & Glossop College of Nursing

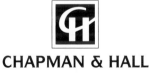

CHAPMAN & HALL

London · Glasgow · New York · Tokyo · Melbourne · Madras

Published by Chapman & Hall, 2–6 Boundary Row, London SE1 8HN, UK

Chapman & Hall, 2–6 Boundary Row, London SE1 8HN, UK

Blackie Academic & Professional, Wester Cleddens Road, Bishopbriggs, Glasgow G64 2NZ, UK

Chapman & Hall Inc., One Penn Plaza, 41st Floor, New York, NY10119, USA

Chapman & Hall Japan, Thomson Publishing Japan, Hirakawacho Nemoto Building, 6F, 1-7-11 Hirakawa-cho, Chiyoda-ku, Tokyo 102, Japan

Chapman & Hall Australia, Thomas Nelson Australia, 102 Dodds Street, South Melbourne, Victoria 3205, Australia

Chapman & Hall India, R. Seshadri, 32 Second Main Road, CIT East, Madras 600 035, India

Distributed in the USA and Canada by Singular Publishing Group Inc., 4284 41st Street, San Diego, California 92105

First edition 1994

© 1994 Chapman & Hall

Typeset in 9.5/11 pt Times Roman by Best-set Typesetter Ltd., Hong Kong
Printed and bound in Great Britain by Hartnolls Ltd

ISBN 0 412 34800 4   0 56593 043 6 (USA)

Contents

Preface

This volume is the third in a series which brings together studies of particular relevance to the care provided by midwives for childbearing women and their families. The series is intended primarily for midwives but we hope that other health professionals involved in the maternity services, as well as those who use the services, will also find the series interesting and useful.

In undertaking this venture we have been fortunate in the support received from colleagues, friends and family. In particular we would like to thank the following: Rosemary Morris, Senior Editor, Health Sciences at Chapman and Hall; all the authors who have contributed to the series; colleagues at both the Nursing Research Unit, London University and the Department of Nursing Studies, Manchester University; and Paul and Rachel Robinson.

Sarah Robinson, *London*
Ann M. Thomson, *Manchester*
March 1993

Contributors

Vanessa Coupland Formerly Research Assistant, Centre for Family Research, University of Cambridge, now a Social Worker, Cambridge

Josephine Green Senior Research Associate, Centre for Family Research, University of Cambridge

Susan A. Kirk Research Associate, Department of Nursing, Liverpool University

Jenny Kitzinger Researcher, Medical Research Council, Medical Sociology Unit, Glasgow

Valerie Levy Principal Lecturer in Midwifery Studies, Institute of Advanced Nursing Education, Royal College of Nursing, London

Rosemary Mander Lecturer, Department of Nursing Studies, University of Edinburgh

Tricia Murphy-Black Research and Development Adviser, Simpson Memorial Maternity Pavilion/Honorary Lecturer, Department of Nursing Studies, University of Edinburgh

Catherine Niven Reader in Psychology, Glasgow Caledonian University

Ann Oakley Director, Social Science Research Unit, Institute of Education, University of London

Contributors

Heather Owen

Formerly Research Associate, Nursing Research Unit, King's College, University of London

Nancy Radford

Formerly Research Fellow, Department of Educational Studies, University of Surrey

Sarah Robinson

Senior Research Fellow, Nursing Research Unit, King's College, University of London

Anne Thompson

Senior Lecturer in Midwifery Studies, Department of Education, Royal College of Midwives, London

Ann M. Thomson

Senior Lecturer in Midwifery, Department of Nursing, University of Manchester/Director, Health Care Research Unit, Stockport, Tameside & Glossop College of Nursing

CHAPTER ONE

Introduction

Sarah Robinson and Ann M. Thomson

As stated in the introductory chapters to Volumes 1 and 2, this series is based on the premise that midwives in Britain are qualified to provide care on their own responsibility throughout pregnancy, labour and the puerperium, to recognize those signs of abnormality that require referral to medical staff, and to provide advice, information and support from early pregnancy to the end of the postnatal period. This is a wide remit and means that in order to function effectively the midwife requires an extensive range of knowledge and skills. This in turn necessitates a high standard of educational preparation for the first level qualification and in relation to continuing education opportunities thereafter. Moreover, if the midwifery component of maternity care is to be effective, then the health service must provide a career structure and conditions of service that encourage recruitment to and retention in the profession, and the maternity services must be organized in a way that enables midwives to deploy their skills to the full.

The aim of the series is to bring together research relevant to these three components of the profession: practice, education and management. We have also included studies of women's views about childbirth and their experiences of the maternity services, as these often have implications for midwifery practice and education. As in the two previous volumes we have included recently reported studies as well as those which are a little older. This has been done for two reasons: firstly some of the older studies are not readily accessible to all midwives and we hope that by bringing them together in a series such as this they will be more readily accessible than hitherto; secondly we stated in Volume 1 that we hoped this series would constitute a comprehensive record of research in this area, to exclude some studies because they are relatively old would defeat that object. There is another reason for having a record of the research that impinges on practice, education and/or management. For a profession to progress there is a need to understand the past so that it can have a view of where it came from. It is only when this view is available that a profession is able to move forward into the future.

Each volume contains only ten studies. This is in order to give authors sufficient scope to review the literature relevant to their area of study, and to write in some detail about their choice of research strategy as well as presenting their findings. For two reasons we rejected an approach that brought together studies pertaining, for example, to antenatal care in one volume, labour in another, and education in a third. In our view such an approach is at odds philosophically with the holistic way in which midwifery should be developing, and indeed is doing with initiatives such as 'team midwifery'. Moreover, many studies do not fit neatly into one category or another; they encompass, for example, care in pregnancy, labour and the postnatal period or relate to experiences of education as well as to subsequent careers.

This volume, like Volumes 1 and 2, demonstrates the wide range of aspects of midwifery that have been the subject of research. Six of the chapters are concerned with midwifery practice. Antenatal care is represented by Ann Oakley's study of the effect of social support during pregnancy provided by midwives for women who have had a previous low birthweight baby (Chapter 3), and by Sue Kirk's study of women who have been hospitalized during pregnancy (Chapter 4). Two chapters focus on labour and delivery; Catherine Niven's work on factors that may modulate pain in labour (Chapter 5) and Ann Thomson's review of several small scale studies on various aspects of care during labour (Chapter 11). Tricia Murphy-Black's chapter is concerned with the extent to which care provided by community midwives meets women's physical, educational and psychosocial needs (Chapter 6), and Valerie Levy reports on a study of the maternity blues and the extent to which this phenomenon exists among postoperative patients (Chapter 7). The second chapter, by Josephine Green and her colleagues, examines the extent to which the level of clinical responsibility exercised by midwives is affected by medical staffing structures, and the relationship that this may have to women's expectations and experiences of childbirth. The division of responsibility between midwives and medical staff is a continuing theme in the series, as represented by Robinson's work in Volume 1 and that of Garcia and Garforth in Volume 2.

Midwifery education is the subject of two chapters in this volume. Rosemary Mander studied the effect of introducing the 18 month post-registration midwifery course in Scotland on students' reasons for entering the course and their confidence and employment intentions upon its completion. The findings from this study plus those from a similar one undertaken in England and Wales (see Robinson in Volume 2) contributed to the decision to introduce pre-registration midwifery education. However, progress to implement these new courses was slow and Radford and

Thompson (Chapter 10) were commissioned to investigate factors affecting the feasibility of direct entry courses. Whatever the route to midwifery education, midwives' careers encompass a variety of professional and personal circumstances, and Robinson and Owen (Chapter 8) present findings from a longitudinal study of events and experiences after qualification.

Although the studies included all relate to midwifery in some way, the authors comprised both midwives (Chapters 4, 6, 7, 9, 10 and 11) and social scientists (Chapters 2, 3, 5, 7, 8 and 10). It is appropriate that all aspects of midwifery are researched by people from a variety of backgrounds, as this enables the knowledge, skills and perspectives of different disciplines to be brought to bear on the problems. There is another advantage: Niven (Chapter 5) found that one of the most important factors which was significantly associated with lower levels of pain in labour was 'trusting the (midwifery) staff'. If a midwife had discovered this it could have been suggested that the midwife had biased the study so that this had been found. The fact that a psychologist found this, and not only had not set out to find this but appeared pleasantly surprised by the finding, is evidence that can be used when midwives are demonstrating the need for an adequately staffed midwifery service.

As well as encompassing a wide range of subjects, the studies in this volume also demonstrate the range of methods appropriate to the study of midwifery. Randomized controlled trials feature in the study of social support in pregnancy (Chapter 3) and in the studies evaluating the birthing chair (Chapter 11). It is not always possible to control a situation such that a randomized controlled trial can be undertaken. In these circumstances researchers have to be content with the less rigorous method of a quasi-experiment and in this volume there are three chapters which report studies using this method. They are the study of the effect of midwives' responsibilities of differing medical staffing structures (Chapter 2), the postnatal blues study (Chapter 7) and the report on the study of management of the third stage of labour (Chapter 11). Surveys have been undertaken to investigate the needs of women admitted to hospital in pregnancy (Chapter 4), pain in labour (Chapter 5), postnatal care in the community (Chapter 6), career patterns of midwives (Chapter 8), midwifery education (Chapters 9 and 10) and women's reactions to caesarean delivery (Chapter 11). Whilst all the studies reported in this volume used research instruments which were designed by the researchers for specific use within that study, some of the chapter authors also used research instruments which had been used in previous studies. Sue Kirk used the Antenatal Hospital Stressors Inventory (Chapter 4); Catherine Niven used the Visual Analogue Scale and McGill Pain Questionnaire (Chapter 5); Tricia Murphy-Black used the Nottingham Health Care Profile in investigating care at home in the postnatal period (Chapter 6); Valerie Levy used Stein's Daily Scoring System to investigate the presence of maternity blues

(Chapter 7); and Ruth Kirchmeier adapted two existing questionnaires in her study of women's reaction to caesarean delivery (Chapter 11). Some of the studies have relatively small samples (Chapters 4, 5, 7, 11) but that does not mean that the findings have no relevance for the midwifery profession. For example Sue Kirk found that one of the major problems for women admitted to hospital in pregnancy is 'boredom'. 'Boredom' has also been associated with an increase in the number of cigarettes smoked by women admitted to hospital in pregnancy (Salariya, 1986; Thomson, 1993). Whilst all three studies had samples of 50 or less there is plenty of anecdotal evidence that women are bored when admitted to hospital during pregnancy and a study investigating the alleviation of this problem is long overdue.

1992 in the UK saw the publication of a very important report on the provision of maternity services – the Winterton Report (House of Commons Select Committee, 1992). Throughout the report there are constant statements on the need to provide care which has been shown to be effective, and some of the recommendations are to research that has been published in this series. For example Bryar (Chapter 3, Volume 2) reported on her study of individualized care in midwifery; Flint described her research into the provision of team midwifery so that women experienced continuity of care (Chapter 4, Volume 2); Thomson described her research into the factors which affected a woman's choice on how she would feed her baby (Chapter 11, Volume 1). The report also recommends that maternity care should be organized in a way that enables the midwife to practise with a greater degree of autonomy than in recent decades, as this will be to the benefit of childbearing women. If midwives are to have the kind of role that the Committee envisaged, then practice and education must be underpinned by high quality research. A number of developments attest to the fact that midwifery research in the UK is firmly established: the growing volume of research as demonstrated by MIRIAD, by collections of research studies such as the series of which this volume is a part, the wide uptake of MIDIRS, by research conferences and study days and an increased willingness by the profession to base practice, education and management on research findings.

REFERENCES

House of Commons Select Committee (1992) Sessions 1991–1992, Second Report. *Maternity Services*. (Chairman: Nicholas Winterton) Vol. 1. HMSO, London.

Salariya, E.M. (1986) A study of smoking habits and attitudes of women in a maternity unit. *Health Bulletin*, **44**, 22–8.

Thomson, A.M. (1993) If you are pregnant and smoke admission to hospital may damage your baby's health. *Journal of Clinical Nursing*, **2**(2), 111–20.

CHAPTER TWO

Midwives' responsibilities, medical staffing structures and women's choice in childbirth

Josephine Green, Jenny Kitzinger
and Vanessa Coupland

INTRODUCTION

The traditional pattern of medical staffing in British hospitals has three tiers. At the bottom is the senior house officer (SHO), the majority of whom are general practitioner (GP) trainees doing an obligatory six months in obstetrics and gynaecology before moving on, maybe never to deliver a baby again. At the top is the consultant, often a remote policy maker who is rarely seen on the labour ward. In the middle is the registrar, the lynchpin of the system, doing everything that the SHO cannot do and the consultant does not want to do.

This chapter starts with some research describing what happens when the registrar grade is removed, leaving just a two-tier hierarchy of consultants and SHOs – and, of course, midwives. The idea of working this way came from the House of Commons Social Services Committee in their second and fourth reports in 1980 and 1981. The restructuring, which was to include doubling the number of consultant posts, was intended primarily as a solution to the career difficulties faced by junior doctors. However it was also argued that improved quality of care would result because more direct patient care would be given by consultants.

The Committee's proposals, although accepted by the Government, were not met with enthusiasm by consultants, as the letters pages of the *British Medical Journal* showed at the time. Nevertheless, one new district hospital opened in 1983 with a medical staffing structure that reflected these proposed changes. Its obstetric staff consisted of four consultants, three SHOs and no registrars, for a projected 2000 deliveries per year. Our initial brief was to assess the implications of this staffing structure for doctors and midwives. Phase 1 of our study therefore set out to examine midwives' and doctors' roles and relationships in this and two other units working without registrars, and also in three traditionally staffed units that served as a comparison. Phase 2, which is described in the second half of the chapter, looked at the expectations and experiences of women delivering in four of these hospitals.

PHASE 1. EFFECTS OF STAFFING STRUCTURES: METHODS

The six hospitals were located in three different National Health Service Regions in the south-east of England. All served semi-rural districts centred on towns in which the major sources of employment were light industry, service industries, agriculture or the Armed Forces. No inner city areas were included although two of the towns had sizeable ethnic minority populations, mainly Asian and Italian. We deliberately avoided teaching hospitals, which is where most reported research is carried out, choosing instead smaller District hospitals. These are the hospitals most likely to be affected by the new staffing proposals and are also where the majority of babies in this country are born.

The focus of our interest was the labour ward and the majority of our data comes from two sources: observation and interviews. We spent over 400 hours in the hospitals, and nearly half of this time was at nights and weekends when we expected that the absence of a resident senior doctor would be most noticeable. Only one of us would be present at any one time, and we usually positioned ourselves near the central desk where most interactions and comings and goings could easily be observed. We did not intrude into delivery rooms. Staff were, on the whole, very tolerant of our presence – the greater the acceptance the more likely we were to be absorbed as an extra pair of unskilled hands when things were busy.

All 18 consultants in the six hospitals were interviewed as well as 30 SHOs and registrars. These interviews were generally prearranged. Arranging appointments to interview midwives, however, was not so easy since the volume of work in labour wards is so unpredictable. Instead, we would arrange to be present on the labour ward on a particular day (or night) taking notes on what was happening when the unit was busy and interviewing staff if and when they had time to spare. This approach also allowed for a great many informal discussions in a relaxed atmosphere, especially at night. We had access to staff rotas and were therefore able to plan our visits to maximize the number of staff that we met. Eighty-five midwives were interviewed formally and we had informal discussions with virtually all other midwives who were on duty at the time of our visits: a further 79. The 'informal' data were used to augment the interview data wherever possible.

The data yielded by these methods obviously lend themselves to a certain degree of crude numerical analysis: so-and-so many doctors said this; X% of midwives thought such-and-such. When appropriate, data are presented in this form. However in practice such an approach ignores the real strength of this kind of data, which lies in its quality rather than its quantity. We therefore present most of the data in the form of quotations from the people concerned, but first explain the process by which these data were analysed.

Once data collection was complete all three researchers re-read all the interviews and observation notes and identified major themes. Some of these themes were topics which had been explicitly built into the interviews, such as reactions to the proposals of the Short Report (Social Services Committee, 1980; 1981) and staffs' perceptions of their own roles. Others emerged from discussions during the research. We then went systematically through all interviews and obervation notes (some hundreds of pages) allocating everything that had been said or observed to one or more of our various analysis categories. We were then able to consider each category in turn, identify predominant attitudes and arrive at some conclusions about majority views. In presenting this information we have then used quotes which we consider to be good illustrations of the point being made. Obviously we have quoted some people more than others if they happened to be particularly fluent, but only if what they had to say appeared to us to illustrate more widely held attitudes. On occasions we have also quoted 'deviant' or atypical remarks, but the individual nature of these is always clearly indicated.

The qualitative data that we will present come almost exclusively from the six study hospitals. Once we had completed the study, however, we collected supplementary data on roles and responsibilities from the only other two-tier unit in England and Wales, and from a further eight three-tier units.

PHASE 1. EFFECTS OF STAFFING STRUCTURES: FINDINGS

Roles and responsibilities

A change as fundamental as working without registrars has many ramifications, not least for consultants, who are required to be much more actively involved on the labour ward (Green *et al.*, 1986; Coupland *et al.*, 1987; Kitzinger *et al.*, 1990). In this chapter, however, we will concentrate on the implications for midwives and, insofar as their roles are inter-related, SHOs.

One of our initial hypotheses was that midwives would have a more extended role in the two-tier system. Many of the two-tier staff believed that, without a registrar, midwives were bound to be given more control in the day-to-day running of the labour ward because they were the most experienced staff in the absence of the consultant. As one two-tier consultant commented:

The midwives have got to, certainly with an inexperienced house-man, regard themselves as far more, infinitely more, experienced at knowing that something's going wrong . . . [where] you've got registrars on the spot . . . you've got the SHOs, midwives, registrars (in order of experience) [but here] you've wiped out that middle tier so the midwives have got to assume more responsibility.

We therefore decided to look closely at the tasks and decisions which midwives took on in the different hospitals. We looked first at 13 key tasks ranging from suturing to performing forceps deliveries. For some of these there was very little variation between hospitals, for example, in none of the hospitals were midwives performing forceps deliveries. We therefore concentrated our attention on the tasks which did vary between hospitals, the two most noticeable being suturing and topping up epidurals. In the original six units it did seem that midwives were more likely to be performing these tasks in the two-tier system. However when we came to consider all 15 hospitals, we found no pattern associated with staffing structure. Therefore, we cannot conclude that two-tier staffing automatically results in midwives performing a wider range of tasks.

Decision making, however, shows a rather more clear cut picture. As one two-tier consultant stated when asked how midwives' roles were different in the two-tier system:

They're making decisions, they're not initiating treatment but it's the decision making behind the treatment that's crucial – and they are making registrar-type decisions.

We are not suggesting that midwives in three-tier hospitals do not also made decisions, but what we see in two-tier units is a greater recognition of that fact. In particular, midwives in two-tier hospitals were more likely to be regarded as responsible for decisions about rupturing membranes, the use of continuous fetal monitoring, and the use of Syntocinon to accelerate labour. Perhaps the most significant decision for which midwives were more likely to have responsibility in two-tier units was the decision to call a consultant. In one unit midwives were expected to ring the consultant directly without going via the junior doctor and the Director of Midwifery in another commented that, while the decision was initiated by the mid-wife, 'if the SHO's around she'll probably get him to phone as it saves her time.'

In all the three-tier units, although midwives obviously had a large in-formal input into the decision, the junior doctors were officially responsible for contacting their seniors and the protocol is that the line of communi-cation is from SHO to registrar to consultant.

Relationships

What we have just described summarizes the differences in the roles of two-tier and three-tier midwives. However this is only part of the story, since changes in roles open up possibilities for changes in relationships.

Midwives and SHOs. The increase in midwives' decision making responsibilities has particular consequences for their relationships with SHOs. In the traditional three-tier system midwives are nearly always formally subordinate to the SHO as far as decisions such as acceleration and calling the consultant are concerned. In the case of a new GP trainee, however, (and three-quarters of the SHOs in our sample were GP trainees), the midwife is obviously the more experienced of the two. This mismatch between the hierarchy of status and the hierarchy of skills is further complicated by a mismatch between midwives' and SHOs' views of each other: the SHO tends to underrate the midwife's skills relative to the midwife's own evaluation, while the midwife views the SHO's training with less respect than the SHO would like.

Since status is conferred in part by the responsibility for making decisions, one would expect that, where midwives are overtly taking more decision making responsibility, SHOs may feel themselves to be demoted. Within the six study hospitals this prediction was indeed borne out. The most fraught SHO-midwife interactions that we witnessed were in two-tier units and it was particularly in the two-tier unit where midwives enjoyed the highest status that SHOs expressed most dissatisfaction. SHOs talked about feeling rather useless in the face of the midwives' efficient assumption of control:

> The unit could run without us – that undermines your status.

They could also feel deprived of the opportunity to learn:

> We need more recognition that the SHO is here to learn especially to make decisions, midwives [should be] geared to informing the SHOs what's going on.

They complained of feeling excluded:

> The midwives don't even want you to go in and say hello to normal women

and resented their lack of status and what they saw as the unit's failure to use their medical expertise:

> I was bleeped to hold a woman's legs while she pushed. I didn't go to medical school for five years for that.

Their resentment was perhaps best summed up by the SHO who stated, 'The midwife's role has been expanded here at the expense of the SHO'.

There is a very real conflict of interest between the SHOs' training needs and the midwives' desire for autonomy and, indeed, the desire of the woman in labour for both privacy and experienced care. However the conflict could also be exacerbated by the SHOs' expectation of what their role should be. In the original study hospital, initially, SHOs were aware that their position in a so-called midwife-dominated unit was unusual and compared it unfavourably to the freedom and responsibility allowed to colleagues in more traditional units. However it is important to say that by the time we came to observe the third generation of SHOs in this hospital the picture had improved considerably. Midwives were more confident and less defensive of their position, and new SHOs knew what to expect and were pragmatic about the restrictions on their role.

> You're always an extra pair of hands at this level and probably get in the way a lot. But it is a training role, you can't expect to jump in and make decisions, they would be all the wrong ones.

Midwives and consultants. In any obstetric unit consultants have a major role in determining policy and influencing attitudes (Robinson *et al.*, 1983; Robinson, 1989; Garcia and Garforth, 1991), but they have a particular importance in two-tier hospitals because they are present on the labour ward much more. Most of the three-tier consultants were rarely seen on the labour ward: 'We don't seen much of Mr X, he doesn't meddle much in obstetrics'.

In contrast many of the two-tier obstetricians would be around on the labour ward and spend time talking to midwives when there was no immediate emergency. This could, of course, mean more medical interference but, in practice, we found that most two-tier consultants had evolved a non-intrusive but supportive relationship with the midwifery team. As one consultant commented:

> You can discuss things over a cup of tea with the midwives – I have a closer relationship with them than (other consultants) do. The midwives . . . really know me and like me.

The midwives in two-tier hospitals were proud of this intimacy; one told how she was chatting to her consultant at a conference and midwives from other hospitals were amazed to see such apparent equality and declared, 'no wonder your system works if you can talk to your consultants like that'. Another midwife, reluctant to leave her two-tier hospital, said, 'I'd hate to return to the almighty system where consultants think they're God'.

Of course the good relationships in the two-tier system were not simply the result of consultants and midwives seeing more of each other but were also built on the consultants' respect for midwives and their attitude towards the midwife's role. Some of the three-tier consultants were very out of touch with midwives and were seen as absentee landlords who imposed policies on the labour ward without knowing anything about what was going on, let alone listening to midwives' point of view. These consultants sometimes did not seem to know what midwives were doing or could do. When we asked one consultant if the midwives in his unit put up drips or took blood he replied that he was not sure but asked: 'Isn't there something against it in their training? I don't think they're allowed to stick needles in people'. It was in this unit that a midwife commented 'We don't see the consultants much on the wards . . . but that's OK as you can gently break the doctor's orders'.

Many three-tier midwives were happy if consultants didn't 'meddle much in obstetrics' because they had little faith in their respect for midwives' autonomy. One consultant was described as wanting 'to turn midwives into obstetric serving hands' while another consultant told us, 'The days of midwives – in my view – of managing cases themselves . . . are gone. I consider the midwives to be my juniors, my deputies'.

The two-tier consultants, on the other hand, showed much greater understanding of and sympathy with the midwife's role. As one two-tier consultant commented:

> It really behoves the midwives to run the show . . . This must be quite a rewarding place to work as a midwife. By and large they get on with it – they are really in charge of the labour ward . . .

The mutually respectful relationship between midwives and consultants was one of the most noticeable features of the two-tier system. It is, of course, impossible to tell whether those consultants who are attracted to the two-tier system are those who already have a high regard for midwives, or whether their attitude has arisen from their dependence:

> In the two-tier structure you're more dependent on the midwives so you have to respect them.

Whichever is the case the result was that the majority of midwives found working in the two-tier structure a highly satisfying experience. The SHO-midwife conflict observed in the two-tier units does not, we suspect, represent an increase in the sum total of interstaff disputes. Instead, the conflict has become more overt because the units attract confident and assertive midwives who know that they have their consultants' respect and are more likely to state their opinions. In addition, conflict that would otherwise be distributed between midwives and all grades of medical staff, becomes concentrated on the SHO in the absence of the registrar.

Unit ethos

An important factor in any obstetric unit (over and above the relationships between staff and the roles that they adopt) is the set of attitudes, assumptions and basic principles that make up what we shall call the unit ethos. This ethos, although rarely stated explicitly, was implicit in many statements and actions by staff and clearly identified by each of the three researchers independently. It was particularly evident in the way staff talked about their jobs, each other and, in particular, the women they were caring for. The form it took in each unit is just as important to that unit as the details of formal policy or structure.

The expression of the labour ward ethos was most easily observed among the midwives, although it was clearly also influenced by the consultants, both directly and indirectly. In contrast, we saw the relatively transient junior doctors as outsiders to the ethos, accepting or rejecting it, but not contributing to it.

Given the diversity of attitudes within any unit, both between and within medical and midwifery staff, it is striking that the ethos of each came across so clearly. There were of course individuals who did not subscribe to particular aspects of their unit ethos, and they were clearly identifiable as 'deviant'. Indeed, it was precisely this treatment of certain attitudes as deviant which helped us to identify the ethos.

We will illustrate what we mean by ethos by describing the dominant attitudes in those four units in which we spent most time and which were also involved in the second phase of our study. We will refer to them by the pseudonyms of Willowford, Exington, Wychester and Zedbury. Willowford and Wychester are two-tier units, Exington and Zedbury have the traditional three-tiers of medical staff. Because the differences between units crystallized most clearly around the idea of women's choice, most of the illustrative quotations concern this topic.

Willowford (two-tier unit): 'Active birth' – 'midwives rule OK'.
'Active birth' and midwives' autonomy were the dominant themes at Willowford and were clearly articulated by both midwives and consultants. In this respect the unit was unusual in being so self-conscious; in other cases the ethos was less clearly stated. The attitude towards women was a consciously courteous one; for example, midwives and doctors would usually knock before entering a woman's room and fathers were generally made welcome.

In keeping with this approach was a positive attitude towards women's choice. 'I want what the patient wants' was a frequently expressed sentiment and many midwives said how much better Willowford was than other places they had worked:

Where I was before was very inflexible, there was no choice for women or for midwives, it's much better here.

In principle there could be a clash between the belief in women's choice and midwives' preference for active birth, and some staff expressed concern about this. We did not witness such a clash of interests but one or two midwives in this hospital did express disappointment when women failed to achieve active births, just as a few others expressed anxiety when women wanted to deliver in alternative positions. However, such midwives were in the minority and were not seen as conforming to the spirit of the unit. As one midwife said:

The beauty of what we're doing here is we've got natural childbirth **and** forceps and epidurals.

Or, as another added:

The policy is good – a woman can come in and lie on a bed and feel she's done the right thing for her and be just as jubilant as if a woman squatted in a corner.

Efforts were made to avoid assigning those few midwives who were seen as having very rigid views on the 'right way' to give birth to women whose own choices might not conform with this. This unofficial policy was presented as being both in the woman's interests and as a recognition of 'the midwife's right to choose'. In this way deviant views within the unit were accommodated and possible conflict avoided.

Wychester (two-tier unit): 'Women's right to choose'. In many ways the attitudes in this unit were similar to those at Willowford: in both, for example, more than half of the midwives made unsolicited comments in favour of women's choice in childbirth. However, the principle of midwife autonomy was not stressed as much at Wychester as it was at Willowford, and neither was there a particular emphasis on active birth. However, as at Willowford, staff at Wychester were keen to stress that they gave priority to what women wanted over and above anything else. As one of the consultants stated:

We try to treat women as individuals and in fact we get more individuals who really want to have as easy a labour as technology will give them, than we do women who want to do it all on their own . . . I think that's where some people get it wrong. Every woman's requirements are different and for every single labour they are different.

Midwives laid great emphasis on women's involvement in decision making:

> It's a sort of partnership – midwives recommend action and discuss it with the woman.

> This unit is so much more progressive – a woman has a say, it's her decision.

> They should have a say – it's their body.

Although, as in other hospitals, women's choice was seen as less viable in an emergency, one midwife did say:

> . . . even if it's unsafe – if she's adamant then we go along with her.

Of course, there were individuals whose views diverged from these. Indeed, one consultant was concerned that not all midwives were in tune with his philosophy of giving priority to women's choice:

> Although I would say that probably two-thirds of the midwives' attitudes I'm happy with, I would also have to say, there are some I am not . . .

Thus the identification of the deviant midwives who failed to respect women's choice was used to reiterate the dominant unit ethos – respect for women's choice.

Exington (three-tier unit): 'The consultants rule the roost'.

Exington was the most consultant dominated of all the units, and the consultants themselves, while differing from each other in a variety of ways, were probably the most orthodox. In many ways Exington was the antithesis of Willowford. Midwives had virtually no autonomy and this created frustration or apathy among many of the midwives. Consequently there was a greater focus on midwives' own grievances than on the needs of women. Indeed the absence of reference to women's needs was striking. Discussions of, for example, the limitations of their labour ward geography concentrated exclusively on the problems for midwives, and the language used tended to be midwife-centred, for example: 'We can't ambulate them' (i.e. women in labour are not able to walk about).

There was also little questioning of routine procedures. One midwife, for instance, when asked why they did perineal shaving, replied 'Well, it doesn't do any harm'. In group discussion, when asked what happened if a woman did not want to sign the General Consent form (i.e. the blanket permission for staff to take whatever action they deem necessary) another midwife quipped: 'They go to Willowford', while a third commented 'If you explain and are reasonable with them they won't be stroppy with you'. Most of the doctors seemed to have a similar attitude. As one of the consultants said:

Most people are fairly sensible. But as to whether they should deliver in various positions, we haven't really got the facilities to cope with that and I'm not sure in my own mind that it is necessary.

He went on to admit:

It's a bit machine-like here. I think perhaps women don't get much say. But . . . it would only be lip-service to pretend – a lot of places pretend they have a lot of say.

Some of the midwives and junior doctors were clearly unhappy about the way women were treated at Exington. As one SHO said 'To be quite honest I don't think the women here get a fair deal'. Other staff worried about specific ways in which women were treated. Some complained about one consultant's policy of removing the baby from the woman at birth to be weighed in a warm room. Others were concerned about the cattle market atmosphere in the antenatal clinic which did not allow them to treat women as individuals. However, staff praised some of the provisions the hospital did make such as a flat for parents to stay in next to the Special Care Baby Unit. In addition, they suggested further improvements that could be made such as the introduction of Birthday beds, and the routine use of birth plans:

If women have birthing plans many midwives are immediately against them. If **all** women have one then it would be accepted as normal.

A few staff made specific comments allying themselves with the principle of a woman's right to choose:

I used to think as a midwife I knew all about labour and I resented being contradicted by women but then I realized it's their bodies, you should listen to women.

However, such views were not generally accepted. The consultant's view that 'I'm not that sure in the majority of cases whether the patient is in the position really to judge', seemed far more dominant.

Zedbury (three-tier unit): 'Who'd have been responsible if he'd dropped it?' Consultants at Zedbury (as in other three-tier hospitals) had little personal labour ward involvement, but neither did they dominate the labour ward via formal policy as much as, for example, their colleagues at Exington. Their contribution to the unit ethos was, therefore, much less evident. As far as midwives were concerned the dominant attitudes tended to be rather negative, with a particular concern about legal liability:

You've got to get a woman's permission (e.g. for episiotomy) because of the legalities.

> We write it down if a woman refuses; you have to cover yourself.

> We should have consent for elective epidurals. So much can go wrong. Something should be signed.

One of the stories we heard was of a father, who had previously been feeling faint, insisting on holding his newborn baby. The midwife had been furious: 'Who'd have been responsible if he'd dropped it?' The interesting aspect of this story was that in all its various tellings there was never any suggestion of sympathy for the father or concern for the baby *per se*. Neither, apparently, did anyone think of sitting the father down or supporting him. The emphasis was entirely on the issue of legal liability and the difficulties created for midwives by the father's wish to hold his own baby.

One midwife remarked sadly on this preoccupation with legal liability as a relatively recent thing:

> In the past if a baby died it was very sad, but just one of those things. Now we have a big investigation with the possibility of being sued etc. . . . That's why some midwives are leaving midwifery, because they are scared of the responsibility and legal implications.

Certainly this emphasis did upset a number of midwives there:

> Everyone's very defensive and the midwife is responsible . . . If things go wrong they're out to point the finger at you. If things go well, nobody says 'well done'.

The resulting attitude towards women in labour was a rather distant one with little evidence of empathy. Very few midwives brought up the issue of women's choice without prompting and the most common reaction to the question on how much choice women had was 'We tell her what we're doing' and 'They don't **have** to accept anything'. Generally speaking, women who wanted control over what happened to them in labour were seen as problems for the midwife. Women who asserted different desires from midwives were written off as 'anti-hospital' and 'problem cases'. Women's views were often portrayed as lacking validity: 'She'll change her mind' (which is inconsistent) or **not** change her mind (which is inflexible). Many staff stated that women should leave it up to the midwives:

> Some lay down their own policies but they should leave it to us. We're the midwife.

Usually the midwives felt they were able to 'talk them round'. One commented 'it's just the way you explain it that helps' – making it clear to us that she would tell the woman that the baby was in trouble. However, for fear of litigation, they would never do anything against the express wishes of the woman, except in the occasional situation when they 'had to'.

Doctors and midwives were surprisingly unselfconscious about their dismissal of women's wishes, and there was little attempt to display any prochoice attitudes for our benefit. Indeed, on several occasions, staff emerged from the delivery room and told us precisely how they were dealing with 'difficult patients'. One doctor, for instance informed us that he had just told a woman 'this is a hospital not a prison, so I can't **order** you'. We were not surprised then that one SHO when asked how much say women had in this hospital replied, succinctly, 'Bugger all', while a deviantly woman-centred midwife was left rather wistfully saying 'I would like to think that if they **really** wanted it they'd get it'.

PHASE 2. THE VIEWS OF CHILDBEARING WOMEN

Having completed the first phase of our research which focused on staff, we then carried out a large scale prospective study of women delivering in four of the original study hospitals. This second phase of the study was mainly concerned with women's expectations and experiences of childbirth (Green *et al.*, 1988), and one of the independent variables under consideration was the unit at which women were booked for delivery. We draw on these data to examine the different perceptions of staff held by women booked for delivery in each of these hospitals.

PHASE 2. METHODS

The sample was drawn from women expecting babies in April and May 1987 in Willowford, Wychester, Exington and Zedbury. Willowford, Wychester and Zedbury each have between 2000 and 2500 deliveries per annum, and virtually all births take place in the consultant units. In the Exington Health District, in addition to the consultant unit in which our Phase 1 observations were carried out, there is also a separate GP unit located in the same hospital and a small satellite unit for low-risk women (Little Exington), approximately 15 miles away. Little Exington is run essentially by midwives with just one resident SHO. In 1987 there were 406 deliveries at the GP unit, 324 at Little Exington and approximately 2800 at the consultant unit. Women booked for delivery in the two subsidiary Exington units were also included in this phase of the research, thus giving us the opportunity to examine women's experiences of two further styles of staffing.

Eight to ten weeks before their expected date of delivery women were sent a letter inviting them to take part in the study, along with a preliminary questionnaire and a prepaid reply envelope. Eight hundred and twenty-five women (73.5%) returned valid questionnaires. There was some variation in response rates between units, with the extremes both coming from within the Exington Health District: 79% at the GP unit (89/113) compared with 67% (84/125) at the consultant unit. Women who returned the first questionnaire were sent the second one four weeks before their expected date of delivery, and the third approximately six weeks after the birth. Response rates at these two stages were 92% and 96%. (One would, of course, expect higher response rates at these stages since questionnaires were sent only to women who had already indicated their willingness to participate.) Three women could not be followed up because they forgot to fill in their address, and a further seven were lost to the study because their babies arrived before the second questionnaire did. Results are therefore based on 751 responses to the second questionnaire and 710 postnatally.

PHASE 2. FINDINGS

Antenatal perceptions

Because both phases of our research focused on events on the labour ward, antenatal experiences had not been our prime concern. Nonetheless, it was evident from the answers that women gave to certain of the antenatal questions that there were differences in their perceptions of the hospitals and the staff even at this early stage. Women at Willowford (two-tier) and Wychester (two-tier), for example, were most likely to be happy about their choice of hospital, to be able to discuss things with professionals and to be as assertive as they wanted to be. Along with women at the Exington GP unit, they were also the most likely to be satisfied with the information that they had been given so far during their pregnancy. Women booked at the Exington consultant unit (three-tier) and Little Exington tended to score worst on all of these indices.

It was also interesting to see that women booked at the different units had different expectations of how the staff would treat them during labour. One set of questions demonstrating this were those concerning the writing of birth plans. Very few women in our sample had had their wishes about labour and delivery put down in writing and the majority (70%) had never even thought of it. Only at Zedbury (three-tier) were birth plans, (called Maternity Care Plans), incorporated into written policy and here 31% of women said that their wishes had been, or probably would be, written down. At all the other units women could, in principle, have their wishes for labour and delivery recorded in writing, but only at Willowford (two-tier) did this seem to occur with any frequency: 19% of women. Anticipating this situation, we had followed our questions on the writing of birth plans by a series of statements about the advantages and disadvantages of birth plans with which women were invited to agree or disagree. Some of these were 'woman centred', such as 'Writing things down helps me to sort things out in my head'. However, the majority were to do with expectations of the staff, for example, 'Writing things down can get you labelled as a trouble maker' or 'I think the staff understand what I want anyway'. The full list of statements, and the proportion of women agreeing with each, is given in Table 2.1 (see page 20). As this table shows, some responses were related to women's level of education and some to parity. In all cases significance was assessed using chi-square tests which compare the observed distribution of responses with those that would be expected by chance if there were no relationship. As is conventional a probability of less than 0.05 was taken as the criterion of statistical signifiance.

Women with a higher level of education were more likely to say that 'writing things down helps me to sort things out in my head' and less likely to say 'decisions should rightly be taken by the staff'; 'I think the staff understand what I want anyway'; and 'there's no need, I don't want anything out of the ordinary'. These differences are in line with what one might expect from women with different levels of education. It is, however, surprising that there are only two differences related to parity: one might have predicted that previous experience would have more effect. 'It's not possible to know what you are going to want . . .' only just reaches the 0.05 level of significance, with first-time mothers (primiparae) being more likely to agree. 'I don't suppose anyone will take much notice of it anyway' is the only statement strongly related to parity with only 4% of primiparae agreeing compared with 11% of women with previous experience (multiparae). This is a rather sad reflection on some women's previous births, but is in line with the greater cynicism of multiparous women that we also observed elsewhere in our data.

The majority of significant differences in agreement with the birth plan statements were not, in fact, associated with education or parity but were between women booked at different units. Table 2.2 (see page 21) shows the distribution of responses for the statements concerned.

These data reveal a very consistent pattern, with Exington women being much more pessimistic (or realistic depending on your point of view) than women at the other units, the marked contrast being between Exington consultant unit and Willowford. Note particularly the sad fact that 22% of women at the Exington consultant unit 'don't suppose anyone will take much notice of it anyway'. This figure is all the more striking because, as we have already seen, this statement is more characteristic of multiparae than of primiparae, yet the Exington consultant unit has relatively fewer multiparae than the other consultant units because low-risk multiparae go to the GP unit and Little Exington. We should therefore expect fewer women at this unit to be agreeing with this statement, not more. It is difficult to interpret the figures for Zedbury, because the fact that it is unit policy to record women's wishes engenders a different point of view. Given this, it is surprising that as many as 10% of Zedbury

Table 2.1 Women's agreement with various statements concerned with recording their antenatal wishes. (Respondents could tick as many statements as they wished)

	(n = 751)	
	% of total sample	No.
1. The advantages of writing down what you want are:		
Even if I don't know the staff who attend me in labour they'll be able to know what I want by reading what I've written	55	416
When I'm actually in labour I won't be in such a good position to tell staff what I want	52	393
If it's in writing the staff are less likely to do things to me that I don't want	35	260
Writing things down helps me to sort things out in my head	34 (E)	253
I want to help myself stick to whatever I decided before I went into labour	6	42
2. The disadvantages of writing things down are:		
If I write things down it might stop me changing my mind during labour	46	346
Writing things down can get you labelled as a trouble maker	14 (U)	102
It might upset the staff	11 (U)	85
It seems a bit of a cheek	10 (U)	77
The decisions should rightly be taken by the staff, it's not up to me to decide what I want	10 (E)	75
3. There is no point in writing down what you want because:		
It's not possible to know what you are going to want during labour in advance	67 (P)	504
I'm sure I can say what I want at the time	45 (U)	335
I think the staff understand what I want anyway	17 (E)	129
There is no need, I don't want anything out of the ordinary	16 (E)	122
I don't suppose anyone will take much notice of it anyway	8 (U,P)	62
I don't like the standard form they gave me to fill in	<1	4

Key: P indicates that responses are significantly related to parity. E indicates that responses are significantly related to education. U indicates that responses are significantly related to unit. (See text for details.)
Source: Compiled by the authors.

Table 2.2 Percentages of women agreeing with each of five statements at each hospital

| | Exington | | | Willowford (two-tier) (n = 184) | Wychester (two-tier) (n = 186) | Zedbury (three-tier) (n = 169) |
	Cons. unit (three-tier) (n = 76)	GP unit (n = 77)	Little Ex'ton (n = 47)			
1. The disadvantages of writing things down are:						
Writing things down can get you labelled as a trouble maker	15 20%	17 22%	13 28%	14 8%	24 13%	17 10%
It might upset the staff	15 20%	11 14%	12 26%	12 7%	24 13%	10 6%
It seems a bit of a cheek	13 17%	14 18%	9 19%	11 6%	13 7%	17 10%
2. There is no point writing down what you want because:						
I'm sure I can say what I want at the time	32 42%	34 44%	18 38%	98 53%	91 49%	56 33%
I don't suppose anyone will take much notice of it anyway	17 22%	8 10%	7 15%	8 4%	10 5%	11 7%

Source: Compiled by the authors.

women thought that is was 'a bit of a cheek' to record their wishes in writing. Zedbury women also have the lowest expectation of being able to 'say what I want at the time'.

Another section of the second antenatal questionnaire asked about various social/behavioural aspects of the birth, such as who would be there and how decisions would be made. For each aspect women were asked, firstly, what they would like to happen or how important it was to them, and, secondly, what they actually expected to happen. There were virtually no differences between units with respect to what women **wanted**, but there were again interesting differences in their expectations of the staff. For example, women were asked whether they expected that there would be lots of people coming in and out during their labour. Table 2.3 shows the different responses by unit.

These figures show very striking (and highly significant) differences: at one extreme 22% of Willowford (two-tier) women were confident of their privacy during labour while at the other over a third of those booked at Exington consultant unit (three-tier) had the opposite expectation. These patterns were also reflected in women's expectations of involvement in non-emergency decision making and of being in control of what the staff do to them (Tables 2.4 and 2.5, see pages 24 and 25).

In every case it is women at Exington consultant unit (three-tier) who had the lowest expectations of their relationship with staff, and women at Willowford (two-tier) who had the highest. At all three Exington units the majority of women expected, at best, only to be 'kept informed' of non-emergency decisions, while at the other hospitals, particularly Willowford (two-tier) and Wychester (two-tier), women were expecting to be rather more involved in decision making. This was reflected also in their answers to the question about being in control of what staff did to them. These differences cannot be explained by differences in the parity or education of women booked at the different units.

It is interesting to see that such differences in women's views and expectations show up at 36 weeks of pregnancy, particularly since they tally with our own perceptions of the 'unit ethos' described above. It is particularly fascinating that these differences should be apparent before many of these women have had any personal experience of their particular hospital's labour ward practice. Most of the women were having at least some of their antenatal care in the community, so they would not even necessarily have had very much experience of the hospital antenatal clinics. Multiparae are presumably drawing largely on their own previous experiences, while the anticipations of primiparae will be based largely on what they have heard from other women who have delivered in these units. Thus it would seem that the 'unit ethos' that we have described exists not only as a researchers' abstraction but also in the local beliefs and ideas about hospitals that women pass on by word of mouth.

Table 2.3 Expectations that there would be lots of people coming in and out during labour at each of the six hospitals

	Exington			Willowford (two-tier)	Wychester (two-tier)	Zedbury (three-tier)
	Cons. unit (three-tier)	GP unit	Little Ex'ton			
Sure there won't be	6	10	4	40	6	11
	8%	13%	9%	22%	3%	7%
Think there probably will/ sure there will be	26	12	6	27	33	36
	35%	16%	13%	15%	18%	22%

Women who thought that there 'probably' would not be or who had no expectations have been omitted from this table
Source: Compiled by the authors.

Table 2.4 Expectations of involvement in non-emergency decision making at each of the six hospitals

	Exington			Willowford	Wychester	Zedbury
	Cons. unit	GP unit	Little Ex'ton			
Expect at least to have decisions discussed	27 36%	33 43%	20 43%	119 66%	111 61%	86 52%
Expect at best to be kept informed	47 63%	41 53%	26 55%	57 32%	66 36%	76 46%

Women with no expectations have been omitted from this table
Source: Compiled by the authors.

Table 2.5 Expectations of being in control of what staff do to you at each of the six hospitals

| | Exington | | | Willowford | Wychester | Zedbury |
	Cons. unit	GP unit	Little Ex'ton			
Think probably will/sure will be	35 47%	46 61%	26 55%	119 67%	119 66%	92 56%
Think probably won't/sure won't be	20 27%	15 20%	13 28%	13 7%	21 12%	24 15%

Women with no expectations have been omitted from this table
Source: Compiled by the authors.

Women's experiences

Naturally the next question of interest was to discover whether the different views that women had of the hospitals antenatally were in fact borne out by experience. The same three questions (concerning non-emergency decision making, control of what the staff do to you, and comings and goings), also distinguished between the units when asked in the postnatal questionnaire, and, broadly speaking, differences accorded with women's expectations. Women at Willowford (two-tier) and Wychester (two-tier) reported the most involvement in non-emergency decision making, while women at all three Exington units experienced considerably less involvement than other women; only 35% of Exington women felt that there had at least been some discussion compared to 59% of women at the other three units. There were also differences between units, consistent with these other findings, in the extent to which women felt in control of what staff were doing, but these were not statistically significant.

Women's reports on comings and goings diverged somewhat from their expectations. Zedbury (three-tier) came out rather poorly, while the hospitals at which women had most privacy were those for 'low-risk' women: Exington GP unit and Little Exington. These results hold true independently for both multiparae and primiparae.

There were also significant differences between the units in **who** women saw during labour. Women at Little Exington were much more likely to have met at least one of the midwives who looked after them in labour: 75% compared to 20% elsewhere. Little Exington women, as well as those at the GP unit and at Willowford (two-tier) were also the most likely to have at least one midwife who looked after them throughout labour and delivery. However, in the case of the two small Exington units this is simply a function of the fact that most of the women were multiparae and therefore had shorter labours. When we look only at multiparae Willowford (two-tier) alone differs from the other units. Willowford women were also the least likely to be seen by a doctor during labour and the least likely to be delivered by a doctor. These differences were true for both multiparae and primiparae. In general the difference between the treatment of multiparae and primiparae was least at Willowford (two-tier) and greatest at Zedbury (three-tier). Thus we find only 13% of Willowford primiparae being delivered by a doctor compared with 40% of those at Zedbury.

There were a number of other significant differences between the experiences of women at the different units. Most noticeably, women's reports confirmed what we already knew or suspected about differences in the use of pain-relieving drugs and various 'minor' interventions: enemas, shaving, glucose drips, episiotomies and electronic fetal monitoring. Related to these, we found significant differences in women's responses to the question: 'Were you able to get into the positions that were most comfortable for you during labour and delivery?', with women at Exington consultant unit (three-tier) and at Zedbury (three-tier) being least likely to have been able to get comfortable. The two main reasons given for this were: equipment, such as drips and monitor leads, hampering movement; and staff preventing women from adopting more comfortable positions.

Perhaps surprisingly, given the variation already reported, we found no significant differences between units in the ways in which women described either the staff or their overall care. There were, however, some significant differences in their satisfaction with their experience of birth. These interact with parity. Primiparae were, in general, less satisfied than multiparae and Zedbury primiparae were significantly less satisfied than others. Satisfaction for multiparae varied more between units; those at Willowford and the Exington GP unit were the most satisfied, those at Exington consultant unit and Little Exington, the least.

We can see a consistency emerging from these data. Overall Willowford (two-tier) comes out well and Exington consultant unit (three-tier) comes out rather poorly. Furthermore the questions that distinguish between units are those which reflect overall staff attitudes towards women in labour: the very same dimension that had been so striking in our assessment of the unit ethos. That this is important to women is reflected in the mean satisfaction scores at each of the units, but we also have more direct evidence, not reported here, showing that such factors as privacy, being able to adopt the most comfortable position possible, and feeling in control of what staff are doing to you, are all related to women's subsequent psychological state (Green *et al.*, 1988).

DISCUSSION

These differences between units give interesting food for thought. Overall our study found a number of factors which were related to women's satisfaction which were **not** functions of the unit booked for delivery. These included parity, anxiety about labour pain, how well a woman felt she coped during labour and her perceptions of the individuals who looked after her. There were, however, a larger number of other factors that **were** related to the unit of booking, including perceived choice about place of birth, involvement in decision making, good communications with staff, adequate and correct information, privacy and continuity of care during labour, being able to get comfortable, and the use of obstetric interventions and pain-relieving drugs. All of these contributed to women's satisfaction and all varied between units. The question is: are they a function of staffing structure or are they simply a reflection of the differing policies and attitudes that we have described above as 'unit ethos'?

Unit ethos need not, of course, be logically linked to staffing structure but might simply be an important independent variable. However there are, we think, two particular features of the two-tier hospitals that we studied that are likely to engender more empathetic, woman-centred attitudes, which give rise to the factors listed. One is the difference in attitudes of the consultants. Consultants who had chosen to work in the two-tier system had attitudes towards their own role and towards midwives which differed considerably from those of their three-tier colleagues. We would suggest that they are also likely to be unconventional in other aspects of their approach to their work, including their attitudes towards women's choice. The other factor which we would see as facilitating a woman-centred approach is the job satisfaction of the midwives; in an environment where midwives are not preoccupied by their own problems it seems reasonable to imagine that they will be more able to devote themselves to the women's concerns. It may also be that the two-tier system directly facilitates a flexible approach to childbirth that is a necessary prerequisite if the woman or her midwife are to make choices during the course of labour. As one two-tier consultant explicitly argued:

> . . . when you have registrars and SHOs acting in a registrar capacity, you have to lay down laws for them to follow . . . You cannot give them the discretion to vary from those rules because they haven't got the depth of experience to know when they are in trouble. So if you are going to avoid a rigid approach to childbirth you cannot have the labour ward managed by junior staff.

Thus, while the two-tier structure does not inevitably lead to more woman-centered care, it evidently has this potential. Results from Little Exington illustrate particularly clearly that the simple absence of registrars from the labour ward does not in itself guarantee increased choice for women or increased satisfaction. Women here had poor communication with staff and low expectations of how they would be treated. Furthermore, although they had relatively straightforward labours and were the most likely to be looked after by a known midwife and to be afforded a higher than average degree of privacy, they did not feel particularly in control of what was happening to them and had lower than average satisfaction scores. Feeling in control was one of the key determinants of women's subsequent feelings and this was in fact much more strongly related to women's perceptions of the individuals who cared for them than to the unit in which they gave birth.

From what we have said it will be clear that we cannot disentangle the effects of the staffing structure from the characteristics of the people who work in a particular unit. The way in which a woman and her midwife interact is likely to be one of the major determinants of how that woman feels about the birth. However that interaction will be influenced by the unit ethos, which in turn is influenced by the attitudes of the consultants both towards midwives and towards childbearing women. The importance of consultants' attitudes should not be under-rated because consultants determine the rules of play. Consequently, we cannot conclude that the two-tier structure is inevitably good news either for midwives or for child-bearing women, but we hope that our study has highlighted some of the ways in which obstetric units can differ and what these differences can mean both for midwives and for the women in their care.

REFERENCES

Coupland, V.A., Green, J.M., Kitzinger, J. and Richards, M. (1987) Obstetricians on the labour ward: implications of medical staffing structures. *British Medical Journal*, **295**, 1077–9.

Garcia, J. and Garforth, S. (1991) Midwifery policies and policy-making. In S. Robinson and A.M. Thomson (eds) *Midwives, research and childbirth*, Vol. 2. Chapman & Hall, London.

Green, J.M., Coupland, V.A. and Kitzinger, V.V. (1988) *Great expectations: a prospective study of women's expectations and experiences of childbirth*. Child Care and Development Group, University of Cambridge. Vols 1 and 2, and appendix.

Green, J.M., Kitzinger, J.V. and Coupland, V.A. (1986) *The division of labour: implications of medical staffing structure for doctors and midwives on the labour ward*. Child Care and Development Group, University of Cambridge.

Kitzinger, J., Green, J. and Coupland, V. (1990) Labour relations: Midwives and doctors on the labour ward. In J. Garcia, P. Kilpatrick and M. Richards (eds) *The politics of maternity care*. Oxford University Press, Oxford.

Robinson, S., Golden, J. and Bradley, S. (1983) *A study of the role and responsibilities of the midwife*. NRU Report No. 1. Nursing Research Unit, Kings College, London.

Robinson, S. (1989) Caring for childbearing women: The interrelationship of midwifery and medical responsibilities. In S. Robinson and A.M. Thomson (eds) *Midwives, research and childbirth*. Vol. 1. Chapman & Hall, London.

Social Services Committee (1980) Second report from the Social Services Committee Session 1979–80. *Perinatal and neonatal mortality* (Chairman: Mrs R. Short). HMSO, London.

Social Services Committee (1981) Fourth report from the Social Services Committee Session 1980–81. *Medical Education: with special reference to the number of doctors and the career structure in hospitals*. HMSO, London.

CHAPTER THREE

Giving support in pregnancy: the role of research midwives in a randomized controlled trial

Ann Oakley

INTRODUCTION

Giving psychosocial support to childbearing women has traditionally been part of the midwife's role. The provision of such support is becoming increasingly difficult in many maternity care settings today, with the growing centralization of care in large centres, and the emphasis on high technology monitoring and intervention at the expense of individual client-based care (Oakley and Houd, 1990). The importance to successful pregnancy outcome of midwife-provided social support was the principal hypothesis behind the Social Support and Pregnancy Outcome (SSPO) study, conducted at the Institute of Education, University of London, in 1985–9. The main study findings are reported in a series of papers (see Oakley, 1989a; Oakley, 1989b; Oakley and Rajan, 1989; Oakley *et al.*, 1990; Oakley and Rajan, 1990; Rajan and Oakley, 1990a; Rajan and Oakley, 1990b; Oakley and Rajan, 1991). This chapter looks at some of the data collected during the study documenting the experiences of the four research midwives who provided the social support intervention, and describing the nature of the intervention they gave. The purpose of the chapter is to explore these experiences both insofar as they throw light on the research process, and because they illuminate some critical issues in maternity care today, including the difficulty under resourced services have in providing good quality care, and the tensions of attempting to provide this to women living in stressed and socially disadvantaged circumstances. The study methods and the findings on health outcomes are described first, in order to provide a context for the findings on the research midwives' experiences.

STUDY METHODS AND FINDINGS ON HEALTH OUTCOMES

The SSPO study was a randomized controlled trial of research midwife-provided social support in pregnancy. The trial was carried out in four centres in England, two in the Midlands and two in the south of England. Women eligible for the study were defined as those with a history of at least one previous low birthweight (LBW) (<2500 g) delivery unassociated with major congenital malformation or elective delivery that might have been responsible for the low birthweight. The criterion of LBW was chosen to select an 'at risk' population who would also (because of the social class distribution of LBW) be socially disadvantaged. The women had to be booking with a singleton pregnancy before 24 weeks gestation and be fluent English speakers as funding for the study did not, unfortunately, cover the provision of interpreters.

Out of 534 women invited to take part in the study, 509 agreed; 255 of these were randomly allocated to be offered a social support intervention provided by four research midwives in addition to their normal antenatal care, and 254 were allocated to the control group who received normal antenatal care only. The design of the study is shown in Figure 3.1 (see page 32). Table 3.1 (see page 33) shows social and medical characteristics of the sample women at entry to the study, and Table 3.2 (see page 33) a breakdown of these by the four centres.

We hypothesized that the effects of the social support intervention on a variety of pre-specified health outcomes would favour mothers and babies allocated to the intervention group. Results showed that babies of intervention group mothers had a mean birthweight 38 g higher than control group babies, and there were fewer very low birthweight babies in the intervention group. More women in the control group (52%) than in the intervention group (41%) were admitted to hospital in pregnancy. Spontaneous onset of labour and spontaneous vaginal delivery were more common in the intervention group, who also used less epidural analgesia. Intervention group babies required less invasive resuscitation methods and used less intensive and special neonatal care. Both mothers and babies in the intervention group were significantly healthier in the early weeks as judged by reported physical and psychosocial health and use of the health services.

The four research midwives were employed in the different centres and worked part time for the duration of the trial. Although each had previous clinical experience, their role in the trial was not to give any clinical care. The purpose of the study was, rather, to examine the effectiveness of the general support component in midwifery. Social support was defined as the provision of a non-judgemental listening ear, discussing with women their pregnancy needs, giving information when asked to, and carrying out

Figure 3.1 Design of the SSPO study.

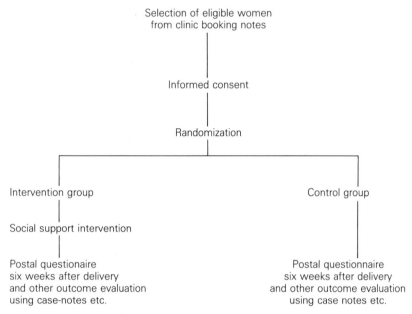

Source: compiled by the author.

referrals when appropriate to other health and welfare professionals and voluntary and statutory agencies. Guidelines were written for the midwives indicating how they should respond to requests for information under such headings as smoking, diet, alcohol, work, and so forth. All these aspects of their roles in the research were covered in detail during induction days held in London before recruitment to the trial started. They were told that there was some suggestion from randomized controlled trials that social support was of benefit, but that the case was not strictly proven.

The midwives were asked to provide a 'minimum support package' for all the women in the intervention group, and in addition as much extra support as the women wanted and their own caseloads would permit. The 'minimum package' was defined as three home visits at 14, 20 and 28 weeks of pregnancy plus two telephone calls or brief home visits between these times. The midwives were provided with radiopagers so they could be contacted by the study women 24 hours a day. Semi-structured interview schedules were written for the home visits, and portions of the home visits were tape-recorded and transcribed. The interview schedules were intended to provide a basis for the interaction between the research midwives and the women, and also to collect data for the study. If the

Table 3.1 Characteristics of women at entry to study

	Intervention (n = 254–255)		Control (n = 253–254)	
	Mean	*SD*	*Mean*	*SD*
Gestational age (weeks)	15.7	3.5	15.6	3.5
Maternal age (years)	27.9	4.9	28.1	5.3
	No.	*%*	*No.*	*%*
Women <20 years of age	9	4	10	4
Previous LBW baby:				
1	220	86	220	87
2	28	11	29	11
3+	7	3	5	2
Smoking at booking	104	41	102	40
Married or cohabiting	214	84	205	81
Working class (partner's occupation)**	194	78	178	75
Partner unemployed**	44	18	46	19
Employed in pregnancy*	77	30	79	34
Ethnicity Afro-Caribbean/Asian***	11	5	12	5

* Information provided by mother postpartum.
** n = 247; 235–238.
*** n = 225; 223.
Source: compiled by the author.

Table 3.2 Sample characteristics by centre

	Centre			
	1	*2*	*3*	*4*
% smokers	42	41	30	43
% working class	73	49	51	79
% unmarried	26	8	9	20
% with parity ≥3	22	13	13	15
% with history of more than one preterm birth	35	26	26	30

Source: compiled by the author.

midwives felt using the schedule would counter the aim of giving support, then the schedule was not used.

One of the research midwives continued to do some part-time clinical work in the hospital during the study. Although asked to avoid delivering women for whom she was providing social support this was not possible in one case; she said she very much enjoyed the delivery.

Throughout the trial the midwives had regular telephone contact with the research team, and monthly meetings were held in London which all the midwives attended. During these meetings the midwives' interpretations of their role were discussed, queries raised and answered, and they had a chance to talk to each other and to the other members of the research team about the complex and at times personally taxing nature of the work involved in giving support to women, many of whom had considerable social and obstetric problems.

Some of these research meetings were tape-recorded and form part of the data drawn on for this chapter. Other data used include questionnaires completed by the midwives about halfway through the study, tape-recorded interviews carried out at the end of the study asking the midwives to evaluate their experiences, the data sheets the midwives completed following any contact they had with the study women, and a 'problem' file kept by the study administrator.

FINDINGS ON THE EXPERIENCES OF THE RESEARCH MIDWIVES

As is clear from the outline of the study above, the research midwives in the SSPO trial were called upon to perform a number of functions critical to the design and content of the study. The main ones were recruitment of eligible women, arranging for randomization, and providing and documenting the social support package. Each of these aspects of the research midwives' roles are explored below. The impact of the research on the midwives themselves is then considered, before the policy implications of these data are drawn out in a final section. In the text the research midwives are referred to as 'RMW1', 'RMW2', 'RMW3' and 'RMW4', and all women's names are pseudonyms.

Recruitment

The research midwives' first task in each of the four centres was to go through the antenatal clinic booking notes, identify women who fitted the eligibility criteria, and then find the women, check their eligibility, explain the study to them, and ask for their consent to take part. A critical aspect of our research design was informing all the women eligible for recruitment about the study **before** randomization. The guidelines the midwives were asked to use when seeking informed consent stressed that agreeing to take part in the study meant accepting a 50% chance of being offered social support in pregnancy, and a 50% chance of not being offered it. Like most aspects of research, recruiting the women proved more complex in practice than in theory, for a number of reasons. Different definition of abortions, stillbirths and live births, and different weighing practices, made interpretation of the criterion of 'at least one previous low birthweight delivery' difficult:

RMW4: There's variation from case note to case note. Sometimes there'll be a 26 week abortion and it'll be weighed, and sometimes it won't be weighed . . . If they're over 26 weeks there's often a query, and then if it's 28 weeks and it's a stillbirth they put it down as a spontaneous abortion. I know **why** they do that, it's to make the hospital figures look better.

RMW1: And to save hassle for the parents.

RMW4: We've got the highest perinatal mortality rate anyway, so I know that if there's one just over 28 weeks they quite often put it down as a spontaneous abortion.

RMW3: As far as our recruiting goes, that's complicated too, because if it's a 27 weeker and it's lived you include it, likewise if it's dead you can't. How far down do you go? I've missed a 24 weeker and it's gone home.

A major problem was the lack of information about obstetric history on the booking notes. Access was sought to notes of women who had previous deliveries at the same hospital, but as found in many other studies (e.g. Davies and Evans, 1991) these were often incomplete or missing. This meant that the research midwives had to wait until after the woman had been seen at the clinic to establish their eligibility and, as some women would then not be due to return to the hospital clinic until 36 weeks, the research midwives had no opportunity to recruit them. A proportion of recruitments was thus done by telephone, or by visits to the women's homes. The research midwives were provided with identification cards they could show to the women.

These procedures raised important questions about the ethics of research, and about the difficulty of recruiting women who will subsequently be denied social support through being allocated to the control group. The following conversation took place at one of the monthly meetings:

RMW1: I hate doing it on the phone. They're very suspicious.

RMW2: Yes they are.

RMW4: I haven't found that, but I don't feel it's fair to ask them to take part on the phone. I mean, they don't know you.

RMW1: That's right, and you get so many weird people trying to sell things.

RMW3: Which is basically what you're doing isn't it?

RMW4: Yes, you are. You're trying to sell them the research.

RMW3: It takes me four and a half minutes to do a recruitment. My husband says I don't give them time to say no.

RMW1: It takes me half an hour.

RMW3: Not on the phone!

RMW1: It does!

RMW3: I'm dreadful. I go far too fast, and they say yes to get rid of me!

At another meeting:

RMW1: I think they feel pressured.

RMW3: Especially if you say you're a midwife – they're not used to saying no to health professionals . . .

The questionnaires the midwives filled in observed that:

Recruiting over the phone is impersonal, doesn't really give the lady a chance to ask questions or retain the information . . . Can't gauge her reaction by facial expression, either . . . (RMW1)

Sometimes when I recruit at their home, I find they are concerned as to how I have got their name, address, etc. and also (despite the ID card) how official I am. (RMW4)

I love the idea of recruiting women at clinic, but find it very time consuming so have done, at most, six women this way. I prefer the telephone to a visit at home. For speed, and to maintain distance between myself and those who are eventually 'control'. . . (RMW3)

The fourth midwife found herself wondering how **she** would react when approached in this way:

I prefer to recruit at the clinic because I feel the women see me in what they might class the 'right setting' for a midwife, even though I am not in uniform. Also I find it far nicer – on the whole easier if speaking face to face. Having said that, I have been amazed at how receptive ladies have been to my recruiting them over the phone, the information they are very free to provide about themselves often without my asking. I often have wondered how I would react to a total stranger claiming to be a midwife telephoning completely out of the blue, who obviously has information about me. (RMW2)

As a result of these considerations, the view was expressed that some of the control women were effectively receiving social support during the recruitment process, despite the midwives' efforts to minimize contact:

RMW1: It must affect them, if you see them at home ... You can't just walk in and out again. They say, oh, are you a midwife? What about this? I try and give a very broad opinion. I say if you're in the intervention group we can talk about that.

RMW3: I say I'm sure that's something your district midwife would love to talk to you about. I think the district midwives will kill me!

The relationship referred to in this last quotation between the research and the work of other health professionals is discussed below.

Randomization

Once women had agreed to take part in the study, the research midwives telephoned London for randomization into intervention and control groups. We have explored the research midwives' experiences in this area in a paper discussing the ethics of the design of randomized controlled trials (Oakley, 1989a), and so will only repeat the main points here. First of all, crucially but unsurprisingly, although all the midwives accepted the need of random allocation as part of the research design, the randomization process was experienced by them somewhat negatively as an aspect of the research over which they had no control, and which allowed neither them nor the women to express a view about which group individual women should be in. These was a general feeling that informing women who would then be allocated to the control group of the availability of social support, and then having to tell them they would not be offered it, was a difficult and unpleasant task. As two of the midwives put it:

For a study such as this it is probably the only fair way – but some ladies obviously need some help, whether just as an outlet for feelings or actual help – but I'm not happy when people I **feel** are in need end up in the control group – perhaps I spend too much time recruiting (average 20–30 minutes I think) so possibly feel their needs and become involved quickly. (RMW1)

Fairly happy about allocation and the implications, although sometimes it is obvious that a lady in the control group would have benefitted from intervention, I accept the need for such a division. (RMW4)

Because of their feelings (encouraged by their midwifery training) that as midwives it was part of their job to assess women's needs for support, it went against the grain to hand over this assessment to the arbitration of a table of random numbers:

It's very hard in that, if this was practice and not research, you would evaluate each woman and decide if she needed the extra care for various reasons . . . It can be shame if, at first, interview, you feel that a woman has no problems, is well informed and supported, and yet you know you will keep on visiting, when you could spend that time with someone who would benefit more. But it's often not until you visit two or three times that problems become apparent. (RMW3)

As this midwife noted, and as the trial progressed, the midwives increasingly recognized that their initial judgements about women's social support needs could be proved wrong. This was particularly the case for middle class women who appeared to have no social problems, but who, as the midwives got to know them, revealed other kinds of problems and considerable support needs. This finding confirms earlier work by Ball (1987).

Providing social support

What did the midwives do? Table 3.3 gives some quantitative information about the structure and content of the social support provided by the research midwives throughout the study. Of the 255 women allocated to be offered the social support intervention, 238 were seen at home for the first interview, 235 for the second, and 224 for the third. (Some women were not interviewed because of difficulties setting up and keeping appointments, and because of hospital admissions and other pregnancy complications.) The mean time in pregnancy for each of these contacts was somewhat later than planned, mostly due to later initial booking times than expected. At each contact most of the women were not referred elsewhere by the research midwives, and did not receive any 'lifestyle' information.

Our broad definition of social support, though more general than the social support definitions operationalized in other studies, for example, the Manchester Family Worker study (Spencer *et al.*, 1989), nonetheless allowed the research midwives to participate in a wide range of very

Table 3.3 Description of the intervention

	Home contact					
	First		*Second*		*Third*	
Structure and content						
Number of women seen	238		235		224	
Intended gestational age (wks)	14		20		28	
Actual gestational age (wks)						
Mean (SD)	17.8 (3.3)		24.0 (4.6)		29.7 (8.5)	
	No.	*%*	*No.*	*%*	*No.*	*%*
Referrals to:						
Health professionals	44	19	58	25	51	23
Welfare agencies	42	18	27	12	19	9
No referral	125	53	129	55	131	59
Information given about:						
Smoking	19	8	12	5	2	1
Diet	24	10	24	10	19	9
Alcohol	12	5	8	3	1	<1
Work	12	5	10	4	4	2
Other	59	25	36	15	30	13
No 'lifestyle' information	142	60	156	66	178	80

Source: compiled by the author.

different kinds of activities under the heading of giving social support. Aside from listening to women's problems and discussing them with them, these included obtaining advice about financial benefits, filling in forms, writing letters to housing departments, accompanying women to the antenatal clinic, providing baby clothes and equipment, going with women to local support groups, taking animals to the vet, and pursuing detailed medical questions raised by the women. The following examples from the 'problem' file give a flavour of some of the work that went on:

1. Angela had a major asthma attack when 18 weeks pregnant and went into hospital to be put on steroids and a respirator. She asked for the research midwife to be contacted as she was worried about the possible effect of the treatment on the baby, and had a general 'phobia' of hospitals. The RMW went to see her and said she would find out about the possible impact of the asthma treatment on the baby ... The hospital doctor asked the RMW for advice about

discharge and after talking to Angela the RMW suggested she be sent home as soon as possible.

2. This lady had a stillbirth in 1973. Macerated, with gross abnormalities. She wants a copy of the stillbirth certificate. Goes to friend's baby's grave on anniversary of death, because she doesn't know where her baby is. Five pregnancies since 1973: two miscarriages, one termination and two children. No proper help to get over stillbirth. Can RMW find out where baby's grave is?

3. Phone call to RMW1 this morning – no money, no food. £89.90 a fortnight, both unemployed. Debts of £800. Threatened with court action by mail order firm. Can't read or write. RMW1 to write letter.

There were many requests for information:

4. This lady's husband rang me up and said what should they do if she had a bleed? I said you should ring the hospital and tell them it's the afterbirth, and as soon as they know that they'll send the flying squad out. He said what will that mean? I said it'll mean that a doctor and a midwife will come to the home in an ambulance, so if she's very poorly they can start to treat her then. So he wrote down what to say. He said shall I drive her in? Oh crikey, driving her in, haemorrhaging all over the place! (RMW4)

And to accompany women to hospital:

5. She's the girl whose husband left her, because he said it wasn't his baby . . . her father was in an accident as well, and was in intensive care. She rang me up one night, said she thought she was in prem labour, could I go into hospital with her, so I did. And she wasn't . . . (RMW4)

Or to other places:

6. I did an interesting thing this week, I had twins. I took Barbara to a twins club. You know, my lady who is expecting twins. I took her to this twins club that we finally got into contact with. And of course all these other mothers either had twins or were having twins and they said what have you got? I said I'm a friend of Barbara's. I don't know whether it will have helped, but she didn't want them to pick her up because they didn't know her. I've told her to keep the contact up because she lives quite a long way out, so she ought to be able to do that now. (RMW1)

In some of these households the research midwives were able to gain an entrée where other 'officials' had not been acceptable. Suspicion of social workers, health visitors and other representatives of the official services

(Mayall and Foster, 1989) did not extend to the research midwives in the same way. The midwives felt this was because they did not present themselves as having any kind of official authority over the women they were visiting, but instead were there in a general 'befriending' role. As one midwife said of a family she was visiting which had multiple problems:

> They're anti everybody. But not me. She's terribly interested in research. As soon as I said research, she said oh come in. She said she told me about this visa card (debt) because I'm not **from** anywhere. That's not the first time I've been told that. It's like husbands having jobs that social security don't know about, and all this sort of thing . . . (RMW1)

The research midwives were also trusted with information that was not made available to those involved in the women's routine care, for example, details of obstetric history, living arrangements and social and material circumstances, and smoking behaviour. This acceptance of midwives was also found in the Newcastle Community Midwifery Care Project, which evaluated the effect of midwifery support for socially disadvantaged women (Davies and Evans, 1991).

There was some evidence that the research midwives altered their behaviour towards the women they were supporting during the study. The data sheets the midwives filled in after any contact with intervention group women recorded the midwives' definitions of the nature of that particular contact (to give advice, support, carry out referrals, etc.). We looked at the amount of advice they gave in the early compared with the later part of the study; in two of the centres, the average number of times advice was given increased slightly and in the other two it decreased slightly. The pattern for the giving of support/reassurance followed the same trend, with the two centres in which advice-giving increased also tending to provide more support/reassurance at the end of the study. The question of how the content of the intervention related to outcome is the subject of a separate analysis, though the analysis is complicated by virtue of the fact that the women with the most problems both had the most intensive interventions and were likely to experience the worst outcomes. For the purposes of the present chapter, we looked at the relationship between the women's social class and the kind of help the research midwives offered. Class was defined on the basis of the woman's own or previous occupation, partner's occupation if appropriate, and the woman's education and housing tenure. There were clear differences in the social class composition of the four centres, with centres 1 and 4 being generally more disadvantaged than centres 2 and 3 (Table 3.2, see page 33). Working class women in general received more advice and more support/reassurance, but less of the research midwives' time. Looking at the four centres separately, three of the four gave advice more frequently to working class women, and the one which showed a reverse pattern was the centre with the smallest overall numbers and the most middle class population. For support/reassurance, three centres gave more to working class mothers, and in the fourth there was no difference by class. Average total amounts of time spent with intervention mothers varied by class, with working class mothers receiving 12% less of the midwives' time overall – six hours for middle class and 5.3 hours for working class women. Most of this difference obtained, not in relation to the minimum package, but in relation to extra time given, where the difference was 33% – 93 versus 62 minutes.

Problems of making contact. All the midwives commented on the practical problems of giving support to women who were living highly stressed lives in socially disadvantaged areas that could be dangerous to visit.

I've tried to find her in six times. The first time I left a card saying when I'd come and she rang back and said it's not convenient so we arranged that I'd see her on the 18th. She wasn't in, so I left her another letter and she did ring me and we made an appointment so I went down ten minutes early thinking ahah and I sat there for ten minutes and nearly got done by a dog . . . (RMW1)

I've got one lady with a very poor obstetric history, she lives on an awful estate and I don't like visiting. She's got four kids under 5, a fifth on the way and the husband says it's not his. He's beaten her up and walked out on her. He's told all his family and friends she's had an affair with someone. And they're coming down at intervals and attacking her, the woman, the children, with physical violence, and they're having to call the police, and she told me all this as the darkness was gathering and the kids were all crowding around and I felt **terribly** unsafe . . . I don't know what we can do because she doesn't want me to go during the day because she feels she can only talk to me when the children are asleep and anyway you can't get a word in edgeways when they're up. (RMW3)

Some male partners were reluctant to get involved in research, although the women they lived with had obvious support needs:

I had one lady – it took me two weeks to recruit her. I went to see her and she was out so I left a letter. Her husband rang me up to ask a little more because she had had a stillbirth, and it was only in February and her LMP was May so there wasn't that much time – because **he'd** found that when she talked about it, it made her depressed and therefore it made it difficult at home. Which was quite a reasonable response from him, he was concerned that I was just going to make her more depressed. So we had quite a chat and he

said he'd talk to her and get back in touch with me. He didn't so I
rang back a week later. He said she was quite willing to take part if it
was only a postal questionnaire. So I had to explain that I couldn't
promise that but I told him the first time and I said it again that I was
quite willing to go and explain it to them. So I did that. And she was
quite happy to take part. And she ended up as intervention. When I
went back to do the interview, it transpired that his attitude is that
when something like this happens the best thing to do is forget about
it. And she feels that's it's better for her to talk about it. So she is
talking about it but not to him. She's talking to her mother and to
friends and she can quite happily talk to me . . . (RMW4)

Another kind of problem was posed by extreme nervousness and initial
inability to communicate and thus make use of the research midwife's offer
to help:

I'm not sure what if anything I can do to help her . . . When I
recruited her on the phone she was so nervous that all she said was
just one word, yes . . . And she is in a complete state of anxiety –
made worse I think at first by my being there . . . It transpired she
was very anxious during her first pregnancy and it's taken her six and
a half years to get the courage up to get pregnant again because she
was so worried about last time. She's got a hospital phobia. She
didn't tell anyone she was in labour – including her husband – so as
far as the hospital are concerned she had a painless labour and
arrived fully dilated but I happened to say something about that to
her and she said well, I did know I was in labour. But she was in
such a state the whole time she wouldn't look at me, she looked out
of the window the whole time . . . The whole time I was there I
didn't get anything spontaneous out of her, but on the doorstep
when I said goodbye she suddenly started talking to me and saying
all sorts of irrelevant things and she asked me how much alcohol she
could drink at the wedding she was going to. And kept me talking
another 15 minutes. (RMW3)

Consciousness-raising and other ethical matters. Because the
research midwives were discussing with the intervention women previous
obstetric experiences and other stressful life events, there was a possibility
that the women might reflect on the meaning of this in a way that they
would not have done had they not been taking part in the research. The
artificial reflexivity imposed by research inquiries is a feature shared by
many types of research (see Oakley *et al.*, 1991). A particularly poignant
example was recounted by one of the midwives. This example also illustrates the severe emotional stress that can be hidden beneath a facade
of material comfort:

She has a beautiful home, a lake – I'm telling you this because money doesn't solve problems – it's like a showhouse. She's got one other child, and then she got pregnant and she thought did I want the child, it died after five hours. They come from the East End of London originally. I think that's relevant. Anyway, obviously it was a terrible shock to her. She was numb. And then after a few months she wanted to talk about it and no one would let her. Her family all said you're over it now, forget it. Her husband told her to go and get a job, that would help her forget it. She's never to this day discussed that baby with her husband . . . She said it was the first time she's ever been able to talk about it, it was very therapeutic. I thought my God what am I doing to her? She was very upset. She said that she felt very guilty that she didn't want the baby, she made it die. Nobody told her the baby was dying. She thought her husband had been told. They'd been to visit the baby because it was doing so well. And they were waiting to see the baby and somebody came over and said it had died. She said the only person she could have discussed it with was her mother. But her mother had had a couple of babies who'd died and she felt she'd passed something on to her daughter for the same thing to happen. So the one person she could have talked to, she couldn't. (RMW2)

Other ethical questions concerned the privileged information the research midwives had about the women they were supporting by virtue of their access to the women's case notes. One woman had an amniocentesis for raised AFP and subsequently miscarried. She asked the research midwife whether the baby had been normal. The research midwife had not read the notes at the time, but subsequently did in order to extract data for the study and discovered that the fetus had had no obvious abnormalities. (She hoped the woman would not repeat her question.) In another case a baby died during labour and the research midwife knew from discussions at the hospital, and from reading the case notes for the study, that there was a real possibility that the stillbirth could have been avoided by a caesarean section. This was confirmed at the hospital internal perinatal mortality inquiry, which the research midwife attended. The parents had asked the midwife for information and for an opinion in this case, and she had found it difficult to be non-committal. Had the social support intervention continued postnatally, this ethical dilemma would have been even more acute than it was.

Sticking to social support. On ocassion, too, the giving of support did not seem sufficient intervention to the research midwives confronted by particular circumstances. One woman allocated to the control group was visited at home by the research midwife for recruitment. The following conversation, which took place at one of the monthly meetings, is interesting because it also shows the value of the midwives being able collectively to discuss and resolve difficult issues:

RMW1:   . . . quite honestly I chewed it over all last weekend and I thought something ought to be done. I've never **seen** social conditions like that at all. There must have been eight or nine pints of milk floating around. Three on the doorstep. Some half used, some whole. I walked through one room, no carpet and the floor had piles of clothes in one corner, piles in the other corner. She'd got a jumper on inside out, perhaps it's neither here nor there . . . She took me through to a room at the back. There was another pile of clothes in the corner, no carpet, a mug tipped over, a birdcage without a bird in with droppings in it, the floor was filthy. I had to sit down, but I perched on the edge. There was a fire that had two of the radiants broken. It reminded me of Trafalgar Square – pigeon droppings all over the floor . . . She told me she can't read, this is an unwanted pregnancy, her husband's not talking to her and she was raped anyway (by her husband). The child she had in 1977 has abnormalities and they haven't talked since then. And then they had one in 1983 (without talking!) I wondered if I should do anything . . .

RMW4:   You can't, she's in the control group.

AO: Well no, but if you feel you have a moral responsibility . . .

RMW1:   That's it. My poor husband and I chewed it over all weekend . . .

AO: What are you worried about?

RMW1:   The home conditions. They're positively unhealthy.

RMW4:   But some homes are like that. That family'll be immune to those conditions. I mean this home I go to, the carpet is black, the whole home is absolutely filthy . . . if the children are well cared for it isn't up to anybody is it?

During the midwives' induction days we emphasized the need for the research midwives to provide generalized social support without behaving in ways that might be dictated by their midwifery training. Responding to pregnancy smoking was an example of this; as Table 3.1 shows (see page 33), about two in five women in the SSPO study smoked during pregnancy. Standard health education practice followed by most health professionals is to advise against maternal smoking. The research midwives were asked not to do this, but only to provide information about pregnancy smoking and how to give up if asked about this by the women they were seeing. As the study progressed, all the midwives discussed how they had come to see antismoking advice as inappropriate, given the context of women's smoking in which the use of cigarettes to cope with stress is a prominent strategy (see Graham, 1987; Oakley, 1989b).

The midwives did not, however, feel quite the same about the injunction that they were not to provide any clinical care:

RMW2: I wonder how different our reassurance or intervention would be if we had a sphygmomanmeter and a pinard . . . the number of women I've had who've been worried about their blood pressure and the baby's heart . . .

RMW1: Oh yes, I've had a quite a few who've said if only I didn't have to sit in the clinic and I knew you were going to come and take my blood pressure. I say I don't think there's any way I can, I say I'm not clinically involved this time. It's talking . . . But yes I wish I'd got one. Particularly a sphyg to be quite honest.

RMW3: With me it'd be the other one. I had one day when three women phoned me up and said they were worried the baby wasn't moving and couldn't I come and listen to them or what should they do? I thought it'd be so reassuring. But I'm sure the local midwives would have a dickey!

Breaking the relationship. The SSPO study was designed to test the effectiveness of a **pregnancy** intervention in improving maternal and infant health. Because of this, the research midwives were asked to provide support in pregnancy only, and not to carry over this support into the postnatal period. This proved extremely difficult in practice. Not only did the women the research midwives had been supporting want to see them afterwards, but the midwives themselves also felt they did not want abruptly to break the relationship that had been established:

RMW1: I usually go and see my ladies and say how are you, it's a super baby. Thank you for helping with the study . . . I think it's quite important. You can't just let them deliver, you've got to have some contact.

RMW2: I **want** to have some contact.

RMW1: Oh I do.

RMW2: Sometimes I think I want to see them, but do they want to see me?

RMW1:   Oh you can tell. Sometimes they want to sit and natter and sometimes it's just yes, I'm fine thank you, and they don't want to talk.

RMW3:   I've had a lot of them say, oh do come and see me when I'm home with the baby.

RMW1:   I try to see them on the postnatal ward because then it is a quickie, if I go home and see them then I'm stuck for at least half an hour. It sounds awful to say it but at that time I don't feel I should be spending that amount of time. It's not that I don't **want** to be there . . .

Sometimes it proved impossible to avoid a prolonged postnatal contact, albeit of an unorthodox kind:

I was trying to be really good and avoid postnatal contact with my ladies, you remember my lovely lady Claudia, who's in a block of flats that's going to be knocked down. Because of damp. We've given her a lot of baby clothes. Just before this baby was born I'd been promised by our local NCT all their nearly new NCT stuff that they didn't sell for babies and I went and picked up four dustbin bags full of baby clothes. You've never seen such a mess in your whole life! Anyway blow me down, she went and delivered before I could get them to her. I visited her in hospital and she was really pleased. She said have you got the stuff yet? And I said yes I'll get it to you. I thought well I don't really want to go and do a home visit on her. So I said to my husband right could you please, if you're going out that way, could you please just drop that bag through the door and say it's from me . . . It took him two hours to get out of the house. Her husband decided he needed some support thank you. He was there for two hours talking about the effect of the baby on the family, how he could cope as a dad. Made him coffee. And Claudia was saying, when's RMW3 going to come and see me again, I want to show her the baby. I thought you'd better know she'd had some postnatal contact. (RMW3)

This midwife's comment flags the role of the research midwives' partners in the research, which was significant in various ways (see below).

The lack of postnatal contact was even more problematic when the outcome of the pregnancy was not a healthy baby. In one case where the mother had a stillbirth due to placenta praevia (she haemorrhaged and got to hospital too late for a caesarean section to save the baby):

She phoned me up again last week she said, oh I've had a reminder (for the postnatal questionnaire), but there's one or two things I really haven't sorted out what you want. They were all things not asking for an opinion, but she said she hadn't understood what we wanted from the question. And so I told her one or two very straightforward bits. I knew it wasn't that, and it took me another 25 minutes to get off the phone. What really came out in the conversation was how bad she felt that I didn't go and see her when the baby died and how she really needed me to go out there and she was desperate for me to talk to her, and nobody else understood because I'd seen her through the pregnancy, and how she'd felt she'd been under quite a lot of extra pressure because I wasn't there. And I . . . felt bad. I had a long chat with her about the effect of the stillbirth. I said, are you going to finish the questionnaire now? Oh yes, she said. I just didn't understand these bits. I think she was just hanging on to it as an excuse to phone me again. I said look if you feel really bad, give me a ring. I don't mind chatting with you. I said if you feel that awful I'll try and pop out and see you. I think probably now I've said that she won't need it. But she was desperate, it was very sad . . . She obviously wanted postnatal help. I know it's not what we're here to do, but in a way I wonder if she felt worse because she'd had the intervention and then nothing, rather than if we hadn't done anything to her.

This question is probably unanswerable. It represents one of the tensions between the need to test scientifically hypotheses about pregnancy interventions, and the need to respect the autonomy and integrity of research participants (see Oakley, 1989a).

Learning about the services. Another central theme highlighted in the research midwives' accounts of their experiences with the research is the relationship between the research and the routinely provided services. During the negotiation with the four centres for the research, the need not to tread on the toes of those already providing antenatal care whether in hospital or in the community had been apparent. There was concern that the research might in some way add to, or otherwise interfere with, workloads. The view that social support was, in any case, being provided under the heading of routine care was also forcibly stated, particularly by community midwives in one of the four areas. Each of the four midwives was dependent to some extent on the goodwill of staff locally towards the reseach, and their experiences were very different, from a very sympathetic attitude in one of the centres, to outright hostility and non-cooperation in another.

I seemed to get the feeling that the senior medical staff had okayed it and not really consulted the ground roots first. (RMW1)

I have been very pleased at how helpful people have been and at the interest shown in the work that we are doing. I have never been made to feel in the way or a nuisance. (RMW2)

(N.B. one reason for this comment might have been that she continued to work at the hospital as a midwife part time during the study.)

One reason why staff locally might have felt threatened was because in the course of the research the research midwives learnt a good deal about the kind of antenatal care normally provided there. The midwives' lessons repeat findings of many surveys of antenatal care (see Macintyre, 1984, for a review) and include lack of communication between different branches of the sevices, the difficulty women experience getting adequate information and/or having their own preferences for care respected, the refusal of staff to recognize women's domestic and other responsibilities and to treat them as individuals in their own right, and the perpetual problem of long waiting times. Examples from the monthly meetings include lack of information, and help for women with heightened anxiety because of past difficulties or present stress:

> She's a lady who had ten years of infertility, got pregnant, had a stillbirth and then got pregnant again and obviously was very concerned about the baby . . . She phoned me up and said she'd been having this pain when she walked, or she couldn't walk because of this pain, when she sat down the pain went away. So I told her to phone her GP immediately to see what he suggested and I said I'd phone her back this afernoon to see what he said. So I phoned her back and she said her told me to take a couple of panadol, and as I'm seeing Mr Cross in a couple of days' time to wait and see what he has to say . . . But the GP gave her the impression that it's that woman again. She said to me they think I'm just panicking about everything, which she's got every right to do in my opinion. I feel now with hindsight I should have said to her phone the midwife and I **know** they would have said come in, and they would have checked her over and she would have seen a doctor . . . Apparently she said to her husband well at least RMW2 asked me questions and I was able to talk to her about it, whereas with the GP it was just take two panadol, he didn't even ask if the baby was moving. (RMW2)

> I've had three phone calls from Diana . . . It's turned out that the baby's a breech, she's under Mr Shrew, she was going to go and see him, but he wasn't in the clinic, so she was going to see him the following week. But he wasn't there. She was a bit fed up, she had a two and a half hour wait. So she was going back on Wednesday, but she rang me on Wednesday night, they'd done an antibodies test. What had they done an antibodies test for? We've got a new lab technician, I suspect it was something to do with that. So I said but this was last week, why are you suddenly worried about this now?

She said a friend of mine had a Down's syndrome baby last week. So I'm sure that was it. So I said I'm sure it isn't anything but I'm going to the clinic tonight, I'll have a look at your notes. I did, and there wasn't anything there, so I rang and told her and said I know, I had a look. (RMW1)

A woman who had a stillbirth and was still seeing the research midwife got extra help from the services as a result:

Because of the intervention she's been having postnatal help. Because I knew her social worker and I happened to say had she been seen, how was she getting on. Just for my own interest. And she said, my God, what's happened, has she lost the baby? What's happened is that the system has broken down. They're meant to have every stillbirth referred straight back to the social work department so they get at least one visit from somebody in the social work department to make sure they've got some counselling help or whatever. And this system had broken down, and people on the wards weren't being referred back. And of course once they'd said that they asked me for her name, and address, and she has had the postnatal counselling and support, but she should have had it anyway. (RMW3)

The manner in which medical care is delivered can cause, as well as relieve, stress:

This lady has a sister who had a stillbirth, her daughter has convulsions, and her husband's in intensive care . . . The same poor lady had the most horrific antenatal experience the other day too. She went in for a routine hospital antenatal and the houseman decided to listen to the baby with an ordinary stethoscope – remember her sister's baby's just been born dead – and he said to her oh I can't hear the baby's heart with a stethoscope, you'll have to go upstairs and be monitored. She went upstairs and this same chap put the things on and after a while he said something's wrong with that trace, something's wrong with that baby. She was climbing the wall. And then an experienced midwife put them on properly. He sat there and he walked up and said to her that's okay then and walked off. Luckily she got hold of him and said come back here and explain to me what's going on (she was a nurse). And he said, well it's all right now. He didn't want to explain but she made him. In the end he said, well I don't think the monitor was on target. (RMW3)

They don't **think**, any of them. They've no idea of the distress and upset they cause. (RMW1)

Differences between the midwives. The qualitative data show considerable variation between the four research midwives in their attitudes to their role in the study. There was also variation in the amount of time they spent providing social support, and in the number of contacts they had with the women in the intervention group. Table 3.4 gives some information on this, taken from the data sheets completed by the midwives following each contact with the mothers in their sample. The first line of the table gives the average of the total amount of time spent by the midwives per intervention woman, including all visits and telephone calls, a total which varies from 4.2 to 6.6 hours. The total time spent in providing the 'minimum package' of three home visits and two phone calls/brief home visits shows less variation, though the total for centre 4 (which had the highest caseload) is rather less than for the other three. There was a general tendency for the length of the visits to decrease from

Table 3.4 The social support intervention: timing and number of contacts by centre

		Centre			
		1	*2*	*3*	*4*
Total amount of time – average					
– (Hours)		5.6	5.0	6.6	4.2
– (N)		(75)	(33)	(57)	(83)
'Minimum package'					
– Visit 1 (hours)		1.8	1.6	1.8	1.3
– Visit 2 (hours)		1.5	1.5	1.5	1.1
– Visit 3 (hours)		1.6	1.3	1.5	1.1
– Phone 1 (mins)		12	9	7	9
– Phone 2 (mins)		10	12	9	10
'Minimum package'					
– Total time (hours)		4.8	4.5	4.7	3.6
– (N)		(75)	(33)	(57)	(83)
Home contacts:	mean	3.8	3.2	4.6	4.0
Telephone contacts:	mean	3.5	3.3	6.8	3.6
Midwife initiated contacts*:	mean	2.1	1.4	4.3	3.6
Woman initiated contacts*:	mean	0.8	0.5	2.2	0.7

* Visits and telephone calls.
Source: compiled by the author.

the first to the third. (This was to some extent determined by the three semi-structured interview schedules the midwives were using for these visits, which decreased in length.) Telephone calls tended to get longer. Mean home contacts go from 3.2 to 4.0 and phone contacts from 3.3 to 6.8 depending on the centre. Midwife-initiated contacts varied threefold: from 1.4 in centre 2 to 4.3 in centre 3. Woman-initiated contacts followed the same pattern. For all these contact variables, centre 2 had the lowest and centre 3 the highest means.

Table 3.5 is also based on the data sheets filled in by the research midwives. Since the midwives varied in the extent to which they took the exercise of filling in these data sheets seriously, the data in the table need

Table 3.5 Nature of the intervention by centre

| | | *Centre* | | | | | | | |
| | | *1* | | *2* | | *3* | | *4* | |
		%	No.	%	No.	%	No.	%	No.
Total advice score (average = 8)	[>8]	17	13	3	1	53	31	64	54
'Someone to talk to'/ reassurance given (average = 5)	[>5]	23	18	0	0	48	28	61	52
Advised to see GP/ obst/MW (average = 2)	[>1]	47	37	55	18	55	32	64	54
Advised to see HV/ other health professional	[>1]	15	12	3	1	10	6	15	13
Gave information/ advice on pregnancy (average = 2)	[>1]	47	37	52	17	79	46	64	54
Advice on benefits, housing, etc. (average = 3)	[>0]	41	32	15	5	29	17	74	63
Advice on smoking		5	4	12	4	31	18	4	3
Advice on diet		13	10	6	2	52	30	22	19

Source: compiled by the author.

to be read subject to the proviso that they represent differences in the recording of aspects of the intervention which may or may not reflect differences in the way the intervention was in fact provided. There are clear differences between centres. It is interesting that the centres ranking highest on advice scores also ranked highest on the 'someone to talk to'/reassurance given factor, and referrals to GP, obstetrician or midwife, and on advice concerning benefits, housing etc. It would thus seem that there is a lack of differentiation between advice, listening/reassurance and referrals, with those midwives doing more of one doing more of the others as well (or at least recording it in this fashion on the data sheets).

The midwives discussed the different ways in which they were interpreting the social support intervention in practice during the monthly meetings. They were also asked to comment on this in their questionnaires and interviews:

> I know my interviews are generally shorter than those of the other midwives. I wonder if this is because I haven't got the right approach, which means the ladies feel less able to 'open up'. (RMW4)

> RMW3 always seemed to have so many problems, it made me wonder if I'd missed them or I hadn't brought them up when I should have done. Or perhaps I don't see them in the same light. Or maybe my mums are coping better. I know I spend a lot longer with my ladies than RMW4 does but then RMW4's got a lot more ladies! (RMW1)

> I wonder if my outlook, lifestyle, is a little less conventional than the others and this could colour my reactions, approaches to situations? (RMW3)

> I feel we were very different. Our characters are different, and the way we handled the women – the character of our caseloads was different, so that even though we were reacting differently, it was to different things . . . I would say I'm very bad at paperwork. I know I am. Often when I'd had a conversation with someone, I'd say oh God, I haven't written that down. I know it had to be done but it was a chore. (RMW2)

The midwives' perspectives: job satisfaction versus role overload?

The role of research midwife on the SSPO study had both a positive and a negative side. Some tension inevitably resulted from the fact that the midwives were employed part time, yet were involved in a task capable of expanding to fill all the time (and more) available. Although they recognized that being on call 24 hours a day, and arranging for 'cover' during holiday periods etc., was an important part of the intervention so far as the women were concerned, this could mean that they were rarely able to feel 'off duty':

> Being on constant call has meant that although I'm only 'working' two days a week, I feel the research is always at the forefront of my mind. (RMW2)

But the fact that the women were able to telephone round the clock did not necessarily mean that they did so:

> It's very valuable, it is often mentioned in conversation, in terms of a 'safety valve' – it may not be needed, but they're glad it's there. Although they like the idea of the pager, they seem to avoid using it if they can, but again say they're reassured by the ease of access it gives them. So far my calls have ranged from 07.30 through to 01.45 . . . In general being on call has not been a problem in itself . . . (but) I remember thinking over the Christmas time that I mustn't drink too much in case I didn't make sense if anyone called! (RMW3)

The mixture of costs and benefits came out clearly in answer to a question about how the research had affected the research midwives' personal lives:

> It has made it easier for me to work while I have a young child. (But) it has been very difficult to give the social support at times of crisis at home, as I felt very guilty giving such personal help to 'outsiders', even if I knew I had done all I could at home. (RMW4)

For another midwife, the research meant that:

> 1. Husband has to go to work on the bus so I can have the car.
> 2. Don't have many evenings in – apart from family social life and activities. I find the best time to check notes and write case histories at the hospital is evenings.
> 3. Clothes – different for work and home depending on who one is going to see – always wore uniform before.
> 4. Days very disjointed – to begin with I found it difficult to adjust to being out for two hours a.m. and two p.m., trying to fit in housework, shopping etc. . . .
> 5. Made me more aware of how fortunate I am.
> 6. More money – increased seniority.
> 7. Learnt a lot about what is available locally. (RMW1)

All four research midwives agreed that their job satisfaction was potentially very high. The degree to which this promise was realized depended on the extent to which it appeared that their support resulted in better outcome for the women and their babies:

(How would you rate your level of satisfaction?)

Very good. I love it. It does vary, because some days are busy and bad and others are great. On the whole more up days than down. However, my husband says I come home frustrated because I've been unable to help. (RMW1)

This does vary. Obviously, if I've been of particular help to a lady with a problem during the pregnancy then yes, there is a sense of achievement. But basically to build up a good rapport with a woman, gain her trust and to support her through the pregnancy in whatever way she needs and at the end of the term to have a live healthy baby (of increased birthweight of course!) then that is sufficient job satisfaction for me. (RMW2)

We asked the midwives to write down the high and low points of the job. High points were:

Meeting the women. (RMW2)

Achieving a type of care not usually possible. Having a chance of acting on your own initiative. (RMW3)

Bigger baby than **all** the others. Where there are previous prems, and this pregnancy has gone full-term . . . Full-term normal delivery and quick discharge. Really getting to know people and families – when they say how good it's been and call me friend or 'mate' and when they've had a lot of problems and involvement and the outcome is very good. (RMW1)

When a lady has a successful outcome to her pregnancy, especially if it is her first living baby. When a lady actually tells me I have helped. (RMW4)

And the low points:

The paperwork. Aggravation over payment of expenses. (RMW4)

(Getting the research midwives' expenses paid on time through the University bureaucracy was a major hassle throughout the study.)

Saying goodbye. When we have a disaster or a baby that's not as big as before . . . (RMW1)

Breaking off contact with the women immediately after delivery. (RMW2)

Working as research midwives, and particularly on a study which had such obvious relevance to the routine provision of midwifery care, the midwives were conscious that the research might have an impact on their conceptions

of what midwives could, and should do, on their own future career plans
and on their ideas about how the routine services might be improved so as
to provide more support for childbearing women. The following conversation took place at a meeting fairly late in the progress of the study:

RMW1:   It's been a tremendous eye opener.

RMW2:   It's made me question the basis of a lot of clinical decision
         making. I think we're inclined to forget the woman
         as a person.

RMW3:   Especially when they tell a woman she's got to come into
         hospital for rest and they don't think of everything else
         at home.

RMW2:   They think about this bump but they forget that there's a
         head up there and feet down the bottom.

RMW3:   Let alone little appendages like children!

RMW1:   And I don't think they realize the effect they have on
         women . . .

One midwife said the research had 'unsettled' her and made her unsure of
the direction in which she wanted to go:

   Where I had, and I hate to admit it, black and white areas, I have
   learnt there are a lot of grey ones. The study has taught me a lot
   about pregnancy, women's needs, lack of services available, lack of
   information imparted, lack of time available for these women, and
   having learnt these things I feel I want to make other personnel
   aware of them and maybe in some small way improve the care these
   women receive. (RMW2)

   I would find it hard to practice as a midwife in a hospital where you
   have little say over how the women were cared for . . . (RMW3)

As to how the services might be improved, and midwives could become
more effective, it would help:

   To be more aware of social problems (i.e. housing, financial, family
   commitments). Midwives in hospital should make more time available
   to discuss these matters with the women, and act accordingly in their
   advice and care. (RMW4)

Another wrote that:

   Relationships are very important. Midwives need more time. They
   have contact with people at one of the most emotional times in
   their lives, so perhaps fewer ladies, more midwives and reduced
   caseloads. (RMW1)

And said, during her interview:

> I think having done the research I'm much more aware of what the mothers actually go through before they come in and have their baby . . . Because you have the contact with the home and the family (as a research midwife) – I mean you're a guest in their home but you can't fail to pick up what's going on in the home. I think they give more because you're in their home and they're confident and happy and their own surroundings. When they come into hospital, they're in a totally alien environment . . . (RMW1)

Communication was regarded as critical:

> For some of the women I was the only midwife they were seeing, so I was answering basic questions like minor disorders of pregnancy and what they should do about them – not that I minded, but I didn't think that was what I was there for . . . More community staff are needed. Maybe this is where we need to centre a lot of the care – out in the community. I feel midwives should go and see the women . . . In an ideal world one midwife looks after you in pregnancy and delivers your baby. (RMW2)

The other side of this coin is strengthening the position of the midwives:

> I'm sure my suggestions would be financially unviable! But provide more continuity of care; work in groups sharing the care of a group of women, with one of you always on call. Make care more flexible – especially the postnatal cut-off. Provide a drop in centre for women with preconceptional through to postnatal advice, information, exercise classes, etc. Give midwives their own clients so that women don't see their care as a back up or poor alternative to GPs. Finally (tongue in cheek) get all midwives to have a baby themselves. (RMW3)

This last, not entirely facetious comment, highlights the importance of personal experience – in more ways than one, as the same midwife thoughtfully reflected in her interview:

> I didn't see the deficiencies before. When you're at the NHS end, you think the system's working, you think you're doing the best you can, but you don't get the women's opinions. You don't find out how long they are actually sitting in the clinic, how many doctors they see in the course of their antenatal care, how often they don't get things explained to them. If you tell them things in the course of your ordinary work as a midwife, very rarely do they say they don't understand. It's made me realize how often people **think** they've explained something which they (the women) don't understand and they don't have anyone to come back and ask so they just go away

and worry... It never occurred to me how much it affects the women. They come to the hospital to see a doctor – the magic consultant – and they don't see him, but it never occurred to me how much it affected them seeing a different person each time. And that's why they don't ask questions. The inconsistencies, the advice that's different every time. It didn't occur to me how often the people working in the same team would tell someone something completely different. The other thing that's struck me is how often people are given advice they can't follow. To actually go home and rest, but there's nobody who's said... does your husband realize he's got to do the housekeeping for you – and very often we blithely say go home and do this, and when they come back they're told off for not having followed that advice... and there's no practical way that they can. (RMW3)

But it was the case that one aspect of personal experience all the midwives felt was relevant to their provision of the social support intervention was the fact that they were mothers.

RMW3:   ... I changed through having a child as well as through the research. I didn't realize what it's like. Several of these women have said to me they only want to be delivered by women who've had children themselves.

RMW1:   Oh, that comes across, especially with health visitors and social workers. Especially with health visitors. Seventeen- and 18-year-old girls going in and telling them what to do with their babies when they don't know anything and it's the practical knowledge you need.

RMW3:   Health visitors only need to do 12 weeks obstetrics. Some women have said to me, she's not a midwife, she's not a children's nurse, she's not a mother – she should really be asking me what to do!

RMW2:   I find a lot of women know. They say, oh you've had children yourself, haven't you? They tell **me**.

RMW3:   Quite a lot have asked me. Otherwise I'll say something and they'll say oh yes, you've had children haven't you? Sometimes you don't even have to say something. Perhaps they've had a baby with colic and you say, oh yes and they know you're not just talking from professional knowledge. It's something you've been through... **I think they know as much about you as you do about them by the end of the research**.

Motherhood was not a selection criterion for the jobs but, as one of the research midwives commented, the flexibility of the work on the study did make it more compatible with motherhood than a clinical midwifery appointment.

CONCLUSION

Different kinds of lessons can be derived from this attempt to draw out the experiences of the research midwives in the SSPO study. One set of lessons concerns the doing of research in the maternity services. This is an activity which requires delicate steering through the politics of the structure within which care is provided, including the control over obstetric work defined and exercised by medical and midwifery hierarchies (Garcia *et al.*, 1988). The limits of the research it is possible to do are often set by other people. But in addition to the normal hazards of maternity care research, the research midwives who provided social support in the SSPO study occupied an ambiguous role inbetween the researchers and the research participants. Although neither of these, they were also both at the same time: participants in the research, and deliverers of a research intervention. They had substantial control over their work, and were required to use their own initiative a good deal of the time, but were ultimately subject to the authority of the London research team and the research design and budget for which the researchers had obtained funding. Thus, the midwives' comments reflect both an appreciation of the autonomy the job offered them, and a dislike of the need to submit their work to the arbitration of preset rules. The clearest examples of this are in relation to the procedure for random allocation, and the termination of the social support at delivery rather than afterwards. Because of the experimental design of the study, and the timing of the informed consent procedure, the research midwives were also led to reflect more, perhaps, than researchers in many other kinds of research, about the ways in which taking part in research may subtly and not so subtly influence the lives of those who agree to do so. The midwives' reflections on the extent to which the study's design meant that women allocated to the control group may have both felt in receipt of support initially and then deprived of it are particularly interesting from the viewpoint of assessing the success of the study. The former observation carries the implication that through designing the study in this way we may have minimized interventioncontrol group differences, and thus statistically significant aspects of social support.

A second set of lessons relates to the meaning of social support. Variably and poorly defined in the literature (see Oakley, 1988 for a review) the concept of social support can mean all things to all people. Our specification of social support at the start of the trial was primarily negative: social support is **not** clinical care, it is **not** health education, it is **not** anti-smoking counselling, it is **not** a device for increasing antenatal attendance, and so forth. Our positive definition of it was minimal: **listening, responding, informing** when asked, helping whenever and however appropriate. Our detailed documentation of the content of the intervention enables us to say that on the whole we were successful in designing an intervention which did offer general social support. One measure of our success is, of course, the way the trial women felt about the study, and this is to be reported on separately. But judging from the records the research midwives kept, and also from the qualitative material we gathered during the course of our team meetings and the interviews and questionnaires the midwives completed, it would be fair to say that the SSPO study was a test of research midwife-provided social support, and not of any of the other kinds of intervention that can masquerade under this heading. As well as the data on the women's views, the links between research midwife-provided social support, and the women's own support resources need to be explored. The relationships between social support, stress and coping in our data are the subject of a new, ongoing study on social support and the health and welfare of vulnerable children which is funded by the Economic and Social Research Council.

Thirdly, the SSPO study throws a good deal of light on the way in which the maternity services currently operate in the four areas where the study was done. Much of this is no surprise to anyone who is acquainted with the 'consumer satisfaction' literature. The importance of continuity of care emerges very strongly: the needs of childbearing women to form a relationship with one care provider, or a small number of these, and to receive care from this source throughout pregnancy and, ideally, through delivery and the postnatal period. Part of this need is being able to count on a reliable source of information concerning medical care and other pregnancy needs and experiences. As the research midwives reported, the maternity services may too often consist of different professionals giving conflicting information and advice, the results of which can increase women's stress. This is particularly the case for a group already exposed to stress, as many of the women in the SSPO study were by virtue of their obstetric histories and current social and medical circumstances. In these respects, as noted above, the findings of the SSPO study discussed here simply confirm other studies – both descriptive surveys of childbearing women's attitudes, and other intervention studies such as the trial of the 'Know Your Midwife' scheme which show the contribution continuity of care can make to improved physical and psychosocial pregnancy outcomes (Flint and Poulengeris, 1987; Flint, 1991). In addition, our study shows how the research role of generalized social supporter can be preferred by women to the scrutiny of social workers and health visitors, who are seen as surveilling and monitoring and not as helping mothers in their childcare work (Mayall and Foster, 1989).

The SSPO study was unusual in that it also contributes to the literature evidence about the change in professionals' perspectives that can be brought about through the taking of a research role. The research midwives said their eyes had been opened through the research – to what it is really like trying to have a baby in conditions of poverty, to how it really feels waiting in line in an antenatal clinic, attempting unsuccessfully to obtain consistent information about one's care, and being treated to unrealistic admonitions about how to behave in pregnancy, as though pregnant women have nothing else to do apart from attend antenatal clinics and listen to health professionals. Visiting the women's homes was seen as particularly crucial to this altered vision.

It is easy to see how developments in the provision of maternity care over the last 30 years have militated against the inclusion within it of the kind of social support the research midwives in the SSPO were trying to provide. It is equally easy to follow some of their suggestions in seeing how it could be put back. More community care, particularly for low-risk women, more midwife-provided care, lower caseloads, more time for individual women, a greater emphasis on social aspects of maternity in midwifery training, more material and other support for disadvantaged women – these are all policy implications which arise out of a series of studies, of which this is only one (see Oakley *et al.*, 1986 and Elbourne *et al.*, 1989, for reviews). The logic of the argument is further reinforced by the evidence that social support is not only nice, but good for health, and cost-effective. The challenge remains one of how to disseminate the results of such research so that health professionals and those who formulate policy in the maternity services take it on board in designing alternatives to the present system. It is a well-known observation that institutional structures and systems can often be subversive of the goals they were set up to meet. As one of the research midwives in the SSPO study put it, 'What I was doing as research was only what I was trained to do'.

ACKNOWLEDGEMENTS

The SSPO study was funded by the Department of Health and the Iolanthe Trust. Grateful thanks are due to all who took part in the study, including the four research midwives and Sandra Stone who provided administrative and secretarial support for the study and who continues to play a key role in organizing its publications.

REFERENCES

Ball, J.A. (1987) *Reactions to motherhood – the role of postnatal care*. Cambridge University Press, Cambridge.

Davies, J. and Evans, F. (1991) The Newcastle community midwifery care project. In S. Robinson and M.A. Thomson (eds) *Midwives, research and childbirth*, Vol. 2., Chapman & Hall, London.

Elbourne, D., Oakley, A. and Chalmers, I. (1989) Social and psychological support during pregnancy. In I. Chalmers, M. Enkin and M.J.N.C. Keirse (eds) *Effective care in pregnancy and childbirth*. Oxford University Press, Oxford.

Flint, C. and Poulengeris, P. (1987) *Know Your Midwife*. Heinemann, London.

Flint, C. (1991) Continuity of care provided by a team of midwives – the Know Your Midwife scheme. In S. Robinson and A.M. Thomson (eds) *Midwives, research and childbirth*, Vol. 2., Chapman & Hall, London.

Garcia, J., Kilpatrick, R. and Richards, M. (1988) *The politics of maternity care*. Oxford University Press, Oxford.

Graham, H. (1987) Women's smoking and family health. *Social Science and Medicine*, **25**, 47–56.

Macintyre, S. (1984) Consumer reactions to present-day antenatal services. In L. Zander and G. Chamberlain (eds) *Pregnancy care for the 1980s*. Macmillan, London.

Mayall, B. and Foster, M.-C. (1989) *Child health care*. Heinemann, London.

Oakley, A., Elbourne, D. and Chalmers, I. (1986) The effects of social interventions in pregnancy. In G. Breart, N. Spira and E. Papiernik (eds) *Proceedings of a workshop on prevention of preterm birth – new goals and new practices in prenatal care*. INSERM, Paris.

Oakley, A. (1988) Is social support good for the health of mothers and babies? *Journal of Reproductive and Infant Psychology*, **6**, 3–21.

Oakley, A. (1989a) Who's afraid of the randomized controlled trial? Some dilemmas of the scientific method and 'good' research practice. *Women and Health*, **15**(2), 25–9.

Oakley, A. (1989b) Smoking in pregnancy – smokescreen or risk factor? Towards a materialist analysis. *Sociology of Health and Illness*, **11**(4), 311–35.

Oakley, A. and Houd, S. (1990) *Helpers in childbirth: midwifery today*. Hemisphere Books, Washington.

Oakley, A. and Rajan, L. (1989) The social support and pregnancy outcome study. In A.M. Thomson and S. Robinson (eds) *Research and the Midwife Conference Proceedings for 1988*. Department of Nursing Studies, University of Manchester.

Oakley, A. and Rajan, L. (1990) Obstetric technology and maternal emotional wellbeing: a further research note. *Journal of Reproductive and Infant Psychology*, **8**, 45–55.

Oakley, A., Rajan, L. and Grant, A. (1990) Social support and pregnancy outcome: report of a randomized trial. *British Journal of Obstetrics and Gynaecology*, **97**, 155–62.

Oakley, A., Brannen, J. and Dodd, K. (1991) Getting involved: the effects of research on participants. Paper presented at the British Sociological Association Conference 1991. Available from the Social Science Research Unit, Institute of Education, London University.

Oakley, A. and Rajan, L. (1991) Social class and social support – the same or different? *Sociology*, **25**(1), 31–59.

Rajan, L. and Oakley, A. (1990a) Infant feeding practices in mothers at risk of low birthweight delivery. *Midwifery*, **6**, 18–27.

Rajan, L. and Oakley, A. (1990b) Low birthweight babies: the mother's point of view. *Midwifery*, **6**, 73–85.

Spencer, B., Thomas, H. and Morris, J.A. (1989) A randomized controlled trial of the provision of a social support service during pregnancy: the South Manchester Family Worker Project. *British Journal of Obstetrics and Gynaecology*, **96**, 281–8.

CHAPTER FOUR

The needs of women hospitalized in pregnancy

Susan A. Kirk

INTRODUCTION

The research described in this chapter was undertaken in part fulfilment for a Master of Science degree at the University of Manchester and was completely self-funded. I spent six months full-time planning the research, conducting the interviews and analysing the data (and of course another two years writing up the study). My interest in the area arose from working as a midwife with women who were hospitalized for long periods during pregnancy. I became aware that these women received little care from midwives apart from 'routine' observations and I was therefore interested in discovering what these women's needs were and what kind of midwifery care would be appropriate for them.

Advances in obstetrics have allowed increasing numbers of women to be identified as having a high-risk pregnancy and it has been estimated that approximately 20% of all pregnant women become high risk by the time of delivery (Curry, 1985). The trend has been to hospitalize this group of women antenatally in an attempt to reduce maternal and neonatal morbidity and mortality. In spite of increasing numbers of women being hospitalized in pregnancy, very little research has been published regarding their needs. It is proposed that these women are unique in that, not only are they experiencing the dual stresses of hospitalization and a high-risk pregnancy but, unlike most other individuals in the hospital setting, they generally feel physically well. Moreover, this situation is superimposed on the normal developmental crisis of pregnancy (Snyder, 1979).

The sociological literature regarding hospitalization of sick people highlights the means through which the hospital depersonalizes individuals and removes their control over most activities (Goffman, 1961; Taylor, 1979). A large body of research has investigated patients' opinions about hospitalization and has highlighted the stress they experience (Volicer and Bohannon, 1975; Wilson-Barnett, 1977). A number of aspects of life as a patient have been identified as causing dissatisfaction and stress, but the area most frequently cited as problematic is that of information giving and communication (McGhee, 1961; Cartwright, 1964; Gregory, 1978).

As previously noted, very little research into the specific experience of antenatal hospitalization has been undertaken, particularly in the United Kingdom. However, three studies in North America have examined women's experiences of hospitalization in pregnancy (Merkatz, 1978; White, 1981; Curry, 1985). These studies have highlighted the stress that such women experience because of their concerns for the health of their unborn baby, the effects of separation on their partner and children, and their own feelings of guilt, low self-esteem and depression. In the United Kingdom, Taylor (1985) examined this area as part of her general survey on women's satisfaction with the maternity services in one District Health Anthority. She identified a number of problems experienced by women hospitalized in pregnancy, in particular those of boredom, uncertainty, loneliness and poor communication of information from health professionals.

The research evidence appears to suggest that hospitalization in pregnancy is a stress-inducing event. This is noteworthy, as stress in pregnancy has been implicated as an aetiological factor in the occurrence of complications in pregnancy, labour and the neonatal period (McDonald *et al.*, 1963; Gorsuch and Key, 1974; Crandon, 1979). Research investigating the relationship between antenatal stress and pregnancy outcome is problematic because of the ethical and practical constraints on the use of experimental research, and because of the interplay of medical, behavioural and socio-demographic factors that contribute to obstetric risk. The research conducted in this area has been criticized because of methodological weaknesses, with the following problems having been identified:

1. the sampling techniques used in some of the studies have been criticized for failing to describe sample characteristics, the use of small samples of convenience and the general methods of sampling (Chalmers, 1982; Lederman, 1984);
2. the absence of control groups (Selby *et al.*, 1980; Norbeck and Tilden, 1983);
3. inadequate definition and assessment of the independent and dependent variables (Carlson and Labarba, 1979);
4. the research studies have frequently used univariate designs which fail to consider the interplay of variables in the causation of obstetric complications (Istvan, 1986);
5. the use of retrospective designs (Istvan, 1986);
6. the use of non-standardized instruments to measure anxiety (Istvan, 1986).

Although much of the research in this area is methodologically weak, there is some evidence to suggest that the hospitalization of women with complications of pregnancy may exacerbate rather than alleviate their condition.

The research described in this chapter aimed to investigate this much neglected area of antenatal hospitalization.

STUDY DESIGN AND METHODS

The research was a small-scale exploratory study undertaken in one maternity hospital. The aims were:

1. to discover pregnant women's experiences of hospitalization;
2. to identify their needs and propose ways in which midwives may meet these needs;
3. to examine the effects (as perceived by the woman) of antenatal hospitalization on the family;
4. to discover the quality of information giving;
5. to discover whether hospitalized pregnant women receive parentcraft and health education.

The aims of the study indicated that a survey would be the most appropriate research method, the method also used by other researchers in the field (White, 1981; Curry, 1985). A survey of women's experiences and views would provide descriptive information on the five aims and also allow for investigation of possible correlations.

The research instruments

The aims guided the development of the two research instruments used in the study, a structured interview schedule and the Antepartum Hospital Stressors Inventory.

A structured interview schedule. For several reasons a standardized semi-structured interview schedule was developed for use in this research rather than a self-completed questionnaire. First it was thought that a higher response rate might be obtained in as short time as possible as response rates for personal interviews are generally higher than those for questionnaires. Second using a standardized schedule in an interview allows for some correction of misunderstandings and probing of inadequate answers. Third the researcher has control over the context in which the schedule is completed; in this study there was concern that, as women in an antenatal ward are a 'mobile' sample, questionnaires might have been completed in a group. Finally, personal interviews allow rapport to be established between the subject and the researcher which can motivate the former to provide full and detailed answers and hence increase the quality of the data obtained.

The development of the schedule was guided by the literature reviewed and the aims of the research. A number of questions in the schedule were replicated or adapted from instruments used in other studies, particularly that of Curry (1985). Information on a wide variety of topics was included:

- the characteristics of the sample, for example, age, length of gestation, obstetric history, smoking behaviour;
- attitudes and opinions regarding issues such as information giving and parentcraft information;
- the feelings and concerns of the women in the sample.

Both closed and open questions were used. A Likert scale was used to collect data on the women's views about information giving. A number of questions used equal interval visual analogue scales to rate the women's concerns about their current pregnancy and family, problems with hospitalization, and to assess the contribution of the individuals comprising their support network.

Due to time constraints, the schedule was not extensively tested for validity or reliability, although it was piloted at a second hospital and a number of alterations were made to improve clarity.

The Antepartum Hospital Stressors Inventory. The Antepartum Hospital Stressors Inventory (AHSI) was developed by White (1981), a Canadian researcher. This instrument utilizes a self-report method of identifying stressors associated with antenatal hospitalization and is based on the Social Readjustment Rating Scale (Holmes and Rahe, 1967) and the Hospital Stress Rating Scale (Volicer, 1973; 1974; 1978). The scale consists of 47 potential stressors for women hospitalized in pregnancy that were identified from the literature and from clinical practice. These 47 potential stressors are assigned to seven stressor categories which are derived from the seven adaptive tasks of illness identified by Moos and Tsu (1977) and from the nine stress factors identified by Volicer (1978).

The seven stressor categories defined by White (1981) are:

1. **Separation** – the change in a woman's relationships and activities outside hospital which occur while she is hospitalized.
2. **Environment** – the experiences resulting from being in a hospital milieu due to an 'at risk' pregnancy.
3. **Health status** – the circumstances, experiences and concerns from increased medical intervention in a hospital setting during pregnancy.
4. **Communications with health professionals** – the experience in relating with health professionals involved in the care of a pregnant woman in hospital.
5. **Self-image** – the changes in perceptions and evaluations of self which occur when a pregnant woman is hospitalized.

6. **Emotions** – those feelings experienced by a pregnant woman in hospital that may be disturbing to her.

7. **Family status** – the family's circumstances resulting from a hospitalized pregnant woman's absence from home.

The 47 stressors are randomly ordered on the AHSI and subjects were requested to respond to each item by assigning a degree of stress on a continuum from 'no stress' to 'a great deal of stress'. The option 'does not apply to me' is also available. For this study two minor alterations were made. The word 'nurse' was changed to 'midwife' and the word 'patient' was changed to 'woman'. White (1981) did not present much information on the tests used to assess the validity and reliability of the instrument. Face and content validity were assessed by a panel of experts (health professionals and women who had experienced antenatal hospitalization). Concurrent validity was said to have been demonstrated by a correlation with a level of significance of $p = 0.001$. Construct validity had not been measured. Reliability in terms of internal consistency was said to have been demonstrated by a split half alpha of 0.91. As with the interview schedule the AHSI was piloted at the second hospital and no problems were identified with the completion of the instrument.

Negotiating access

The hospital chosen for the study was a large maternity hospital which serves as a regional referal centre for obstetrics, gynaecology and neonatology. It is a teaching hospital involved in the education of midwives, nurses and doctors. The proposed design entailed recruiting a sample of convenience from all the maternity wards in the hospital. Random sampling was not considered appropriate because of the limitations of time and study size. The size of the sample required for statistical analysis was determined to be 50 and a number of inclusion criteria for the subjects were fomulated for the study:

- gestation of 20 weeks or more;
- hospitalized for three days or more;
- intending to keep the baby;
- able to read, write and understand English.

The process of gaining access to the study area took three and a half months. It involved gaining approval at three levels: the Director of Midwifery Services; the Division of Obstetrics and Gynaecology for the hospital, and the District Health Authority Research Ethics Committee. At each stage a research proposal was submitted together with examples of the instruments to be used. Ethical approval was obtained for the study with the proviso that potential subjects were to be excluded from the study if it was assessed by the midwives, medical staff or researcher that their participation might prove detrimental to themselves.

Data collection

The desired sample of 50 was obtained in a period of three weeks. There was no attempt to recruit women at a specific point after admission, providing that they met the inclusion criteria of having been hospitalized for a minimum of three days. Therefore, as this study used a sample of convenience, there was a wide variation in the length of hospitalization of women recruited to the sample in the earlier stages of data collection. In the later stages, however, the majority of the women recruited had been hospitalized for three days (Table 4.1). In the final days of data collection the researcher had to wait for some subjects to meet the inclusion criteria regarding length of hospitalization.

The procedure for data collection was as follows. On arrival in each ward the researcher introduced herself to the midwife in charge and ensured that staff were aware of the research. Names and bed numbers of women meeting the inclusion criteria were requested and enquiries made regarding their suitability for recruitment into the study (e.g. whether they were at risk of emotional distress by participating). No problems were experienced in using ward staff to identify suitable subjects. The researcher

Table 4.1 Number of days respondents had been admitted to hospital prior to interview

No. of days in hospital	No.	%
3–5	34	68
6–8	8	16
9–12	1	2
13–16	3	6
17–19	0	0
20–22	0	0
23–25	2	4
26–28	0	0
29–32	1	2
44	1	2
	50	100

Source: Kirk, 1990.

introduced herself to potential subjects as a student studying for a nursing degree and a standard written format was read to each subject. This was used to introduce both the researcher and the research and to obtain informed consent for participation. The subjects were assured of confidentiality and given the opportunity to ask questions. The written format was left with the subjects for their information.

The majority of interviews took place beside the woman's bed. The opportunity was always given to use a single room for the interview to ensure privacy for those sharing a room and this offer was generally accepted. The women's preferences for time and location were always respected. On two occasions the interviews had to be abandoned until later in the day when visitors arrived unexpectedly.

The structured schedule was administered as an interview conducted by the researcher. Following the completion of the interview the woman was then asked to complete the AHSI alone and it was collected later by the researcher. A response rate of 100% was obtained. Generally the women appeared to welcome the opportunity to discuss their experiences even though the schedule was structured.

During the period of data collection three women were excluded from the study. One woman did not meet the inclusion criteria as she did not speak English. Another woman was awaiting induction of labour on the morning of the interview and it was decided by the researcher that it was inappropriate to ask her to participate in the study. The third woman who was excluded had experienced a fetal death *in utero*.

Analysis of data

Data obtained from the interview schedule and the AHSI were numerically coded, either at the time of interviewing or following completion of the data collection phase. These data were then statistically analysed using the Statistical Package for the Social Sciences (SPSSx) computer program. As the data were not normally distributed, non-parametric statistical tests were used – Kruskal-Wallis, Mann-Whitney U (Seigel, 1956). A p level of 0.05 was accepted as a level of statistical significance.

Most of the analysis of the data from the interviews was descriptive although some correlational tests were performed. Descriptive analysis of data from the AHSI was undertaken and these data were also converted into both intensity and identification scores. The intensity scores are the mean intensity of stress for each of the seven stressor categories and the identification scores represent the percentage of stressors in the category that were assigned a degree of stress. Both these scores are calculations that were originally made by White (1981). Some correlational analysis was performed and this is described later in the chapter.

FINDINGS

The main findings from the study are included in this chapter and relate to the following: characteristics of the sample; the women's experiences of hospital life; the effects of hospitalization on their families and on smoking behaviour; the women's feelings about themselves and their pregnancy; and their experiences of information giving and parentcraft information. The above data were collected during the interview. The stress that the women were experiencing during hospitalization is also discussed. This information was gathered from both the interview and the AHSI. Readers are referred to associated work (Kirk, 1990) for a description of all the findings from the study.

Characteristics of the sample

The mean age of the 50 women in the sample was 27.6 years and the majority were married or cohabitating. Twenty-six (52%) of the sample had children at home (i.e. this excludes multiparae with no living children). Twenty-four (48%) were working before becoming pregnant, mainly in social class IIInm and social class IIIm occupations. Twenty-nine (58%) of the sample had left school with some form of educational certificate.

The mean gestational age of the pregnancies was 34 weeks and for the majority of the sample the pregnancy was 'planned'. The most frequent reason for admission to hospital was intra-uterine growth retardation (IUGR). For 21 (42%) the present admission to hospital was not their first in the current pregnancy and 19 (38%) of the sample had been admitted to hospital in a previous pregnancy.

The majority of the women (27, 54%) were admitted to hospital suddenly, with little or no time to prepare themselves or their family for the admission. There was a wide range in the length of hospitalization from 3–44 days, with 34 (68%) having been hospitalized for up to five days (Table 4.1, see page 69).

The sample's obstetric history was poor. Among the 50 women there was a total of seven previous stillbirths, four neonatal deaths, and six preterm deliveries. Twelve (24%) of the sample had experienced at least one spontaneous abortion.

Experience of hospital life

Nineteen (38%) of the sample described their reaction to their admission to hospital as 'not surprised', which may reflect the finding that a significant proportion of the sample had previously been admitted to hospital. However, 21 (42%) described themselves as feeling 'shocked', 'angry', or 'depressed' at the time of their addmission. The remaining ten women reported feelings of helplessness, resignation and relief at the time of their admission. Nineteen (38%) of the women still reported negative feelings about the need for hospitalization at the time of the interview.

The women were asked to rate various aspects of hospital life on a scale of 1 to 5, with 1 meaning that it was not a problem to them and 5 meaning it was a great problem to them; the findings are shown in Table 4.2. The major problem for the women in this sample was boredom, with 35 (70%) assigning it a score of 4 or 5 (indicating that they regarded it as a great problem). Twenty-seven (54%) felt that their stay in hospital could have been improved and their suggestions for how this might be achieved fell into the following five categories:

1. the provision of more recreational activities/facilities;
2. the provision of facilities to make drinks;
3. more flexible visiting hours;
4. improvements to the quality and quantity of food;
5. improvements in information-giving by professionals.

Twenty-nine (58%) of the sample reported that their partner and family were the most important individuals in helping them to cope with being in hospital.

Table 4.2 Women's ratings of potential problems associated with hospitalization

Potential problem	Mean score
Boredom	4.12
Having little freedom to make drinks/snacks	3.12
Lack of recreational activities	3.12
Uncertainty about condition	3.10
Having little freedom to leave ward/go outside	2.68
Loss of control over sleeping and waking times	2.38
Being woken too early	2.20
Having fixed mealtimes	2.14
Having to sleep with others	2.12
Noise at nights	2.02
Lack of privacy	1.98
Wearing night clothes in the daytime	1.78
Having babies on the ward	1.78
Staff being in too much of a hurry	1.68
Seeing and being with other women who have problems	1.54

Source: compiled by the author.

The effect of hospitalization on smoking behaviour

Sixteen (32%) of the sample smoked cigarettes and information was collected regarding the alteration, if any, in their smoking behaviour following admission to hospital. All of these 16 women had been smoking on admission to hospital. The average number of cigarettes smoked per day increased from 11 before admission to 18 following admission. While four (25%) were smoking 20 or more cigarettes per day before admission, eight (50%) were smoking this amount following hospitalization. Thirteen (81%) of the smokers had increased the number of cigarettes they smoked, eight (50%) having increased the number of cigarettes they smoked each day by 100% or more following hospitalization. The mean percentage increase in smoking for this sample was 78%. The women were also asked what time of day they had their first cigarette, both prior to and following admission to hospital, so that some assessment could be made of duration of smoking in the day as well as the quantity of cigarettes smoked. As the half-life of carboxy-haemoglobin is seven hours, the only time that the baby has a potential period of no carboxy-haemoglobin is the long period over night. If the first cigarette of the day is moved forward this reduces the time of unattached haemaglobin. Thirteen of the women (81%) were smoking their first cigarette earlier in hospital than at home with 12 (75%) smoking their first cigarette of the day before 9 a.m.

The effect of hospitalization on the family

Data regarding the effects of hospitalization on the women's family were obtained entirely from the women themselves and, therefore, reported findings reflect the women's perception of these effects, rather than the views of the family itself. As noted earlier in the chapter, 45 (90%) of the women had a partner and 26 (52%) had children at home.

The women's anxieties about their family. During the interview the women were asked to rank various worries and concerns that they may be experiencing about their family, on a scale of 1 to 5 (with 1 meaning that it was of 'no worry or concern' to them and 5 meaning that it was of 'great worry or concern'). Both the items and the scale were derived from Curry (1985). The findings (Table 4.3, see page 74) indicate that the women's main concern about their family related to their children at home, particularly the effect that their absence may have on them. The women were also concerned about their children's care arrangements and a number expressed feelings of guilt for the strain and worry that they felt they were putting on their family.

Table 4.3 The women's concerns about their family

Concern	Mean score
The effect of the separation on the children	4.31
Being unable to see the children	4.04
Care of the children	3.85
Being separated from your partner	3.60
Finances	2.32
Being separated from other family members	2.25
Unhappy about the way partner is managing things at home	1.53

Source: compiled by the author.

The effect of the hospitalization on their partner. Forty-four (88%) of the women said that they were depending most on their partner for help while they were in hospital. The women perceived that their partner was very concerned, about both the health of the unborn baby, and the health of the woman herself. The women described their partner as being under stress with the extra responsibilities of child care and housework, as well as with their own anxieties over the pregnancy. Consequently, the women often felt a need to protect their partner from the severity of their own condition and the anxiety they themselves were experiencing, by withholding information and not discussing their own fears.

The effect of hospitalization on the children. The children of the women in this sample were generally cared for by a combination of people; usually their father and grandparents. When the 26 women with children were asked how they felt their children were adjusting to their (the women's) hospitalization, 22 (85%) felt that the children were coping well at home. However, when the women with children were asked specifically about behavioural problems following the woman's admission to hospital, 20 (77%) identified at least one problem (with two women identifying five problems).

The women's feelings about the pregnancy

The majority of the women expressed positive feelings, such as happiness and excitement, about the pregnancy. For example:

I'm really happy about the pregnancy even though it has meant me having to come into hospital.

However, 12 (24%) expressed negative feelings, such as depression and anger. For example:

I don't like it (the pregnancy). I feel uncomfortable, fed up and angry that it has caused me to come into hospital.

A theme that emerged from some women was a feeling of ambivalence over the outcome of the pregnancy. They wanted the pregnancy to be over for their own sake, but also had a strong desire for the pregnancy to continue to ensure the wellbeing of the baby. This ambivalence appeared to lead to feelings of guilt for the women, as their own desires conflicted with the needs of the baby.

The women's feelings about the baby

Twenty-eight (56%) of the women expressed positive feelings about the baby, for example:

I'm so excited. I just can't wait to see the baby.

However, nine (18%) women expressed negative feelings, for example:

I'm angry. I feel great animosity towards it. I feel guilty about it, but I just can't help it.

The remaining 13 (26%) reported neutral feelings or said that either they could not express their feelings or did not know what they felt about the baby. Seven (14%) of the total sample had a pregnancy of less than 28 weeks at the time of the interview and a number of these women focused on reaching 28 weeks gestation when they believed the baby could be born without danger. Until they reached this 'milestone', they would engage in attempts to calculate the risks to the baby if it was born. To some extent, it appeared that the women viewed the pregnancy and the baby as two separate entities.

Feelings about themselves

It was noticeable that some women found it difficult to express their thoughts and feelings about themselves. Thirteen (26%) replied that they had no thoughts about themselves and two said that they did not know what they thought about themselves. Curry (1985) also reported this phenomenon. Twenty-one (42%) of the sample reported negative feelings – largely ones of low self-esteem and negative body image:

I feel a failure as a woman and a mother. I can't even have a baby without having problems.

I feel fat and ugly.

The self-descriptions of 'fat', 'ugly', and 'a failure' emerged a number of times. Only nine (18%) women expressed positive feelings about themselves. As previously noted, a number of the women reported feeling guilty about the strain they felt they were putting on their family. The majority of the sample did not feel that they themselves were to blame for the occurrence of pregnancy complications.

Stress experienced during hospitalization

The women's anxieties and stress during hospitalization were identified using both the structured schedule and the AHSI. Data from the structured schedule were expressed as mean rating scores (from 1 to 5) and items that had the highest average rating were as follows:

1. the effect of the separation on their children (4.31);
2. concern that something may be wrong with the fetus (4.06);
3. being unable to see the children (4.04);
4. concern that the baby won't live (3.90);
5. care of the children (3.85).

The data obtained from the AHSI were converted into intensity scores – the mean intensity of stress reported for each of the seven categories (e.g. separation). The scales on the AHSI were graded from 0 to 4 for the degree/intensity of stress. Table 4.4 shows the mean scores for each stressor category in a hierarchical order. The findings from the AHSI also suggest that the women in the sample experienced the most stress in relation to separation from their family. The relationship of some of the sample characteristics to these intensity scores was investigated using non-parametric statistical tests. The correlational analysis is discussed in detail in Kirk (1990).

The statistical analysis indicated that there were no significant relationships between intensity scores and the following variables: age; diagnosis; obstetric transfer; and previous experiences of hospitalization (not in this pregnancy). However, a number of significant relationships were discovered and are as follows.

Stress related to the 'Separation' category. Women with a low educational attainment and those with children at home reported the greatest stress regarding this category ($\chi^2 = 14.198$, $p = 0.006$ and $U = 211.5$, $p - 0.05$ respectively). It also appeared that as the gestation of the pregnancy increased the amount of stress regarding separation decreased ($r = -0.2809$, $p = 0.02$).

Stress related to the 'Emotions' category. There was a positive correlation between the length of hospitalization and the intensity of stress

Table 4.4 Intensities of stress reported for stressor categories

Category	Mean intensity score*
Separation	1.922
Emotions	1.578
Family status	1.547
Health status	1.484
Self-image	1.174
Communications with health professionals	0.969
Environment	0.950

* Friedman's two-way analysis of variance indicated that there was a significant difference ($p < 0.05$) in the amount of stress assigned to specific categories by this sample.
Source: compiled by the author.

for the emotions category, indicating that the longer the hospitalization, the greater the stress experienced ($r = 0.3571$, $p = 0.005$). However, there was also a negative correlation between length of gestation and stress regarding this category, suggesting that as gestation increased stress related to emotions decreased ($r = -0.2652$, $p = 0.03$).

Stress related to the 'Family status' category. Women who experienced the greatest stress relating to the family status category appeared to be those who were married ($\chi^2 = 5.939$, $p = 0.05$) had a lower educational attainment ($\chi^2 = 11.723$, $p = 0.01$), were classified as housewives or who occupied social class IIInm occupations ($\chi^2 = 16.942$, $p = 0.01$) or who had children at home ($U = 143.0$, $p = 0.0009$).

Stress related to the 'Health status' category. There was a negative correlation between gestation length and stress related to health status ($r = -0.2415$, $p = 0.04$). Women who had experienced a number of miscarriages also reported a greater amount of stress with regard to this category ($r = 0.2515$, $p = 0.03$).

Stress related to the 'Communications with health professionals' category. Women who had previously been hospitalized in this pregnancy reported significantly less stress related to communications with health professionals than those for whom this was their first admission ($r = -0.2872$, $p = 0.02$), suggesting that the more admissions a woman had experienced, the less stress she felt with communications with health professionals. Women in the later stages of pregnancy also reported less stress with communications with health professionals ($r = -0.3683$, $p = 0.004$).

Stress related to the 'Environment' category. Women who were on partial or total bed-rest experienced the greatest stress related to the environment ($\chi^2 = 6.0271$, $p = 0.04$), as did those, perhaps not surprisingly, who had felt that improvements were required in the hospital ($\chi^2 = 5.9256$, $p = 0.005$).

Parentcraft information

Only nine (18%) women in the sample had attended parentcraft classes before they were admitted to hospital, despite the fact that the majority were in the late stages of pregnancy and had only been hospitalized for five days or fewer. The women were shown a list of topics generally accepted as part of a parentcraft programme and asked if they had received any information on any of these whilst in hospital. Twenty-three (46%) had received parentcraft education on a formal or informal basis during hospitalization. When the women were asked to identify which parentcraft topics they had received information about, the most frequently cited areas were relaxation exercises and baby feeding. None of the sample reported receiving information about the dangers of alcohol, physical and emotional changes to expect following childbirth, or the realities of caring for a baby at home.

The physiotherapist was identified as the professional providing most parentcraft information in hospital. When the women in the sample were asked to single out their main overall source of parentcraft information in the pregnancy to date, 37 (74%) identified non-professional sources, such as books, magazines, etc. Only 3 (6%) reported that the midwife was the main source of parentcraft information.

Eight (16%) of the women has been shown around the delivery unit and the majority had found the experience useful. Women admitted to hospital before the 36th week of pregnancy will be more likely to have their baby admitted to a special care baby unit (SCBU) and it would therefore appear to be particularly beneficial to this group to be given the opportunity to visit this area. Although 36 (72%) had a pregnancy of 36 weeks gestation or less, only eight (16%) had visited the SCBU. The majority of these women had found the visit useful. Of the 42 who had not visited the SCBU, 25 (60%) said that they would have found such a visit useful, 12 (29%) reported that a visit would not be useful and five (12%) did not know.

Information giving and communication

The women's opinions on information giving and communication were collected using a Likert scale, which was scored from 1 = strongly agree to 5 = strongly disagree. The women were asked to assign a level of

Findings 79

agreement to a series of statements that were either negative or positive in their attitude toward information giving from health professionals. Table 4.5 shows, for each item, the percentage expressing a level of agreement (i.e. strongly agreed plus agreed) and a level of disagreement (i.e. strongly disagreed plus disagreed). The findings suggest a generally positive attitude towards information giving. The sample were particularly positive regarding: receiving information about what was going to happen to them; and being given explanations they could understand. However, the findings do indicate areas in which there was dissatisfaction:

Table 4.5 Attitudes towards information giving and communication (*n* = 50)

Statement	Total in agreement		Total in disagreement	
	No.	%	No.	%
While I've been in hospital I've received as much information as I've wanted	31	62	17	34
I have not been able to ask all the questions I wanted to	14	28	33	66
Things are explained to me in a way I can understand	38	76	9	18
I have not been told anything about what is going to happen to me	8	16	41	82
Any tests and their results are always explained to me	33	66	16	32
I am always involved in making decisions about what is going to happen to me	16	32	27	54
I feel I have no control over what is happening to me	13	26	31	62
I always have to ask if I want to find out what is happening to me	34	68	15	30
I receive different information and opinions from different members of the staff	20	40	28	58

Source: compiled by the author.

34 (68%) felt that they always had to ask to find out information;
27 (54%) reported that they were not involved in decision making;
20 (40%) received conflicting information;
17 (34%) felt that they had not received as much information as they
would have liked.

Thirty-one (62%) of the sample identified the doctor as the professional
providing most information, while 15 (30%) identified the midwife in
this role.

The women in the sample were asked several specific questions relating
to midwives and information giving. In particular, they were asked to
assess (subjectively) the quantity of information they had received from
midwives in the ward. As shown in Table 4.6, 30 (60%) reported that they
had received a little or no information from the midwives.

Women with a lower level of educational attainment appeared to be
more likely to feel that they had not received sufficient information from
the midwives ($r = 0.2247, p = 0.05$). The women were questioned about

Table 4.6 Women's views of the amount of information
received from midwives

Response	No.	%
A lot of information	20	40
A little information	26	52
No information	4	8
Total	50	100

Source: compiled by the author.

Table 4.7 Expectations regarding the quantity of
information received from the midwives

Response	No.	%
Same as expected	33	66
Expected more	13	26
Expected less	2	4
Don't know	2	4
Total	50	100

Source: compiled by the author.

their expectations of the amount of information that they might receive from midwives. The findings in Table 4.7 indicate that the majority of the sample received the amount of information that they had expected. However, this question does not allow for women with low expectations. It is notable though that 13 (26%) had expected to receive more information from the midwives.

When asking the women about the midwife's role in information giving, two disturbing and unforeseen comments were made. Firstly, 10 (20%) women stated that they had not seen a midwife. Further questioning revealed that this was because they did not identify the ward 'nurses' as midwives. Secondly, 16 (32%) stated that they always had to ask the midwives for information.

DISCUSSION

This study suggests that certain aspects of hospital life are problematic for women hospitalized in pregnancy. Boredom was the main problem associated with hospital life identified by the women and was also identified by Taylor (1985). The finding that the sample's smoking behaviour changed significantly following admission to hospital may relate to the boredom and stress that they were experiencing. Not only were the women found to have increased their consumption of cigarettes, but the majority were also smoking their first cigarette of the day earlier than when at home. Salaryia (1986) and Thomson (1993) reported a similar increased consumption of cigarettes for women hospitalized in pregnancy and they also reported that the most frequently given reason for this was boredom. The finding that smoking increases following hospitalization is disturbing, particularly for women with a high-risk pregnancy, as it appears that an already compromised fetus is being exposed to an increased amount of cigarette smoke, for a longer period in the day. It is also notable that the most frequent reason for admission to hospital for this sample was intra-uterine growth retardation, a condition frequently associated with smoking in pregnancy (Black, 1985).

The major concern and source of stress for the women in this study appeared to be the effect of the separation on their children at home and their own separation from their family. This is consistent with the findings of both White (1981) and Curry (1985). The health of the fetus was another major concern and the primary concern for those women without children.

Emotionally, the women appeared to be experiencing several problems. A number of women experienced conflicting desires about the pregnancy. Whilst they wanted the pregnancy to be over, they also wanted the pregnancy to continue to increase the baby's chance of survival. Twenty-one (42%) reported experiencing negative feelings, especially related to their own self-esteem and body image. These findings were also reported by Kemp and Page (1987) and appear in personal reports (Galloway, 1976; Snyder, 1979); these authors suggest that such feelings arise from the women's sense of guilt for the occurrence of complications and their own loss of role function within the family. In this study the longer the women were hospitalized, the more stress they felt concerning their emotions.

The majority of the women did not define themselves as being ill as they did not experience any physical symptoms of illness, a similar finding to that of MacDonald (1991). As Galloway (1976) has noted, it is precisely the absence of symptoms that leads to the difficulty for women with a high-risk pregnancy in accepting the reality of the situation. But it also means that their hospital care must be based on an alternate philosophy to that of general hospital patients.

The women saw their partner as their most important source of help and support. They perceived their partner as being under stress in coping with family duties and anxieties about the pregnancy. These findings were also reported by Curry (1985) and Mercer *et al*. (1988). According to reports by the women of behavioural problems exhibited by their children following their (the women's) admission to hospital it seems that the children may also have been stressed by the admission. What is evident, however, is the need to examine, in more detail, the impact of the woman's hospitalization on the family, particularly from the family's point of view.

The overall findings regarding information giving reveal a number of specific aspects about which the women in the sample were dissatisfied. It is of concern that the majority of women reported receiving so little information from the midwives. This seems to apply particularly to those women with a low educational attainment, and this may relate either to the problem of midwife identification or, as shown in other studies, to socially disadvantaged women wanting information, but having less success in obtaining it (Cartwright, 1979; Jacoby, 1988). The findings suggest that previous experience of hospitalization in this pregnancy reduces the stress relating to communications with health professionals.

The women appeared to have received little, if any, parentcraft information both prior to and during hospitalization, in that only nine (18%) had attended classes and/or received information before admission and 23 (46%) during hospitalization. The involvement of midwives in the provision of parentcraft education is disappointing as this is a major part of the midwife's role. Moreover, she is ideally placed to co-ordinate the provision of antenatal education to women hospitalized in pregnancy. The finding that the sample acquired most parentcraft information from non-professional sources, such as books, supports Jacoby's (1988) findings.

In spite of the majority of the sample having a gestation length of less than 36 weeks, very few had been shown around the SCBU. Such a visit was found to be useful and many of those not given the opportunity for a preparatory visit felt it would have been helpful. Visits to the delivery unit were also regarded as being useful, particularly for those women in their first pregnancy.

IMPLICATIONS FOR MIDWIFERY PRACTICE

A number of implications arising from the findings of this study are suggested in this section of the chapter. However, it has to be remembered that a sample of convenience, consisting of 50 women at one hospital, was used in this study, therefore no claims can be made for the generalizability of the findings. Another limitation of the study is that the data on the family's response to the woman's hospitalization were collected entirely from the woman's perspective.

It is proposed that the central issue is the need for individualized, family-centred care and this was endorsed by the recently published House of Commons Health Committee on the Maternity Services (The Winterton Report) (House of Commons Select Committee, 1992). Individualized, family-centred care requires recognition of the stress hospitalization places on all family members. Assistance may be needed with practicalities, such as child care arrangements, finances, transportation or household duties and the midwife may be able to help directly with these or refer the family to an appropriate agency. The woman's partner may need the opportunity to discuss his own feelings or anxiety and any difficulties he is experiencing in coping alone. A major concern for the women in the study was their separation from their children and they need help in coping with these anxieties. Children should be encouraged to visit and an unrestricted family visiting policy implemented. Despite the fact that 'lack of privacy' received a low score (Table 4.2, page 72) privacy is particularly important in the maintenance of the woman's relationship with her partner. Ideally, this may mean creating a family visiting room. Provision of privacy would encourage communication between the couple, help them to maintain their intimacy and discuss any problems in private, rather than in the company of other room-mates and their visitors.

These women need assistance to adapt to the dual crises of pregnancy and hospitalization. They need opportunities to explore their feelings, fears and frustrations. Consequently, it is proposed that counselling should be a major part of the care that midwives provide for these women. This counselling may occur on an individual or family basis. A number of authors have noted how useful support groups may be for women hospi-talized in pregnancy (Halstead, 1974; Dore and Davies, 1979; Snyder, 1988), as in these groups, women can share experiences with others who have confronted the same issues. The midwife's role should include that of group facilitator who can provide professional support and act as a resource person.

A major need for both the women and their partner is for clear and consistent information. The partner's need for information should not be underestimated nor can it be assumed that it is adequate to leave this area to the woman to provide. Some of the women indicated that they tended to keep their partner 'in the dark' in an attempt, as the women saw it, to reduce stress. Information regarding the woman's condition and treatment has to be given jointly to both members of the couple by professionals if that is what the couple indicate they would prefer. Information giving should be planned to ensure adequate information is provided, and the opportunity to ask questions is given. As far as possible, both partners need to be involved in decision making about proposals for the woman's care and treatment as shared decision making helps to increase the family's sense of control of the situation. On admission it may be helpful to provide anticipatory guidance about the stresses involved, the need for mutual support and the possible progress of the condition. At the same time, however, there is a need to emphasize the normal physiological and psychological aspects of pregnancy. An approach to care such as primary nursing, and recently advocated in the Patients' Charter, would be helpful as it would promote individualized care, planned information giving and continuity of care (Marram *et al.*, 1979).

This study has shown that a major problem for women hospitalized in pregnancy is boredom. A variety of activities need to be available with which these women can occupy their time, for example, occupational therapy. Types of ward-based activities suggested for general ward patients in the literature are gardening, arts/crafts, videotapes of films, cards/games and keep fit (Langrehr, 1974; Savitz and Friedman, 1981; Thompson, 1983). It will be a creative challenge for the midwifery team to devise suitable activities for pregnant women. The women also need to be involved in planning recreational activities in order to optimize their sense of control. Relief of boredom may help to reduce the large increase in smoking found in this study and others (Salariya, 1986; Thomson, 1993).

Findings showed that the sample women received little, if any, parentcraft education either before or during hospitalization. Ward-based parentcraft sessions should be available for both partners to attend and such provision should be part of the midwife's role. The development of a parentcraft course for women at high obstetric risk in hospital has been outlined by Avery and Olsen (1987) and includes standard topics plus those, such as caesarean section, medical therapies, and breast feeding and the preterm baby, which may be of particular relevance to women at high obstetric risk. Moreover, Avery and Olsen (1987) report that the teaching of relaxation techniques may be useful as a means of stress reduction.

Women hospitalized in pregnancy are different to most other adults in hospital in that they generally do not feel ill (MacDonald, 1991). Consequently the institutional aspects of hospitalization need to be decreased. The general appearance of the ward could be made less clinical by use of wallpaper, colourful fabrics, plants, etc. Although the women in this study did not appear to consider it problematic, it is recommended that women hospitalized in pregnancy should be encouraged to wear their normal day clothes. Having to wear night clothes was identified as a problem by the women in Taylor's (1985) study and it has been associated with promoting dependence and depersonalization (Darcy, 1980; Milner, 1982). The ward routines need to be relaxed, and those such as bed making and physical observations should be planned according to the needs of the individual. Waking and sleeping times should be flexible and under the woman's control.

A number of women in this study appeared to desire improvements in the quality and quantity of food and for the provision of facilities whereby they can make drinks and snacks. Food could be brought in from home and then reheated in a ward microwave, although, the removal of 'Crown Immunity' from hospitals in the United Kingdom has made the possibility of creating these facilities more difficult. Special diets should be provided, as a number of women were dissatisfied that Kosher meat but not Halal meat was provided.

The sense of prison confinement could be avoided by allowing women who do not have a life-threatening condition (e.g. severe pregnancy induced hypertension) to visit other parts of the hospital or go outside. Outdoor facilities could be utilized, if available.

Options to hospitalization for some women experiencing complications in their pregnancy need to be examined. There is some evidence to suggest that treatments, such as bed rest, commonly used for complications of pregnancy, are ineffective (Diddle *et al.*, 1953; Mathews, 1977; Weekes *et al.*, 1977; Grant *et al.*, 1982; Crowther *et al.*, 1992) except in cases of extreme maternal and fetal pathology (Mathews *et al.*, 1982). A number of schemes have been described in which women with a high-risk pregnancy have received care on an 'outpatient' basis (Butters, 1987; James, 1988; Lambkin, 1991) and others in which certain observations are recorded in the woman's own home by telemetry. These observations include the fetal heart rate (Currie and Dalton, 1986; James *et al.*, 1988), glucose levels (Dalton *et al.*, 1987) and blood pressure (Swindells *et al.*, 1990). Middlemiss *et al.* (1989) have described a scheme, known as the 'Cardiff integrated antenatal care system', which provides intensive individualized care at home to women with a high-risk pregnancy. Care is provided by a hospital-based midwife and it has been shown to decrease the duration and frequency of hospital admissions. Women receiving care at home are reported to experience less anxiety than those cared for conventionally in hospital. Provision of social support by a midwife to women with a history of delivering a low birthweight baby has also been shown to significantly reduce the incidence of hospital admissions (Oakley and Rajan, 1989; the chapter by Oakley in this volume).

Providing care at home for some women experiencing pregnancy complications would be more cost-effective and less stressful for the women and their families. These schemes can only be implemented, however, with adequate services in the community and need careful evaluation.

Recognition is needed of the uniqueness of the situation for women hospitalized in pregnancy as opposed to other adults in hospital. Firstly, they do not generally feel ill and, secondly, the stressors they experience are influenced by the co-existing crises of hospitalization and pregnancy. Admitting women with pregnancy complications into hospital may exacerbate the underlying condition, as it appears to lead to increased stress and increased smoking. Many admissions to hospital may also be unnecessary and costly in both human and financial terms because of problems of over diagnosis of certain complications such as intra-uterine growth retardation (Hall *et al.*, 1980) and hypertension (Hall and Chng, 1982). In a randomized controlled trial comparing admission to hospital with care at home for women with non-proteinuric hypertension, Crowther *et al.* (1992) have shown that the group of women provided with care at home had a significantly better outcome than women in the group admitted to hospital.

Although the study reported in this chapter was small scale and exploratory, it has identified a number of issues that have implications for midwifery care, such as the stress and boredom experienced by women admitted to hospital in pregnancy and alterations in their smoking behaviour. Findings showed that they and their families have a number of needs of which midwives should be aware. Care of these women should, it is suggested, be based on a health model which would include individualized, planned midwifery care and education, and maternity wards should discard their traditional ethos of illness and patienthood. The impact of hospitalization on the family from the family's perspective needs to be investigated and a qualitative study would also be useful to examine in depth these women's experiences of hospitalization and having a high-risk pregnancy. Longitudinal studies could also be employed to study the long-term effects of hospitalization on factors such as postnatal adjustment.

REFERENCES

Avery, P. and Olsen, I.M. (1987) Expanding the scope of childbirth education to meet the needs of hospitalised high risk clients. *Journal of Obstetric, Gynecological and Neonatal Nursing*, **16**(6), 418–21.

Black, T. (1985) Smoking in pregnancy revisited. *Midwifery*, **1**(3), 135–45.

Butters, L. (1987) The midwife and high risk pregnancies: experience in an obstetric medical clinic. *Midwives Chronicle*, **100**(1,194), 199–202.

Carlson, B. and Labarba, R.C. (1979) Maternal emotionality during pregnancy and reproductive outcome: a review of the literature. *International Journal of Behavioural Development*, **2**(4), 343–76.

Cartwright, A. (1964) *Human relations and hospital care*. Routledge and Kegan Paul, London.

Cartwright, A. (1979) *The dignity of labour. A study of childbearing and induction*. Tavistock, London.

Chalmers, B. (1982) Psychological aspects of pregnancy: some thoughts for the 80s. *Social Science and Medicine*, **16**, 323–31.

Crandon, A.J. (1979) Maternal anxiety and obstetric complications. *Journal of Psychosomatic Research*, **28**, 109–11.

Crowther, C.A., Bouwmeester, A.M. and Ashurst, H.M. (1992) Does admission to hospital for bed rest prevent disease progression or improve fetal outcome in pregnancy complicated by non-proteinuric hypertension? *British Journal of Obstetrics and Gynaecology*, **99**, 13–17.

Currie, J.R. and Dalton, K.J. (1986) Fetal home telemetry. *Midwifery*, **2**(4), 202–5.

Curry, M.A. (1985) Antenatal hospitalisation: maternal behaviour and the family. Final project report, Department of Family Nursing, Oregon Health Sciences University, Oregon, USA.

Dalton, K.J., Alban-Davies, H., Edwards, O.M. and Nicholls, J. (1987) Computerised home telemetry of maternal blood glucose levels in diabetic pregnancy. In K.J. Dalton and R.D. Fawdry (eds) *The computer in obstetrics and gynaecology*. IRL Press, Oxford.

Darcy, L. (1980) The wearing of day clothes by patients in hospital. *The Lamp*, **37**(7), 45–7.

Diddle, A.W., O'Connor, K.A., Jack, R. and Pearse, R.L. (1953) Evaluation of bedrest in threatened abortion. *Obstetrics and Gynaecology*, **2**, 63–7.

Dore, S.L. and Davies, B.L. (1979) Catharsis for high risk antenatal patients. *American Journal of Maternal and Child Nursing*, **4**(3), 96–7.

Enkin, M. and Chalmers, I. (1982) *Effectiveness and satisfaction in antenatal care*. William Heinemann, London.

Galloway, K. (1976) The uncertainty and stress of a high risk pregnancy. *Maternal and Child Nursing*, **1**(5), 294–9.

Goffman, E. (1961) *Asylums*. Penguin, Harmondsworth.

Gorsuch, R.L. and Key, M. (1974) Abnormalities of pregnancy as a function of anxiety and life stress. *Psychosomatic Medicine*, **36**, 352–62.

Grant, A., Chalmers, I. and Enkin, M. (1982) Physical intervention intended to prolong pregnancy and increase fetal growth. In M. Enkin and I. Chalmers (eds) *Effectiveness and satisfaction in antenatal care*. William Heinemann, London.

Gregory, J. (1978) *Patients' attitudes to the hospital service: a survey carried out for the Royal Commission on the National Health Service*. Research Paper No. 5. HMSO, London.

Hall, M.H., Chng, P.K. and MacGillivray, I. (1980) Is routine antenatal care worthwhile? *Lancet*, **12**(7), 78–80.

Hall, M.H. and Chng, P.K. (1982) Antenatal care in practice. In M. Enkin and I. Chalmers (eds) *Effectiveness and satisfaction in antenatal care*. Spastics International Medical Publications/William Heinemann, London.

Halstead, L. (1974) The use of crisis intervention in obstetrical nursing. *Nursing Clinics of North America*, **9**(1), 69–76.

Holmes, T.H. and Rahe, R.H. (1967) Social readjustment rating scale. *Journal of Psychosomatic Research*, **11**(8), 213–18.

House of Commons Select Committee (1992) Sessions 1991–1992, Second Report. *Maternity Services* (Chairman: Nicholas Winterton) Vol. 1., HMSO, London.

Istvan, J. (1986) Stress, anxiety and birth outcomes: a critical review of the evidence. *Psychological Bulletin*, **100**(3), 331–48.

Jacoby, A. (1988) Mothers' views about information and advice in pregnancy and childbirth: findings from a national study. *Midwifery*, **4**(3), 103–10.

James, D., Peralta, B. and Porter, S. (1988) Fetal heart rate monitoring by telephone. *British Journal of Obstetrics and Gynaecology*, **95**(10), 1024–9.

James, D.K. (1988) Hypertension in pregnancy: do we need to admit all mothers to hospital for assessment and management? *Journal of Obstetrics and Gynaecology*, **8**(4), 314–18.

Kemp, V.H. and Page, C.K. (1987) Maternal self-esteem and prenatal attachment in high risk pregnancy. *Maternal Child Nursing Journal*, **16**(3), 195–206.

Kirk, S.A. (1990) The experience of antenatal hospitalisation. Unpublished MSc thesis, Department of Nursing, University of Manchester.

Lambkin, A. (1991) An acceptable alternative. *Nursing Standard*, **6**(7), 20–21.

Langrehr, A.A. (1974) Social stimulation. *American Journal of Nursing*, **74**, 1300–1.

Lederman, R.P. (1984) Anxiety and conflict in pregnancy: relationships to maternal health status. *Annual Review of Nursing Research*, **2**, 27–61.

McDonald, R.L., Gynther, M.D. and Christakos, A.C. (1963) Relations between maternal anxiety and obstetric complications. *Psychosomatic Medicine*, **25**, 357–63.

MacDonald, S.J. (1991) Antenatal admissions: women's perception of the experience. In S. Robinson, A.M. Thomson and V. Tickner (eds) *Proceedings of the 1990 Research and the Midwife Conference*. Department of Nursing, University of Manchester.

McGhee, A. (1961) *The patients' attitude to nursing care*. Livingstone, Edinburgh.

Mathews, D.D. (1977) A randomized control trial of bedrest and sedation or normal activity and non-sedation in the management of proteinuric hypertension during pregnancy. *British Journal of Obstetrics and Gynaecology*, **84**, 108–14.

Mathews, D.D., Agarwal, V. and Shuttleworth, T.P. (1982) A randomised controlled trial of complete bedrest versus ambulation in the management of proteinuric hypertension during pregnancy. *British Journal of Obstetrics and Gynaecology*, **89**, 128–31.

Marram, G., Bennett, B. and Bevis, E. (1979) *Primary nursing: a model for individualised care*. C.V. Mosby, St Louis.

Mercer, R.T., Ferketich, S., DeJoseph, J., May, K. and Sollid, D. (1988)

Effect of stress on family functioning during pregnancy. *Nursing Research*, **37**(5), 268–75.

Merkatz, R. (1978) Prolonged hospitalisation of pregnant women: the effects on the family. *Birth and the Family Journal*, **5**, 205–6.

Middlemiss, C., Dawson, A.J., Gough, N., Jones, M.E. and Coles, E.C. (1989) A randomised study of a domiciliary antenatal care scheme: maternal psychological effects. *Midwifery*, **5**(2), 69–74.

Milner, J. (1982) Clothes maketh a patient. *Nursing Mirror*, **154**(11), 30–1.

Moos and Tsu (1977) As cited in White (1981) (see below).

Norbeck, J.S. and Tilden, V. (1983) Life stress, social support and emotional disequilibrium in complications of pregnancy: a prospective multivariate approach. *Journal of Health and Social Behaviour*, **24**(1), 30–46.

Oakley, A. and Rajan, L. (1989) The social support and pregnancy outcome study. In S. Robinson, A. Thomson and V. Tickner (eds) *Proceedings of the 1988 Research and the Midwife Conference*. Department of Nursing, University of Manchester.

Salariya, E.M. (1986) A study of smoking habits and attitudes of women in a maternity unit. *Health Bulletin*, **44**, 22–8.

Savitz, J. and Friedman, M.I. (1981) Diagnosing boredom and confusion. *Nursing Research*, **30**(1), 16–20.

Seigel, S. (1956) *Nonparametric statistics for the behavioural sciences*. McGraw-Hill/Koga Kusha Ltd, Tokyo.

Selby, J.W., Calhoun, L.G., Vogel, A.V. and King, A.H. (eds) (1980) *Psychology and human reproduction*. Free Press, New York.

Snyder, D.J. (1979) The high risk mother viewed in relation to a holistic model of the childbearing experience. *Journal of Obstetric, Gynecologic and Neonatal Nursing*, **8**, 164–70.

Snyder, D.J. (1988) Peer group support for high risk mothers. *Maternal and Child Nursing*, **13**(2), 114–17.

Swindells, H., Mooney, P., Cartwright, W. and Dalton, K.J. (1990) Blood pressure telemetry from home. *Midwife, Health Visitor and Community Nurse*, **26**(3), 8888–90.

Taylor, A. (1985) In for a rest. *Nursing Times*, **81**(36), 29–31.

Taylor, S. (1979) Hospital patients' behaviour: reactance, helplessness or control. *Journal of Social Issues*, **35**(1), 156–84.

Thompson, J. (1983) Caring and sharing: ward based activities. *Nursing Times*, **79**(19), 62–3.

Thomson, A.M. (1993) If you are pregnant and smoke admission to hospital may damage your baby's health. *Journal of Clinical Nursing*, **2**(2), 111–20.

Volicer, B.J. (1973) Perceived stress levels of events associated with the experience of hospitalisation. *Nursing Research*, **22**, 491–7.

Volicer, B.J. (1974) Patients' perceptions of stressful events associated with hospitalization. *Nursing Research*, **22**, 491–7.

Volicer, B.J. (1978) Hospital stress and patients' reports of pain and physical status. *Journal of Human Stress*, **4**(2), 28–37.

Volicer, B.J. and Bohannon, M.W. (1975) A hospital stress rating scale. *Nursing Research*, **24**(5), 325–59.

Weekes, A.R., Menzies, D.N. and DeBoer, C.H. (1977) The relative efficacy of cervical suture, bed rest and no treatment in the management of twin pregnancies, *British Journal of Obstetrics and Gynaecology*, **84**, 161–4.

White, M. (1981) Stressors reported by hospitalised antepartum women. Unpublished Master's thesis, Dalhousie University, Halifaxs Nova Scotia, Canada.

Wilson-Barnett, J. (1977) Patients' emotional reactions to hospitalisation. Unpublished Ph.D. thesis, University of London.

CHAPTER FIVE

Coping with labour pain: the midwife's role

Catherine Niven

INTRODUCTION

The research study described in this chapter forms part of a larger study on 'Factors affecting labour pain' (Niven and Gijsbers, 1984; Niven, 1985; 1986) and was particularly concerned with the role played by psychological factors in modulating labour pain. The study was informed by current theories of pain perception, such as the gate theory (Melzack and Wall, 1965; 1988), which predict that psychological factors as well as physiological ones can affect pain perception. Accordingly the study examined the effects of obstetric factors such as parity, induction of labour, duration of labour and weight of the baby as well as the effects of psychological factors such as the desirability of pregnancy, expectations of childbirth, antenatal education, and the presence of the partner during labour. Other factors examined included analgesic use (pethidine and Entonox), social class and previous pain experience. These factors were examined in the first phase of the study which involved 101 labouring women. In the second phase of the study the coping strategies of 51 of these women were examined in some detail.

While many of the factors examined in the first phase of the study will be of considerable interest to midwives, this chapter concentrates on those which emanate from the second phase. Details of the intensity of labour pain, the midwife's perception of that intensity and the use of pharmacological analgesics, which derive from the first phase of the study, will be included as they relate closely to the midwife's role in helping the client to cope with labour pain. Information on other aspects of the first phase of the study is available elsewhere (Niven and Gijsbers, 1984).

The use of pain coping strategies has been investigated in clinical and experimental studies. Clinical and experimental research has established the efficacy of psychological analgesia, the use of coping strategies to modulate pain. For example experimental pain studies have demonstrated that relaxation training was effective in increasing pain tolerance (Stevens and Heide, 1977); that distraction was effective in increasing pain thresholds and tolerance (Barber and Cooper, 1972; Stone *et al.*, 1977); that the use of pleasant imagery as a focus of distraction was more effective than the manipulation of expectations of pain reduction in reducing self-reports of pain (Stone *et al.*, 1977); and that 'reversing the affect' of pain, i.e. thinking of the sensations associated with pain as positive rather than negative, was more effective than distraction in reducing the distress associated with prolonged experimental pain (McCaul and Haugtvedt, 1982). The use of Lamaze type breathing techniques, the rigorous form of controlled breathing exercises, has also been shown to be effective in reducing experimentally induced pain (Worthington, 1982).

Experimental pain is not, of course, the equivalent of clinical pain. It is, of ethical necessity, mild in intensity, short in duration and can be terminated at will. Studies of clinical pain have shown that relaxation is effective in relieving tension headache (Cox *et al.*, 1975); that the use of pleasant imagery was effective in reducing self-reported discomfort in dental care (Horan *et al.*, 1976); that the reinterpretation of pain stimulation (a process akin to reversal of affect) was more effective in reducing ratings of the quality and quantity of chronic pain experience than distraction (Rybstein-Blinchik, 1976); and that Lamaze breathing techniques were effective in reducing labour pain (Worthington, 1982).

The aim of the second phase of the labour pain study was to examine the use and effectiveness of the strategies discussed above, i.e. relaxation, distraction, use of imagery and reversal of affect during labour. The use of structured breathing techniques as taught in British antenatal classes was also examined. Two further aspects of coping with pain were included. The first concerned the normalization of the pain which occurs during childbirth. Misattribution of pain to a harmful source has been shown to increase pain perception (Nisbett and Schacter, 1966). As the pain of childbirth could be attributed by a woman to harmless sources, or to some abnormality in herself or the baby, the former might be expected to be related to lower levels of pain than the latter. The second aspect concerned control. Bowers (1968) showed that if a subject believed that she or he had control over noxious stimulation, then the pain and anxiety levels associated with such stimulation were lower than when no perception of control existed. Subjects experiencing noxious stimulation in childbirth may vary in their perception of being 'in control' and this perception might therefore affect their levels of labour pain.

Numerous writers have disapproved of the helplessness imposed upon labouring women by modern hospital-based obstetrics and have encouraged women to take a more active part in the birth, believing that activity – being 'in control' – rather than passivity, will improve the woman's experience of childbirth and thus perhaps modulate the pain associated

with it (e.g. Kitzinger, 1962; Oakley, 1979). Hospitalization and intervention during labour can, it is predicted, have the effect of removing the
locus of control from the woman and placing it in the hands of the attendant medical, midwifery and nursing staff (Wolkind and Zajicek,
1981). Thus the perception of personal control should be associated with
less pain in labour than the perception of being controlled by hospital
personnel.

The use of strategies other than those listed above was of particular
interest. While many spontaneously generated strategies may be classifi-
able as relaxation, distraction, etc. others may be idiosyncratic. The nature
and usage of idiosyncratic strategies was therefore included in the study.

Although this chapter reports on the use of coping strategies during
labour, it focuses particularly on the effects that a positive relationship
between care givers and labouring women can have on the woman's
experience of pain. The study did not initially set out to examine this
relationship. Its examination emerged from an interest in how women
coped with labour pain and in particular how their coping affected their
perceptions of control during childbirth. As will be seen in the following
pages, this interest led to a realization that issues of control were complex
and were often affected by the woman's perceptions of, and feelings about,
the care givers. Analysis of the relationship between the labouring woman
and care givers showed that it was one of the most significant variables in
the entire study, being associated with considerably lower levels of labour
pain **and** with the effective use of pharmacological analgesics, psychological coping strategies and attendance at antenatal classes – all of which are
in turn associated with lower levels of labour pain. 'Trusting the staff', as
a positive relationship between care givers and labouring women was
labelled, came out top in both categories.

The next section discusses the assessment of pain, and the two measures
that were used in this study.

Pain assessment measures

Pain of all kinds is a subjective experience. 'A personal, private sensation
of hurt' (Sternbach, 1968, p. 12). As such it is not available for direct
measurement. An outside observer can never experience another person's
pain but can gain some information about it through the sufferer's behaviour, physiological responses and reports of the pain.

We commonly infer knowledge about another's pain through observing
his or her behaviour. Cries, screams, groan, grimaces, rigidity, 'guarding'
all communicate that the subject is in pain. However, such behaviours are
difficult to quantify and are susceptible to social pressure, cultural norms
and individual differences (Bond and Pearson, 1969). Pain behaviours and
the behaviours which accompany great physical effort are rather similar

(witness a tennis player serving or a weight lifter lifting). Therefore the pain behaviour and the effort behaviour of women in labour could be confused and thus observation of labour pain behaviour is not a suitable method of assessing labour pain.

The stress of being in pain invokes the normal bodily response to stress of any kind – increased adrenalin secretion, heart rate, respiration, etc. These physiological responses can be objectively measured but do not give information about the pain itself, only about pain as a stressor. In labour there are multiple potential stressors, both physiological (e.g. the effort of delivery) and psychological (e.g. anxiety). Therefore, physiological measures of heart rate, etc. obtained during childbirth would reflect the effects of all these stressors, not just the effects of pain.

The most common assessment technique used by pain researchers involves the use of structured numerical or semantic scales. There are a large number of such scales – 3, 5, or 10 point numerical scales with or without accompanying descriptors such as 'no pain', 'mild pain', 'severe pain', but all that these pain scales measured was the intensity of the pain. Such scales have been used in labour pain research (e.g. Klopfer *et al.*, 1975; Nettlebladt *et al.*, 1976). Labour pain, however, like pain of any other kind, is not simply experienced along a dimension of intensity. Pain has many different qualities, both in its sensory nature – the dull ache of a headache, the cramping of period pain, the crushing pain of angina – and in its non-sensory qualities – how frightening it is, how sickening, how unbearable (Melzack and Torgerson, 1971). Thus pain is multidimensional in nature and it is desirable that the assessment of pain should reflect this complexity. It could be particularly important to measure labour pain in a way which reflects its multidimensional nature. Not only is childbirth a very complex psychophysiological event, but it is one in which positive and negative aspects are mixed and to a certain extent co-exist. 'The agony and the ecstasy' as Ann Oakley summarizes it (Oakley, 1979, p. 86), or as one of the participants in this study said, 'Giving birth was excruciating. It was like a red hot poker going through my spine. It was the most wonderful experience of my whole life'. That kind of mixture of sensations cannot be summed up on a 1–10 scale.

Developments in pain research have lead to the construction of a pain assessment scale which reflects the multidimensional nature of pain, the McGill Pain Questionnaire (MPQ). The MPQ is based on the pain transmission and perception theories of Melzack and Wall (Melzack and Wall, 1965; 1988). These regard pain as a multifaceted perception which reflects the differing brain areas involved in the reception of noxious stimulation. According to this model, pain has **Sensory**, **Affective** and **Evaluative** components and these dimensions of pain experience are assessed by the MPQ (Melzack, 1975). The MPQ utilizes word descriptors of pain which the subjects select from groups of words derived from the clinical literature and the work of Dallenbach on pain qualities (Dallenbach, 1939). These words have been grouped into a number of categories divided into **Sensory**, 'the temporal, spatial, pressure, thermal and other sensory qualities of pain experience'; **Affective**, 'the tension, fear and autonomic properties of pain experience'; and **Evaluative**, 'the subjective overall intensity of the total pain experience', sections (Melzack and Wall, 1988, p. 38). The words within a category are ranked in intensity, the first word representing the lowest intensity.

The grouping and ranking of words was achieved by presenting the list of pain descriptors to groups of subjects (medical doctors, patients and students). A substantial and significant level of agreement was found on the grouping of words into categories presenting the same quality of pain and on the rank ordering of these words. In one group of Evaluative words the increase in intensity was constant between each word and these words:

mild, discomforting, distressing, horrible, excruciating.

These were therefore used separately as a scale of the overall intensity of pain experience. This scale, the Present Pain Intensity (PPI) scale, uses both the pain descriptors and numerical markers of each point on the scale (e.g. 1 = mild), whereas the remainder of the MPQ uses only semantic descriptors.

Quantification of assessed pain is achieved through totalling the rank values of the Sensory, Affective and Evaluative descriptors selected by the subject to describe his or her pain (Melzack and Torgenson, 1971; Melzack, 1975). These measurements are known as the Pain Ranking Index (PRI). Thus the MPQ can be used to provide a number of different measures of pain, yielding a more complex assessment of the subject's pain experience than is available from simple intensity scales. It can produce a pain profile, a description of the individual or average pain experienced in a certain condition, derived from the words or categories selected to describe the pain. The total intensity of pain experienced can be calculated from the sum of the ranks of the words selected by the subject – the total PRI – and the relative contribution of Sensory, Affective and Evaluative components of pain to that total score can be calculated from the sum of the ranks of the words selected from the Sensory, Affective and Evaluative categories. The PPI yields a 5-point intensity scale.

The MPQ has been used to describe different pains. It has been used to evaluate different treatments and has been found to differentiate between different pain groups. It shows a high level of agreement on the intensity relationships between the pain descriptors in subjects from different cultures, classes and educational backgrounds (Melzack, 1975). A critical appraisal of the MPQ has concluded that it displays 'acceptable reliability and face, construct, discriminant and concurrent validity' (Reading, 1983, p. 59). Thus it should produce a qualitative and quantitative assessment of the sensory and non-sensory dimensions of labour pain which can be related to variations in the independent variables which were examined. The MPQ has been used to assess labour pain (e.g. Melzack *et al.*, 1984; Reading and Cox, 1985) and has been found to be satisfactory. It was therefore used in the study reported in this chapter.

Some doubt has been cast upon the accuracy of the Present Pain Intensity scale in assessing the overall intensity of clinical pain (Melzack, 1975). So another measure of the overall intensity of pain was also used. The measure selected was the Visual Analogue Scale. Visual Analogue Scales (VAS) have been widely used in pain research as they provide a simple, quick method of assessing the intensity of pain free from the problems (e.g. clustering) associated with numerical scales (Scott and Huskisson, 1976). Respondents are asked to indicate the intensity of their pain along a 10 cm scale (Figure 5.1). The MPQ is comparatively time consuming in use (5 min) and is dependent on a reasonable level of verbal comprehension. The VAS can be administerd in seconds and requires no verbal or numerical comprehension at all. It has been used to assess pain during labour (Revill *et al.*, 1976). The VAS thus provided an alternative method of assessing pain to the MPQ and also yielded complementary data on the intensity of labour pain.

In this study the MPQ and VAS were used to assess labour pain recorded during the first stage of labour and 24 to 48 hours postnatally. Whilst it would have been desirable to have recorded the women's assessments of labour pain at various times throughout childbirth, and in particular in the second stage of labour as well as in the first stage, it was considered that the effort involved for the women in the first stage of labour was too great to undertake assessments at intervals and that nothing should be done to distract women from their efforts in delivery. Therefore, the women were required to recall the pain they experienced throughout labour and delivery, 24 to 48 hours after birth, when the immediate euphoria/exhaustion of the birth should have worn off and the 'fourth day blues' would not yet have set in. Recall of pain, assessed on the MPQ has been found to be accurate for up to five days (Hunter *et al.*, 1979). The 'recall reliability' of the VAS has also been established (Revill *et al.*, 1976). Therefore recall of labour pain should yield a useful measure of total labour pain experience.

Figure 5.1 Visual analogue scale.

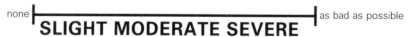

Source: Scott and Hudson, 1976.

METHODS

Phase 1

The aims of Phase 1 were to assess the effects of obstetric factors, such as parity, induction and duration of labour and weight of the baby, and the effects of psychological factors, such as the desirability of pregnancy, expectations of childbirth, antenatal education and the presence of the partner during labour, on pain perception. Other factors assessed included the use of analgesia, pethidine and Entonox, social class, as assessed on the Registrar General's Classification, and previous pain experience. This phase had two parts and pain was assessed using two methods (see Figure 5.2). In the first part the labouring women were asked to complete the McGill Pain Questionnaire (MPQ 1) and a Visual Analogue Scale (VAS 1). The midwife caring for each individual woman was asked to complete a Visual Analogue Scale at the same time as the woman, but without knowledge of the woman's VAS 1 score. At the end of labour the midwife was asked to provide information on the amount and type of analgesia used, duration of labour, unforseen complications which occurred, baby's weight, sex and Apgar score. In the second part of this phase the women were interviewed 24 to 48 hours after giving birth. They were again asked to complete the McGill Pain Questionnaire (MPQ 2) and the Visual Analogue Scale (VAS 2) recalling the pain they had experienced (Hunter *et al.*, 1979) throughout labour and delivery. Information on social class (assessed using the Registrar General's classification), any previous births or miscarriages, previous pain experiences, expectations of labour, antenatal education and partner's presence during labour and delivery was obtained at this time.

The study took place in a modern, well staffed and well equipped maternity unit in central Scotland. The author undertook the data collection. All women fulfilling the inclusion criteria who were in the labour

Figure 5.2 Time in relation to delivery when pain and coping strategies were assessed.

In labour
McGill Pain Qestionnaire 1
Visual Analoge Scale 1 by labouring women
Visual Analogue Scale by midwives

24–48 hours after labour
McGill Pain Questionnaire 2
Visual Analogue Scale 2 Interview

3–4 months after delivery
Interview on coping strategies

Source: compiled by the author.

ward when the author visited the labour ward during weekday afternoons were invited to participate. The inclusion criteria were that the women were to be having at least two contractions in every 10 minutes and the cervical os was to be at least 3 cm dilated. Women were not approached and invited to participate or were excluded from the study if any of the following conditions existed: the woman was approaching or was in the transition stage of labour; there was an anticipated complication of labour and/or birth in either the woman and/or the fetus; the woman was using epidural analgesia; or if the woman, despite having agreed to partici- pate, appeared worried or upset about the study. Of the 105 women approached, 101 agreed to participate. The author administered the MPQ 1 and the VAS to the midwife. The author interviewed the women in the VAS 1 to the woman and the postnatal ward 24 to 48 hours post delivery. At the end of this interview the women were asked if they would be willing to take part in Phase 2 of the study.

Phase 2

The principle aim of the second phase of the study was to elicit the women's use of coping strategies during labour, and relate their use to levels of labour pain and to their previous use of coping strategies. A semi- structured interview schedule was designed. This had been developed following discussions with the first 30 women who took part in Phase 1. Two to three months after delivery the next 60 of the 101 women in the study were phoned and asked to participate in a further interview at home, three to four months after the birth. Five women had moved out of the area by that time and five refused to participate further because of lack of time (2), they were back to work; lack of privacy (2), they were living with relatives; and illness in the baby (1). This left 51 women participating in Phase 2 of the study. Before commencement of the interview the women were informed about its nature and format, confidentiality was assured and permission was sought to use a tape recorder. The interview was conducted as a dialogue and consisted of a number of open-ended ques- tions regarding previous pain experience; strategies used in response to previous pain, stress and labour pain and the desirability of pregnancy. These questions were followed by a number of probes designed to clarify, extend or help in the categorization of the primary responses. An attempt was made to ascertain whether the women had acquired their coping strategies through direct teaching by others such as parents, or through imitating (modelling). It was considered essential that the interview should be conducted in a friendly, relaxed and non-judgemental manner. Quanti- fiable data was required, but the method by which it was acquired had to facilitate free recall of strategy use and avoid any embarrassment to the women.

Data analysis

Analysis of the interview data was based on methodologies developed by Markova (see Markova *et al.*, 1980). The tape recorded responses were analysed by the author and, in 50% of cases, by an independent rater. The information obtained from the women's responses to the principal and subsidiary questions was assessed on the basis of predetermined criteria. Classification of strategies and strategy used during labour was agreed upon by the two raters in at least 96% of cases. Disagreements were resolved by discussion.

The statistical tests used were one and two way analysis of covariance (Dixon and Massey, 1969) the student's *t* test and Pearson's correlation, Levene's test for equal variances was used in the analysis of variance (Brown and Forsythe, 1974a). When variances were unequal an analysis of variance, which does not assume equal variances, the Welsh statistic (see Brown and Forsythe, 1974b) was computed. Bonferroni corrections were used to test for the significance of multiple *t* tests.

FINDINGS AND DISCUSSION

Findings relating to the three main areas are presented and discussed here:

1. intensity of labour pain and effects of pharmacologic analgesics;
2. the use of coping strategies;
3. control in labour.

First the characteristics of the sample as a whole and the sub-sample who were interviewed in Phase 2 are briefly described.

All 101 women were English speaking and of Caucasian origin. The average age was 26 years (range 15–39). Social class was 1 – none; social class 2 – 11 (11%); social class 3 – 37 (37%); social class 4 – 34 (34%); social class 5 – 18 (18%). Fifty nine (58%) women were primiparous. The average cervical dilatation, as assessed at the nearest vaginal examination, on recruitment into the study was 5 cm (range 3–7 cm). The sub-sample of 51 women were representative of the women in the main sample (Table 5.1, page 100).

The intensity of labour pain: findings

Assessment of pain by labouring women. The average intensity of labour pain assessed by the women in Phase 1 of the study on the Total Pain Ranking Index of the MPQ during the first stage of labour was 26.8 (SD = 12.0, $n = 101$). Recall of the pain of labour and delivery 24 to 48 hours later was assessed on average as 32.4 (SD = 14.1, $n = 94$). This difference between the two scores was statistically significant ($t = 5.43$,

Table 5.1 Comparison of characteristics of women in main and sub-samples

	Main sample (n = 101)	Sub-sample (n = 51)
Age (yrs)		
Average	26	27.4
range	15–39	15–38
Social class		
1	—	—
2	11 (11%)	6 (13%)
3	37 (37%)	22 (43%)
4	34 (34%)	15 (30%)
5	18 (18%)	7 (24%)
Parity		
Primiparous	59 (58%)	30 (59%)

Source: compiled from Niven (1986).

$p < 0.001$). When compared with PRI scores reported by people with various different clinical disorders (Figure 5.3), the pain of labour represents severe pain. Sixty per cent (60) of the women reported that labour pain was the most severe pain they had ever experienced. However, pain scores varied considerably, first stage scores ranging from 5 to 59 on the McGill Pain Questionnaire (MPQ) and from 4 to 67 on recall. Scores on the Visual Analogue Scale (VAS) also varied considerably; from 0 to 9.5, average 5.5, for first stagge scores and from 1.5 to 10, average 7.9, for recall scores. This difference between the two scores was again statistically significant ($t = 7.40$, $p < 0.001$). As indicated in the section on 'Pain assessment measures' this difference could be because the women had not experienced transition or the second stage of labour when they completed MPQ 1 and VAS 1.

The MPQ was found to be more satisfactory for labour pain assessment than the VAS. Twenty-two per cent (22) of the women could not complete the VAS 1 during labour because they found it too difficult to focus on the line when in severe pain and under the influence of potent analgesic drugs. When the women recalled labour pain during the postnatal interview some difficulty was experienced with the restricted nature of the VAS, a number of subjects wanting to put their rating of pain beyond the end of the line. These problems with the VAS may have reduced its sensitivity. Therefore the MPQ results are regarded as the more reliable. Further details of pain

Figure 5.3 Levels of labour pain compared with levels of clinical pain.

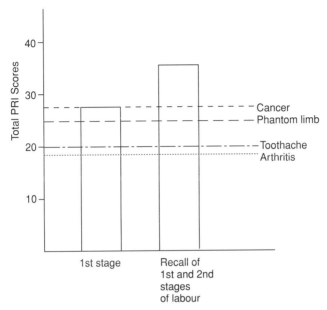

Source: complied by the author using data on clinical disorders from Melzack, 1975.

assessment and of the methodology of the main study are available in Niven (1986) and Niven and Gijsbers (1984).

Assessment of labour pain by midwives. The midwives' assessment of the pain, using the VAS, experienced by the women correlated highly with the women's scores, i.e. where the woman recorded a high pain score so to did the midwife. However, the midwives' scores were always lower than those of the women ($t = 2.2$, df $= 76$, $p < 0.05$) (Figure 5.4, page 102).

Effects of pharmacological analgesics on labour pain: findings

Pethidine. Eighty-six women received pethidine (150 mg) at some stage during labour; 27 of them during the first quarter of the first stage or before the cervical os was 4 cm dilated (here defined as 'early' in labour).

Figure 5.4 Labouring women's and midwives' assessment of labour pain.

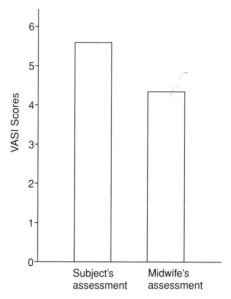

Source: compiled by the author.

Sixty-eight per cent (40) of the women who received pethidine later in labour reported that it gave them some relief from pain, compared with 54% (14) of the women who received it earlier but this difference was not statistically significant ($\chi^2 = 1.24$, df = 3, $p = 0.74$). Women who did not use pethidine had significantly lower levels of pain. As can be seen in Table 5.2 the difference in pain levels between these groups was particularly marked on the Affective component of pain for MPQ 1 when those women who had not received pethidine early in labour (group 2) were compared with the women who had not received any pethidine (group 1).

Entonox. The most commonly used inhalational analgesia in labour in the United Kingdom is a mixture of 50% nitrous oxide and 50% oxygen. Midwives may administer this via a machine named 'Entonox'. The latter word is used as a shorthand in the midwifery profession instead of the longer '50% nitrous oxide and 50% oxygen'. Eighty women received Entonox during labour; 12 of them during the earlier part of the first stage. Ten (91%) of the women who had received Entonox early in labour reported that it had been beneficial in some way, whereas only 49

Table 5.2 Pethidine use and levels of labour pain

Labour pain measure	No pethidine (n = 15)	Early pethidine (n = 27)	Late pethidine (n = 59)	F	df	p	Probability values for t-tests		
							1/2	1/3	2/3
During 1st stage									
Sensory 1	17.0	22.3	19.7	1.9	2, 96	0.14	0.06	0.29	0.1
Affective 1	1.7	6.3	3.8	7.7	2, 96	0.0007	0.003***	0.06	0.01*
Evaluative 1	2.3	2.2	2.4	0.1	2, 96	0.88	0.98	0.75	0.65
Total PRI 1	21.1	31.0	26.2	3.3	2, 96	0.04	0.01*	0.1	0.8
PPI 1	2.1	3.1	2.5	4.3	2, 91	0.01	0.008*	0.27	0.01*
VA 1	5.1	6.3	5.3	1.3	2, 74	0.27	0.1	0.1	0.74
At recall									
Sensory 2	16.6	27.3	22.9	4.9	2, 91	0.009	0.002*	0.04*	0.06
Affective 2	4.5	7.9	5.5	4.9	2, 91	0.009	0.01*	0.39*	0.008*
Evaluative 2	2.0	3.6	3.2	3.6	2, 91	0.03	0.008*	0.02	0.33
Total PRI 2	23.2	38.8	31.3	6.1	2, 91	0.003	0.001*	0.06*	0.01*
PPI 2	3.1	3.1	3.0	0.1	2, 90	0.92	0.89	0.73	0.79
VA 2	8.1	8.1	7.7	0.6	2, 79	0.56	0.99	0.46	0.35

Key: PRI = pain ranking index; PPI = present pain intensity; VA = visual analogue.
Significance level:
  * p < 0.05;
  ** p < 0.01;
  *** p < 0.001.
Source: compiled by the author.

Table 5.3 Entonox use and levels of labour pain (pethidine as co-variant)

Labour pain measure	Early Entonox*			Later Entonox*			No Entonox*		
	n	Pain levels	SE	n	Pain levels	SE	n	Pain levels	SE
Sensory 1	12	18.6	2.3	68	19.8	0.9	16	20.9	2.1
Affective 1	12	4.7	1.0	68	3.9	0.4	16	4.5	0.9
Evaluative 1	12	3.1	0.4	68	2.2	0.2	16	2.3	0.4
Total PRI 1	12	26.5	3.3	68	25.9	1.3	16	27.6	2.8
PPI 1	11	3.3	0.3	65	2.3	0.1	15	2.4	0.3
VA 1	8	7.1	0.8	55	5.2	0.3	12	5.5	0.6
Sensory 2	12	17.8	2.9	67	24.5	1.2	15	23.2	2.6
Affective 2	12	5.1	1.1	67	6.1	0.4	15	6.6	1.0
Evaluative 2	12	3.6	0.5	67	3.2	0.2	15	2.9	0.4
Total PRI 2	12	26.5	4.1	67	33.5	1.7	15	32.8	3.6
PPI 2	12	3.0	0.3	66	3.0	1.4	15	3.4	0.3
VA 2	11	7.9	0.5	59	8.0	0.2	11	7.5	0.5

For abbreviations see key to Table 5.2. Numbers do not add up to 101 (total number of women in Phase 1) as some data were missing.
* Adjusted means.
Source: compiled by the author.

(73%) of the women who had received Entonox in late first or early second stage reported as positively. However, this difference was not statistically significant ($\chi^2 = 1.84$, df = 3, $p = 0.6$). The majority of women who had received Entonox had also received pethidine. When the effect of pethidine was controlled statistically by an analysis of covariance, the difference between these groups was as shown in Table 5.3. Women who had received Entonox early in labour had more **Evaluative** pain during the first stage of labour ($t = 1.7$, df = 92, $p = 0.08$) and had higher PPI ($t = 2.2$, df = 87, $p = 0.01$) and VA 1 scores ($t = 2.2$, df = 71, $p = 0.03$) than those women who had Entonox later in labour. They also had higher PPI scores ($t = 2.1$, df = 98, $p = 0.03$) than women who used no Entonox. When the women who had received Entonox early in labour recalled their labour pain they reported marginally, but not significantly, less pain in total (Total PRI 2) than women who received Entonox at a later stage ($t = 1.6$, df = 90, $p = 0.1$).

The intensity of labour pain and effects of pharmacological analgesics on labour pain: discussion

The average level of pain experienced by the women in this study was very high. However, the midwives consistently under-estimated this pain. Under assessment of pain by health professionals has also been reported by DeKornfeld *et al.* (1964) and Seers (1989). This is puzzling. The puzzle may be resolved by looking to the midwives' behaviour when asked to assess the pain of the women in their care. Typically they first palpated the woman's abdomen during a contraction, presumably basing their assessment on the strength of the uterine contraction. Modern theories of pain perception have demonstrated that the amount of pain a person experiences is not equal to the amount of noxious stimulation they are encountering (in the case of labour pain, the amount of noxious stimulation emanating from the contraction of the uterus and consequent dilatation of the cervix). Instead it is influenced by a complex interaction between psychological and physiological mechanisms which may serve to exacerbate or modulate the effects of noxious stimulation (Melzack and Wall, 1988). In labour the amount of pain experienced is likely to be affected by a substantial number of factors in addition to the effects of uterine contraction and cervical dilatation (Bonica, 1975). Physical factors, such as the size and position of the baby, and the resistance and elasticity of the musculature of the uterus and birth canal, will influence the amount of noxious stimulation occuring but these cannot be directly detected through abdominal palpation during labour. Psychological factors, such as the woman's attitudes, expectations and anxieties about childbirth, may modulate that noxious stimulation (Melzack and Wall, 1988); again information about these may not be available to the midwife and certainly will not be elicited by abdominal palpation. Therefore the midwife's inaccuracy in assessing the woman's pain may have been the result of lack of information and a mistaken belief that labour pain is influenced by relatively simple physiological factors. However, analysis of the inaccuracy shows that it is biased in one direction only – the inaccuracy lies in the underestimation of pain levels. Not one midwife, female or male, nulliparous or parous, over-estimated labour pain. Perhaps there is a protective mechanism operating here. Perhaps when a midwife is faced with a woman in severe pain in labour, when there is a limited amount that can be done to relieve the pain, it is better for the midwife to imagine that the pain is not so intense. This would lessen the midwife's distress; however, it is unlikely to lessen the woman's. This may be a general human tendency rather than one peculiar to midwives and nurses (having recently experienced a sore back I feel that humanity is not predisposed to empathize with pain). But it may be more apparent in midwives who, during their nursing career, were used to having access to potent analgesics to relieve their patients' pain and who are therefore relatively unprepared for the stress of working closely with labouring women whose pain cannot be entirely relieved.

The findings of this study showed that the effects of pethidine and Entonox were regarded as fairly satisfactory by the majority of the women. Pethidine use was not associated with lower levels of pain. It is suggested that this was because it was only used when labour pain became severe. However, Entonox was associated with non-significantly lower levels of pain. Its use early in labour did not seem to be effective just as pethidine use at that time also appeared ineffective. However, when the women recalled the pain they had experienced throughout labour and delivery, those who had received Entonox early in labour recorded the lowest levels of pain and the highest levels of satisfaction with its effectiveness. This suggests that it was a relatively effective analgesic when used repeatedly from early on in labour. Some authorities have suggested that the use of Entonox has been waning since the introduction of 'epidurals on demand'. The findings of this study suggest that its usefulness might be re-evaluated, especially as nitrous-oxide inhalation is regarded as comparatively free of side effects (Bonica, 1967), is under the woman's control and seems to be conducive to her use of psychological analgesia – breathing techniques, distraction, etc. (Niven, 1986).

While the majority of the women expressed some satisfaction with the pain relief obtained from pethidine and/or Entonox, it should be noted that some women reported that they did not have any relief from these drugs. These women were over-represented in the 'early pethidine' group; a group (27% of all women in the study) characterized by youth, inexperience and anxiety (70% primiparous, 25% teenagers, 44% with 'fearful/terrified' expectations of childbirth, 62% no previous experience of severe pain). The midwives reported that the principal reason for administering pethidine early in labour was to alleviate anxiety and excessive early labour pain. It appears that, as such, it was unsuccessful.

Although some women were satisfied with the pain relief obtained from pethidine and/or Entonox overall the group experienced considerable pain when compared with pain from other origins (Figure 5.3, page 101). This reinforces the impression that total relief from labour pain is not sought by all women – an impression supported by the findings of research carried out in London (Morgan *et al.*, 1982) which found a negative relationship between the effectiveness of obstetric analgesics and ratings of overall satisfaction with childbirth.

The use of coping strategies

Information about the coping strategies that the women had used was obtained during the interview 3 to 4 months post delivery. The coping strategies that the women were asked about were relaxation, distraction, imagery, reversal of affect, breathing techniques, normalization of pain and idiosyncratic strategies. This information was then related to the pain scores recorded by the women in labour and 24 to 48 hours after delivery.

Relaxation. Relaxation was used during labour by 17 of the 51 women who participated in the second phase of the study. They used the structured relaxation techniques (Jacobsson, 1929) that they had been taught in antenatal classes. Twenty other women reported that they had tried to use these techniques but failed. For them relaxation was unattainable. Women who could use relaxation techniques during labour had significantly lower levels of labour pain than women who did not successfully utilize relaxation, as assessed by the Sensory, Affective, Evaluative and total measures of the MPQ recorded after childbirth (Table 5.4, page 108).

Distraction. Thirty-four women used some form of distraction during childbirth. Physical distractors, such as 'doing the ironing', were used by 10 women to cope with labour pain before admission to hospital. Reading, watching television and chatting to others were effective distractors for many in early labour, but were reported to be useless (and in the case of 'small talk' often irritating) once active labour was established. Eleven women used mental distractors, such as counting the ceiling tiles, at that time. Many women complained about the lack of suitable distractors in the labour room. 'There's nothing to watch but the clock', except when squirrels could be seen playing in the tree tops outside the labour room's high windows; a very effective source of distraction but unfortunately not one that could be produced 'to order'. Levels of labour pain were significantly lower as measured by the Sensory 2 scale of the MPQ for women who used distraction (Table 5.4, page 108).

Table 5.4 Strategy use and levels of labour pain

Labour pain measure	Strategy used in labour			Strategy not used in labour			t	p
	No.	X score	SD	No.	X score	SD		
PART A – Significant differences between use and non-use of coping strategies								
Relaxation								
Sensory 2	16	19.9	8.7	33	25.2	9.0	1.95	0.05*
Affective 2	16	3.8	3.6	33	6.6	3.3	2.6	0.01**
Evaluative 2	16	2.5	1.8	33	3.5	1.3	2.29	+0.02*
Total PRI 2	16	25.6	12.4	33	35.1	12.2	2.5	0.01**
Distraction								
Sensory 2	32	21.5	8.6	17	27.0	9.4	2.04	0.04*
Reversal of affect								
Affective 1	11	1.5	1.9	39	4.5	3.7	3.6	+0.001***
Affective 2	10	3.2	2.9	39	6.3	3.6	2.56	0.01**
Evaluative 2	10	1.6	1.7	39	3.6	1.3	4.06	0.0002***
Total PRI 2	10	24.4	10.1	39	34.1	13.1	2.16	0.03*
Breathing techniques								
Affective 2	36	5.1	3.8	13	7.3	2.8	1.87	0.06
VAS 2	18	7.29	2.0	12	9.11	0.8	2.84	0.007**
PART B – Non-significant differences between use and non-use of coping strategies								
Imagery								
Normalization								
Personal control								
Staff control								
Idiosyncratic strategies								
Focusing								

The + represents separate variance *t*-test used because of unequal variance. For remaining key see footnote to Table 5.2.
Source: compiled from Niven (1985).

Imagery. Imagery was used by 17 women during labour. The image used was typically related to the baby, e.g. of taking the baby home, of dressing the baby, of how the baby would look. Only 23 women utilized images of holiday scenes; basking in the sun, listening to the waves, etc. and yet this is the type of imagery typically used by subjects who have participated in studies which have demonstrated that imagery is effective in reducing pain.

The use of imagery by the women in this study was not associated with any significant reduction in labour pain (Table 5.4).

Reversal of affect. Eleven women utilized a coping strategy which was categorized as reversal of affect. These women positively and enthusiastically welcomed the pain of their contractions as evidence of a healthy and rapid progress in labour. These women experienced significantly lower levels of labour pain as assessed by the Affective and Total PRI scales of the MPQ recorded during the first stage of labour and by the Affective, Evaluative and Total PRI scales recorded after the birth (Table 5.4).

Breathing techniques. Breathing techniques were used by 38 women during labour. Thirty-four women used deep, slow thoracic breathing during contractions and panting during crowning. Four women who had attended National Childbirth Trust classes used Lamaze-type techniques. Their data were not analysed separately because of the small numbers involved. Women reported that breathing exercises (apart from panting) helped them to relax and were also a source of distraction because they had to concentrate on their breathing. The use of breathing techniques was associated with lower levels of labour pain recorded on the VAS after labour (Table 5.4). It was associated with a marginal reduction in the MPQ's Affective score only.

Normalization of pain. Thirty-two women regarded labour pain as being a normal part of childbirth. The remaining 19 women felt that something must be wrong since the pain was so bad. Nine women thought that they were dying because the pain was so severe. Despite this clear and dramatic difference between these two groups of women, those who normalized labour pain did not experience significantly less of it.

Idiosyncratic strategies. Thirty-one women used strategies which did not fit into the above categories and were thus labelled 'idiosyncratic'. Ten women reported that they focused their mind on the pain they were experiencing rather than seeking to distract themselves from it. Nine women reported that the presence of their partner made the pain easier to cope with. Three women used a kind of 'time limiting' strategy in which they concentrated on the idea that 'it will be all over by tomorrow'.

Many idiosyncratic strategies had been used previously by the women to cope with pain or stress. For example, Mrs A always talked to one of her four children when she was in pain or under stress. She brought a picture of this child into hospital with her and 'talked to her in her head' during labour. Prayer had helped Mrs B to cope with the chronic pain she suffered and with the many stresses she had experienced in life. During labour she 'prayed her way through each contraction'. Some idiosyncratic strategies were related to specific experiences of the women, for example, Mrs C was a concert pianist and played symphonies in her head during labour; Mrs D was a policewoman and thought about the agony that some accident victims she had attended must have felt, this she contrasted with her own pain, allowing her to conclude that her own pain 'can't be that bad'. These strategies could not be analysed individually. Taken as a whole, idiosyncratic strategies were not related to significantly lower levels of labour pain (Table 5.4, page 108).

The women in this study used a tremendous range of coping strategies in labour. Table 5.4 shows that the use of many of these was associated with significant pain reduction. This is quite remarkable given the intensity of the pain that the women were experiencing. However, it should be

Figure 5.5 Levels of labour pain associated with the use of varying oping strategies during labour.

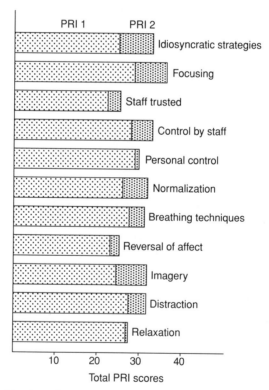

Source: compiled by the author.

noted that even the most successful of these strategies, reversal of affect, did not totally abolish the pain (Figure 5.5). Thus in this study there is no evidence of 'painless childbirth'. Instead there is evidence of strategies used during labour which often, though not invariably reduced the pain that the women experienced. Further details of the use of coping strategies are given in Niven (1986).

Control in labour

Personal control: findings and discussion. Nineteen women reported that they felt 'in control' during labour. Twenty women reported that they had felt 'out of control' at some stage during labour. The remaining 12 women could not categorize their feelings as either 'in' or 'out' of control. Perceptions of control were associated with varying aspects of childbirth. For five women their concept of control in childbirth was concerned with control over its processes, for example, its duration; for six women it involved some participation in the decisions which were made about the management of labour and delivery, for example, the choice of analgesics or the use of an episiotomy; and for 10 women it concerned not being 'out of control' which they defined as 'not giving myself a showing up'. There was no significant difference in levels of labour pain between the subjects who felt 'in control' (i.e. a sense of personal control) during labour and those who did not (see Table 5.4, page 108).

It was evident from these findings that control is not a simple concept. It clearly meant different things to different people and as such it is hardly surprising that it was not clearly related to lower levels of pain. A study by Scott-Palmer and Skevington (1981) which looked at Locus of Control in labour produced similar findings. Locus of Control (LOC) is defined by psychologists as a tendency within individuals towards an internal LOC, i.e. a belief that they were in charge of their own destiny, that they are 'in control'; **or** towards an external LOC, believing that things happen by chance or luck or through the control of others (Rotter, 1966). Scott-Palmer and Skevington showed that labouring women with an internal LOC had higher levels of labour pain than those with an external LOC, thus demonstrating that feeling 'in control' in labour is not necessarily helpful. Researchers involved in the study of stress (e.g. Folkman, 1984) have suggested that striving for direct personal control may not be beneficial in situations in which the amount of control that can be exercised is limited. Childbirth may be just such a situation (see the section on 'Staff control' below). In such situations an individual may retain an element of control by allying him or herself to a person who can exercise control. The midwife is such a person (see the sections on 'Staff control' and 'Trusting the staff').

Staff control: findings and discussion. Twenty-six women reported that they felt that the staff were 'in control' during labour, 16 of whom reported that they themselves were also 'in control'. Six women reported that they felt that neither they nor the staff were in control, but overall there was no clear dichotomy between staff control and personal control. There was no significant relationship between staff control and low levels of labour pain (Table 5.4, page 108).

One particular point that is notable about these findings is the comparatively small number of women who perceived that the staff were in control. This is in a way surprising since the control odds during childbirth are in fact weighted in favour of the staff. The staff control the environment, they control access to professionals (doctor, sister, etc.) and to loved ones – it would be a brave husband who would insist on staying with his wife if the staff asked him to 'just wait outside for a minute', and the minute can be a long one. The staff control access to analgesia; they have the power and the knowledge to strongly influence decisions made about induction/acceleration of labour, monitoring, analgesia, position, episiotomy, etc. In contrast the labouring woman is relatively helpless and could feel vulnerable (supine, naked, attached to various machines and in pain). Yet only half of the women acknowledged this reality (i.e. perceived the staff as 'in control'). Perhaps it was because the staff were very tactful in their exercise of control, allowing the women to participate in decision making and to maintain as much self-control as possible. But it may also reflect the fact that childbirth is a very unpredictable event, the precise progress of which cannot be influenced by doctors, midwives and technology in the way that most medical procedures can (compare, for instance, childbirth with surgery). It may have been this feeling which underlay the responses of the six subjects who felt that neither they nor the staff were in control. It would be deeply worrying if they felt as helpless and abandoned as their responses suggest.

The second notable feature of the findings is that perceptions of staff control are neither associated with significantly higher **nor** significantly lower levels of pain. The literature which criticises the medicalization of childbirth emphasizes the negative effects of staff control. These are not apparent in this study. Staff control was not associated with higher levels of labour pain and as already detailed, neither was it associated with a lack of personal control. In a study which related antenatal expectations with perinatal experiences, Brewin and Bradley (1982) found that women who expected that staff would be in control of their (the women's) discomfort had lower levels of pain in childbirth. This might suggest that staff control would be associated with lower levels of labour pain but this is not so.

'Trusting the staff': findings. Twenty-one of the twenty-six women who felt that the staff were in control were happy about this. This combination of variables was labelled as 'trusting the staff' as it was felt that this best characterized the positive nature of the woman's attitude towards staff control. The majority of the women regarded 'the staff' as being synonymous with midwifery staff, not medical staff. 'Trusting the staff' was associated with significantly lower levels of labour pain on a large number of measures of pain (Table 5.5). The differences between the pain levels of the women who 'trusted the staff' and those who did not (i.e. who did not perceive the staff to be in control, or who did, but were unhappy about the staff control) were highly significant (Table 5.5). 'Trusting the staff' was significantly associated with attendance at antenatal classes ($\chi^2 = 4.02$, df $= 1$, $p = 0.04$), which was in turn associated with significantly lower levels of labour pain (Affective 1, $F = 9.1$, df $= 99$, $p = 0.003$; Affective 2, $F = 4.08$, df $= 99$, $p = 0.04$).

There were a number of significant interactions between trusting the staff and the use of analgesics, both pethidine and Entonox. These statistical interactions signify that the effect of 'trusting the staff' cannot be separate from the effects of the analgesics which were administered by the staff.

The effects of trusting the staff were not solely due to the pharmacological properties of pethidine and Entonox. An analysis of co-variance which controlled statistically for analgesic effects showed that trusting the staff had an effect over and above that of the analgesics and in half of the measures this reached a level of statistical significance (Table 5.6, page 114). 'Trusting the staff' was associated with the use of coping strategies, in that women who felt positive about staff control used a larger number of

Table 5.5 Trusting the staff and levels of labour pain (significant results only)

Labour pain measure	Staff not trusted			Staff trusted			*t*	*p*
	n	*Pain levels*	*SD*	*n*	*Pain levels*	*SD*		
Sensory 1	29	22.2	8.9	21	17.3	6.6	4.40	0.04*
Affective 1	29	4.9	3.8	21	2.1	1.9	11.80	+0.001***
Total PRI 1	29	29.6	12.3	21	22.0	8.2	6.90	+0.01**
Sensory 2	29	26.2	9.1	21	19.0	6.7	9.04	0.004**
Affective 2	29	6.8	3.2	21	3.9	3.3	9.63	0.003**
Evaluative 2	29	3.6	1.3	21	2.6	1.7	5.37	0.02*
Total PRI 2	29	36.4	12.3	21	25.1	9.5	11.83	0.001***

The + represents separate variance *t*-test used because of unequal variance. For remaining key see footnote to Table 5.2.
Data not available for one woman.
Source: compiled by the author.

Coping with labour pain

Table 5.6 Trusting the staff and levels of labour pain (pethidine and Entonox as co-variants)

Labour pain measure	Staff not trusted			Staff trusted			t	p
	n	Pain levels	SE	n	Pain levels	SE		
Sensory 1	29	21.8	1.6	21	17.2	1.7	1.89	0.06*
Affective 1	28	4.9	0.6	21	2.3	0.7	2.76	0.008**
Evaluative 1	29	2.5	0.3	21	2.4	0.4	0.10	0.91
Total PRI 1	29	29.3	2.1	21	22.0	2.4	2.21	0.03*
PPI 1	28	3.0	0.4	20	2.4	0.3	1.79	0.07
VA 1	22	6.0	0.9	16	5.2	0.8	1.02	0.28
Sensory 2	27	25.8	1.5	21	19.5	1.8	2.58	0.01**
Affective 2	27	6.8	0.6	21	4.0	0.7	2.86	0.006**
Evaluative 2	27	3.6	0.3	21	2.7	0.3	2.03	0.04*
Total PRI 2	27	35.9	2.1	21	25.8	2.4	3.03	0.004**
PPI 2	27	3.2	0.4	20	2.9	0.4	1.14	0.25
VA 2	27	8.4	0.8	20	7.7	0.7	1.54	0.16

For key see footnote to Table 5.2.
Numbers do not add up to 51 (total numbers women in Phase 2) as some data were missing.
Source: compiled by the author.

coping strategies in labour ($r = 0.56$, $n = 51$, $p = 0.001$). The number of coping strategies used in labour was negatively correlated with levels of pain (Figure 5.6); i.e. the larger the number of strategies used, the lower the levels of pain.

'Trusting the staff': discussion. The relationships between the variable entitled 'trusting the staff' and other variables is complex. Stated simply the data show that a positive attitude to staff control was associated with effective pharmacological analgesia, with effective psychological analgesia and with antenatal class attendance. Each of these variables in turn is associated with lower levels of labour pain. These inter-relationships suggest that attendance at antenatal classes facilitates the development of a positive relationship between the labouring woman and the staff. The labour ward staff involved in this study did not regularly participate in antenatal education so the development of these good relations was not due to their antenatal establishment. Either women who attend antenatal classes are different from those who do not, or attending antenatal classes would appear to lay some general foundation of goodwill which makes positive relationships between staff and labouring women more likely to occur. This is likely to involve both the woman being more positively

Figure 5.6 Levels of labour pain correlated with the number of coping strategies used in labour.

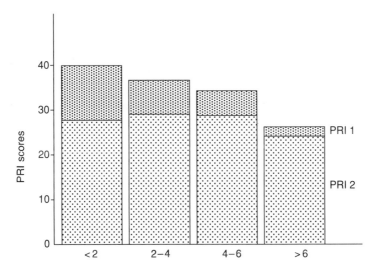

Source: compiled by the author.

predisposed towards the staff in general and the staff being more positively predisposed towards women who have attended classes.

The limited effects of analgesic drugs in labour has already been discussed. The interaction between analgesic use and trusting the staff suggests that the drugs are more effective (associated with lower levels of pain) when administered by staff who are trusted by the woman **and** that efficient administration of analgesia enhances perceptions of staff competence. These findings may be analogous to those of Brewin and Bradley (1982). In their study, women who had positive expectations of staff control over pain had lower levels of labour pain. In this study, positive perceptions of staff control were related to lower levels of labour pain. These positive perceptions may be related to positive expectations built up through attendance at antenatal classes.

Labouring women who had a good relationship with the staff used a larger number of coping strategies. Although the women who had not attended antenatal classes were sometimes taught breathing exercises by the attendant midwife (Niven, 1986), there was little evidence in general that the staff deliberately encouraged the use of coping strategies. Indeed, when discussing the use of psychological coping strategies with midwives, they often gave the impression of being somewhat hostile to the use of such fanciful 'NCT' type techniques. However powerful and effective strategies, such as relaxation and reversal of affect, may be much easier for the labouring woman to achieve when she is being attended by staff that she trusts.

CONCLUSIONS AND IMPLICATIONS OF THE FINDINGS FOR MIDWIVES

This study was undertaken in one maternity unit in Scotland and used a daytime only sample of 101 women. Although not totally representative, the study raises a number of important implications for midwives. It appears that labour pain is hard to cope with. It is (on average) very intense; its duration, distribution and quality are unpredictable; and it can only be partially relieved by the use of analgesic drugs such as pethidine and Entonox. If these difficulties are acknowledged by the midwife, the labouring woman will benefit. She will realize that the midwife appreciates the pain she is experiencing and will therefore do everything possible to alleviate that pain. This will contribute to the development of a good relationship between midwife and labouring woman which, as shown in this study, will in turn tend to alleviate labour pain. Furthermore it will allow both the midwife and the labouring woman herself to recognize the achievement inherent in coping successfully with such a demanding situation.

However, acknowledging that childbirth is typically severely painful and that analgesic drugs will at best modulate that pain, not reduce it to insignificant levels, may cause some distress to midwives. They may feel rather helpless and inadequate. Such feelings will benefit neither midwife nor labouring woman. The data presented in this chapter show very clearly that the good midwife is neither helpless nor inadequate. On the contrary she or he is uniquely placed to help the woman to cope with labour pain and consequently to experience less pain. The midwife does this by administering analgesic drugs skilfully **and** more importantly, by facilitating the development and maintenance of a good midwife/woman relationship. This allows the woman to utilize her own coping skills to the full.

Relatively little is known about the factors which are involved in the complex interactive dynamics of establishing good midwife/woman relationships. Clearly much more research is needed in this area. The findings of the study discussed in this chapter strongly suggest that anything which can be done to facilitate and enhance good midwife/woman relationships, should be done.

ACKNOWLEDGEMENTS

I would like to thank the Nuffield Foundation, who supported this study in part financially; the senior medical and midwifery staff of the maternity unit who gave me permission to carry out the study; and especially the midwives in the labour suite whose co-operation and support was greatly appreciated and whose skills and expertise greatly admired. This study comprised part of a Ph.D. thesis supervised by Dr Karel Gijsbers at Stirling University.

REFERENCES

Barber, T. and Cooper, B. (1972) Effects on pain of experimentally induced and spontaneous distraction. *Psychological Reports*, **31**, 647–51.

Bond, M.R. and Pearson, B. (1969) Psychological aspects of pain in women with advanced cancer of the cervix. *Journal of Psychosomatic Research*, **13**, 13–19.

Bonica, J.J. (1967) *Principals and practice of obstetric analgesia and anaesthesia*. Davis, Philadelphia.

Bonica, J.J. (1975) The nature of pain of parturition. In J.J. Bonica (ed.) *Obstetric analgesia and anaesthesia; recent advances and current status*. WB Saunders, New York.

Bowers, K. (1968) Pain, anxiety and perceived control. *Journal of Consulting and Clinical Psychology*, **32**, 596–602.

Brewin, C. and Bradley, C. (1982) Perceived control and the experience of childbirth. *British Journal of Clinical Psychology*, **21**, 263–9.

Brown, M.B. and Forsythe, A.B. (1974a) The small sample behaviour of some statistics which test the equality of several means. *Technometrics*, **16**, 129–32.

Brown, M.B. and Forsythe, A.B. (1974b) Robust tests for the equality of variances. *Journal of the American Statistics Association*, **69**, 364–7.

Cox, D.J., Freudlich, A. and Meyter, R.C. (1975) Differential effectiveness of electromyographic feedback, verbal relaxation instructions and medication placebo with tension headaches. *Journal of Consulting and Clinical Psychology*, **43**, 892–8.

Dallenbach, A. (1939) Somesthesis. In J. Boring (ed.) *Introduction to psychology*. John Wiley, New York.

DeKornfeld, T.J., Pearson, J.W. and Lasagna, L. (1964) Methotrimeprazine in the treatment of labour pain. *New England Journal of Medicine*, **270**, 391–4.

Dixon, W. and Massey, F. Jr (1969) Analysis of co-variance. In W. Dixon and F. Massey Jr (eds) *Introduction to statistical analysis*, 3rd edn. McGraw-Hill, New York.

Folkman, S. (1984) Personal control and stress and coping processes; a theoretical analysis. *Journal of Personality and Social Psychology*, **42**, 839–52.

Horan, J.J., Layng, F.C. and Purcell, C.H. (1976) Preliminary study of effects of 'in-vivo' emotive imagery in dental discomfort. *Perceptual and Motor Skills*, **42**, 105–6.

Hunter, J., Phillips M. and Rachman S. (1979) Memory for pain. *Pain*, **6**, 35–46.

Jacobsson, E. (1929) *Progressive relaxation*. University of Chicago Press, Chicago.

Kitzinger, S. (1962) *The experiences of childbirth*. Gollancz, London.

Klopfer, F., Cogan, R. and Henneborn, W. (1975) Second stage medical intervention and pain during childbirth. *Journal of Psychosomatic Research*, **19**, 289–93.

McCaul, K. and Haugtvedt, C. (1982) Attention, distraction and cold pressor pain. *Journal of Personality and Social Psychology*, **43**, 154–62.

Markova, I., Lockyer, R. and Forbes, C. (1980) Self perception of employed and unemployed haemophiliacs. *Psychological Medicine*, **10**, 559–65.

Melzack, R. (1975) The McGill Pain Questionnaire; major properties and scoring methods. *Pain*, **1**, 277–99.

Melzack, R. and Torgerson, W. (1971) On the language of pain. *Anaesthesiology*, **34**, 50–59.

Melzack, R. and Wall, P.D. (1965) Pain mechanisms; a new theory. *Science*, **150**, 971–3.

Melzack, R. and Wall, P.D. (1988) The challenge of pain, 2nd edn. Penguin, Harmondsworth.

Melzack, R., Kinch, R., Dobkin, P., Lebrun, M. and Taenzer, P. (1984) Severity of labour pain; influence of physical as well as psychologic variables. *Canadian Medical Association Journal*, **20**, 215–21.

Morgan, B., Bulphit, C.J., Clifton, P. and Lewis, P.I. (1982) Effectiveness of pain relief in labour; survey or 1000 mothers. *British Medical Journal*, **285**, 689–91.

Nettlebladt, P., Fagerstrom, C.F. and Uddenberg, G. (1976) The significance of reported childbirth pain. *Journal of Psychosomatic Research*, **20**, 215–21.

Nisbett, R.E. and Schacter, S. (1966) Cognitive manipulations of pain. *Journal of Experimental and Social Psychology*, **2**, 227–36.

Niven, C. (1985) How helpful is the presence of the husband at childbirth? *Journal of Reproductive and Infant Psychology*, **3**, 45–53.

Niven, C. (1986) Factors affecting labour pain. Unpublished Ph.D. thesis, University of Stirling.

Niven, C. and Gijsbers, K. (1984) Obstetric and non-obstetric factors related to labour pain. *Journal of Reproductive and Infant Psychology*, **2**, 61–78.

Oakley, A. (1979) *Becoming a mother*. Robertson, Oxford.

Reading, A. (1983) The McGill Pain Questionnaire; an appraisal. In R. Melzack (ed.) *Pain measurement and assessment*. Raven Press, New York.

Reading, A.E. and Cox, D.N. (1985) Psychological predictors of labour pain. *Pain*, **22**, 309–15.

Revill S., Robinson, J., Rosen, M. and Hogg, M. (1976) The reliability of a linear analogue for evaluating pain. *Anaesthesia*, **31**, 1191–8.

Rotter, N. (1966) Generalised expectancies for internal vs. external control of reinforcement. *Psychological Monographs*, **80**, 1–28.

Rybstein-Blinchik, E. (1976) Effects of different cognitive strategies on chronic pain experience. *Journal of Behavioural Medicine*, **2**, 93–101.

Seers, K. (1989) Patients' perceptions of acute pain. In J. Wilson-Barnett and S. Robinson (eds) *Directions in nursing research*. Scutari Press, London.

Scott, J. and Huskisson, E.C. (1976) Graphic representation of pain. *Pain*, **2**, 175–84.

Scott-Palmer, J. and Skevington, S. (1981) Pain during childbirth and menstruation; a study of locus of control. *Journal of Psychosomatic Research*, **3**, 151–5.

Stevens, R.J. and Heide, F. (1977) Analgesic characteristics of prepared child-birth techniques; attention focusing and systematic relaxation. *Journal of Psychosomatic Research*, **21**, 429–38.

Sternbach, R.A. (1968) *Pain: a psychological analysis*. Academic Press, New York.

Stone, C.I., Demchik-Stone, D.A. and Horan, J.J. (1977) Coping with pain; a component analysis of Lamaze and cognitive-behavioural procedures. *Journal of Psychosomatic Research*, **21**, 451–6.

Wolkind, S. and Zajicek, E. (1981) *Pregnancy; a psychological and social study*. Academic Press, London.

Worthington, E.L. Jr (1982) Labour room and laboratory; clinical validation of the cold pressor as a means of testing preparation for childbirth strategies. *Journal of Psychosomatic Research*, **26**, 223–30.

CHAPTER SIX

Care in the community during the postnatal period

Tricia Murphy-Black

INTRODUCTION

Midwives have three main areas of responsibility during the postnatal period: physical, educational and psychosocial (Rider, 1985). Although some aspects of the care entailed in these three areas can be separated and easily defined, many of them are interdependent. Midwives are qualified to monitor the physical health of mother and baby to ensure they make normal progress in the immediate post-delivery period and during the first days of life and to recognize those abnormalities that require referral to a medical practitioner. The midwife's educational role may also be undertaken at the same time as she is providing physical care, as the woman may need advising as well as assisting with the care of both herself and her baby. During the early postnatal period while the family is developing, and adjusting to its new member, women, both in hospital and at home, may need educating, counselling and supporting so they can care for the baby as well as for the rest of the family (Rider, 1985). The establishment of sound infant feeding is also seen as an essential part of postnatal care (Ball, 1984). Ideally, the work which has started in hospital will be continued when the newly delivered woman and her baby are transferred home.

Despite the concentration in recent years on antenatal monitoring and on the management of labour, midwives have always seen the postnatal period as an essential component of maternity care (Royal College of Midwives, 1987). It is during this time that a woman's return to normal health requires both support and care, so that adjustments within the family can be made to achieve a good outcome from this and subsequent pregnancies. The provision of an appropriate pattern of care for a woman and her child, and the approach taken to them at this time can contribute to the future health not only of the baby but of the whole family (Royal College of Midwives, 1987).

The study described in this chapter focused on womens' perceptions of postnatal care at home; it formed part of a wider research programme concerned with women's views of the maternity services, based at the Nursing Research Unit of Edinburgh University. The research sought to answer the following question:

> Does the care provided by midwives meet the physical, educational and psychosocial needs of women following transfer from hospital to home?

In order to provide a context for the study, the next section describes some of the changes that have occurred in the provision of postnatal care and some of the research that has focused on this aspect of the role of the midwife. As the study took place in Scotland, reference is made to developments and research relating to Scotland as well as those relating to England and Wales.

THE DEVELOPMENT AND ASSESSMENT OF POSTNATAL CARE

Changes in the midwife's role in the provision of postnatal care

Postnatal care at home has been a well established part of midwives' work particularly since the passing of the first Midwives' Act of Parliament in England and Wales in 1902 and in Scotland in 1915. During the first 30 years of this century, when at least three-quarters of births were at home, care was only provided during labour and immediately afterwards. The period of time for which care was provided after delivery was, however, subsequently increased. Following the Midwives Act of 1936, which entitled every woman having a baby to the services of a qualified midwife free of charge, care after birth was extended in England and Wales from 10 to 14 days. The pattern of home visits by midwives was specified by the profession's statutory bodies (Central Midwives Board for Scotland, 1944, 1965; Central Midwives Board, 1962). The postnatal period in Scotland was defined as ten days in a normal case and, although the midwife could visit as often as necessary, the minimum was laid down as visits twice a day for the first three days and daily thereafter unless there were special circumstances and this has been the norm.

A recent Scottish study showed that women delivered by caesarean section were visited until the thirteenth day (Askham and Barbour, 1987). In England and Wales, the situation has always been slightly different as midwives have greater flexibility to visit up to 28 days after delivery (Central Midwives Board, 1962, 1980). However, it is not always possible for midwives to carry on visiting until the twenty-eighth postnatal day even when they felt it to be necessary (Royal College of Midwives, 1987). Twenty-eight day visiting has never been the policy in Scotland but was reported to be the practice in 12 of 93 Health Districts in England (Mugford *et al.*, 1986). Women themselves have indicated a need for support after birth by turning to lay self-help groups, such as the breast feeding counsellors of the National Childbirth Trust (Seel, 1987). The Royal College of Midwives (Royal College of Midwives, 1987) has recommended sufficient community staffing levels to provide midwifery care up to 28 days on a 24 hour basis, so that advice, support and visiting can be offered to those women who need it. A personal handover to the health visitor on the twenty-eighth day is also recommended.

In recent decades, the nature of the community midwife's work in the postnatal period has been characterized by two major changes. First, the fragmentation of maternity care between hospital and community settings and between many different health professionals has meant that, whereas community midwives used to provide postnatal care for women for whom they had cared during pregnancy and labour, this is now rarely the case. It is much more likely that either they will be meeting women for the first time following discharge after a hospital confinement, or that they will have met them during antenatal visits at a general practitioner's surgery, but not cared for them during delivery. Secondly, the nature of the work during the postnatal period has changed from an emphasis on physical aspects of care to a greater concern with the educational and psychosocial aspects of caring for a new baby.

The process by which continuity of care by midwives during pregnancy, labour and the puerperium gradually became eroded has been documented by a number of authors (e.g. Walker, 1954; Bent, 1982; Robinson, 1990) and so just the main developments in relation to postnatal care are outlined here. In the early decades of the century when the majority of births took place at home, there was considerable continuity of care. Women in labour were attended at home by a midwife they knew, who would then spend much time providing physical care for them over the next ten days. The work of the domiciliary midwife was rewarding but demanding; women in labour had to be cared for during the day and often throughout the night, with antenatal and postnatal visits to be undertaken the next day. The institutional confinement rate was rising rapidly however; figures for England and Wales showed a rise from 15% in 1927 to 36% by 1937 (Walker, 1954). This was due primarily to two factors; first, the Local Government Act of 1929 placed hundreds of poor-law hospitals under municipal control, which removed the stigma of giving birth in a poor-law hospital; second, many of the leading obstetricians of the day were advocating hospital delivery on the grounds of greater safety for women and their babies (Robinson, 1990). The Second World War provided a further impetus for institutional delivery, as evacuation of women led to an increase in the number who had babies in hospital or maternity homes, a trend which continued post war.

The introduction of the National Health Service in 1948 meant that women could, for the first time, have a doctor in attendance without paying a direct fee (Wood, 1963). Although initially limited to those fulfilling specific criteria, there was an increased demand for hospital delivery. Figures for Scotland show that 36% of births took place at home in 1950 compared with 0.5% in 1980 (Information Services Division, 1970, 1988). The rise in hospital confinement coincided with the need for additional antenatal beds (Theobald, 1959). This, combined with a rising birth rate, lack of hospital beds and earlier ambulation, resulted in earlier discharge from hospital. From 1958 some women were discharged as early as 48 hours after delivery (Theobald, 1959), although the majority still stayed for ten days. The Peel Report (Department of Health and Social Security, 1970) advocated provision for 100% hospital delivery for women in the UK and so extra maternity beds were provided during the next 10 to 15 years.

The increase in hospital births changed the position of the community midwife. Initially women who delivered in hospital stayed for at least ten days and had little or no postnatal care at home. Following the move towards early discharge home, community midwives were then involved in the postnatal care of women whom they may not have met previously. The present pattern of care is that nearly all women have their babies in hospital and are transferred home to the care of the community midwife. The mean postnatal stay in Scotland was 5.3 days in 1980 (Information Services Division, 1980) compared with 4.4 days in 1986 (Information Services Division, 1988) and 5.0 days in 1982 compared with 4.1 days in 1985 in England and Wales (Department of Health and Social Security, 1988). These mean figures represent a range from planned transfer soon after birth (between 6 and 12 hours) to discharge at any time up to 7 to 10 days according to the condition of the woman and her baby.

The history of antenatal care also shows a similar fragmentation between hospital and community (Robinson et al., 1982; Robinson, 1990). The consequence of the move to hospital confinement and the fragmentation of both antenatal and postnatal care between hospital and community staff, meant that midwives no longer cared for women throughout pregnancy and childbirth. Nowadays they have to provide only some of the care, but for a greater number of women, most of whom they may not know. Recent years have seen a desire to recreate continuity of midwifery care by means of team midwifery schemes (e.g. Flint, 1991). However, the majority of women will be cared for postnatally at home by midwives whom they may or may not have met during pregnancy.

Changes in the pattern of postnatal care provision have also been accompanied by changes in the nature of the care itself. The work under-taken by midwives has been controlled by statute since both Midwives Acts of 1902 and 1915 and the original pattern of care was established during a time of high perinatal and maternal mortality and morbidity. Maternal mortality, for example, stood at around 3000 deaths per annum in the 1920s (Campbell, 1923, 1924, 1927). Puerperal sepsis was the major cause of maternal deaths and the number and type of visits to women, the observations to be undertaken and the care to be given was based on the need to prevent or detect both puerperal and neonatal infection. The maternal mortality rate started to fall steadily from the end of the 1930s (Wood, 1963) when both aseptic techniques and treatment with sulpho-namides became common.

During the 1950s onwards, postpartum care was characterized by a move away from carrying out detailed procedures for lying-in women, and towards early ambulation and independence in self-care and baby care. These changes, as well as those occurring subsequently, have been in response to changes in the demographic and social patterns of society as well as changes in the management of pregnancy and childbirth. Grand multiparae are rarely seen today but in the past these women, and those with severe anaemia, took a long time to recover during the postnatal period. Lengthy labours, measured in days rather than hours, followed by a difficult delivery could leave both the woman and her baby in very poor condition. Complicated postnatal periods were common and the baby, cot nursed for 48 hours and probably starved for the first 24, was not in the best state to establish breast feeding (Barnett, 1984). The nursing care of a woman 'lying-in' in bed for 10 to 14 days is no longer required. Instead of developing poor muscle tone, today's women are up within hours of giving birth and looking after their own babies and this has reduced the midwives' involvement both with the newborn baby and the physical care of women. There has however been an increased need for supervision, teaching, counselling and support (Barnett, 1984), as community midwives now visit women who may have had no previous experience with babies, and their own mothers are not readily available to provide them with support.

The fragmentation of the postnatal period between hospital and com-munity settings, the changing nature of postnatal care and the limited number of home births, have meant that the workload in the community is very different in the 1980s and 1990s compared with what it was some 20 to 30 years ago. There is less time to spend with individual women, yet many more to be visited. In the Short Report (Social Services Committee, 1980) the importance of ensuring that there is job satisfaction for the community midwife was noted. It was maintained, however, that the care and support of women during the antenatal and postnatal period provided both variety and fulfilment for community midwives. The Committee went on to recommend schemes, such as integration between hospital and community or 'domino' schemes, which allowed community midwives to maintain a full range of midwifery skills, including that of delivery. As noted earlier, a number of such schemes have now been adopted.

Assessment of postnatal care

Although a considerable volume of research now exists on the postnatal period, it is perhaps less well researched than either the antenatal or intranatal period; and the Royal College of Midwives has advocated the need for further research into postnatal care (Royal College of Midwives, 1987). A number of both national and local consumer surveys of maternity services have been undertaken that include views on postnatal care (Boyd and Sellars, 1982; Amos *et al.*, 1988; Farleys, 1988; Williams, 1988). These surveys have, however, tended to focus on hospital rather than community-based services, with data collection limited to postal questionnaire. There has been a considerable body of work, by midwives and others, on topics such as breast feeding (Thomson, 1989), perineal care (Sleep, 1991), team care (Davies and Evans, 1991; Flint, 1991), the role of the midwife (Robinson *et al.*, 1983; Askham and Barbour, 1987) and many projects on the organization of care have included aspects of the postnatal period. Two projects concerning postnatal care are of particular relevance to the study described in this chapter. First, Laryea's (1989) study of 44 primiparae in the first month after delivery using both observation and interviews: this author focused on the midwives' and womens' views of motherhood and suggested there were fundamental differences in the perspectives of both groups in defining the meaning of motherhood. Second, an extensive study by Ball (1987) examined the effects of psychological and social factors and the care given by midwives on the emotional needs of women during the first six weeks after delivery. A similar study by Woollett and Dosanjh-Matwala (1990) focused on the experiences of Asian women.

Despite the acknowledged importance of the postnatal period for both the woman and the baby, it has often been regarded as the 'Cinderella' of the maternity services (Ball, 1987; Royal College of Midwives, 1987). A range of criticisms has been voiced arising both from research findings and from professional, statutory and lay organizations. One of the complaints by the Maternity Services Advisory Committee for England and Wales (Maternity Services Advisory Committee, 1985) is that postnatal care is given low priority, is often inadequate and provided by unqualified staff. Some writers have suggested that postnatal care has a low priority because it is low status (Ball, 1987) and because it does not need 'hi-tech' medical interventions (Rider, 1985). Yet the first few days of a baby's life are important in the development of maternal-child relationships and the

Royal College of Midwives (1987) felt that this ought to be recognized in postnatal wards by having staffing levels that allow midwives to foster such relationships. Other criticisms have been that midwives seem to focus on the baby (*NT News*, 1985) and that women found it difficult to get information that they required (Jacoby, 1988).

Two areas of criticism focus on the deleterious effect that the hospital setting in particular can have on the provision of postnatal care. First, the nature of the environment itself maybe a major barrier to the initial success of postnatal care (Rider, 1985). Sleep, for instance, is difficult for the newly delivered woman, whether disturbed by her own or other babies, and drug induced sleep is a poor substitute. Unfamiliar surroundings with little privacy, and a diet possibly lacking in variety and attractiveness do not help the restoration of other physical functions. Moreover, the false atmosphere of hospital facilities makes teaching baby care unrealistic and it is difficult to involve the partner and other members of the family.

The second area of criticism relating to care in hospital concerns the increase in medical control of the postnatal period, despite the fact that it falls within the midwife's recognized sphere of responsibility. Large scale research studies undertaken in England and Wales (Robinson *et al.*, 1983; Robinson, 1985) and in Scotland (Askham and Barbour, 1987) have documented the extent to which the midwife's role has been eroded by medical staff, in particular by doctors undertaking clinical assessments of normal postnatal women. Askham and Barbour (1987) observed in their Scottish study that midwives exert considerable influence over decision making by medical staff and maintain that this accounts for the acceptance of the situation by midwives. Rider (1985) has argued that this medical dominance has hampered hospital postnatal care being organized so that the non-physical needs of women can be given proper attention, and that this in turn has prevented the midwifery profession from facing up to its responsibility to research and develop a system of postnatal care which reflects the educational, emotional and psychosocial needs of the woman and her family. She recommended that decision making authority should be given to midwives in charge of postnatal wards and that the necessity of routine rounds by doctors should be reviewed (Rider, 1985).

The importance of assessing women's needs postnatally has been stressed by Laryea (1989); she saw a need for more staff on the postnatal wards so that the detailed assessment required to discover individual women's needs can be made. Despite Laryea's doubts about the likelihood of such changes being implemented, Lewis (1987) has reported the successful implementation and evaluation of such a system, noting, in particular, that women were given information about follow-up care in the community.

The need for research on the extent to which community midwives meet women's needs in the postnatal period

As described earlier, the Midwives Rules originally specified the pattern of care to be provided by community midwives during a time when a large proportion of births were undertaken at home, there were levels of high perinatal and maternal mortality, and social conditions for many women were different from those usually prevailing today. It could be argued that women who leave hospital after one or two days need less care than those of 50 years ago, who may have been in poorer health at the start of their pregnancies, had many more pregnancies and were more likely to live in less suitable surroundings than the majority of women today. Unlike their earlier counterparts, however, women in the 1980s and 1990s may have only limited experience of child care, as they are likely to have grown up in one nuclear family and are now part of another. Their needs are more likely to be educational than physical and, perhaps having little support from an extended family, they might well envy those who were able to call on a relative at any time of day.

Although the Midwives Rules have been revised, and the organization of postnatal care has altered considerably with the mean length of postnatal hospital stay reducing steadily over the years, there has been little research on the extent to which postnatal care provided by community midwives has been meeting the needs of women in the 1980s and 1990s. Other reasons for undertaking the study at this time include consumer group criticisms of postnatal care, many of which have been supported by research evidence. Moreover, the pattern of postnatal care may have to be adjusted in the future in response to demographic changes, and information about women's views on present provision will help in planning such developments. Finally the hospital in which the study was undertaken was in the process of upgrading, resulting in a halving of the number of postnatal beds, and information was needed on the effect that this might have on the work of the community midwives.

AIMS AND METHODS

The aim of the research was to investigate whether daily visits of community midwives are providing women with the confidence, knowledge and skills to cope with the 24-hour demands of a newborn baby after they have been transferred home from hospital, and to focus in particular on the balance between the provision of physical care on the one hand and education and psychosocial support on the other. The research design was a descriptive study of a cohort of 645 women delivering in selected months in one hospital in Scotland, with information obtained from nursing records, questionnaires and interviews.

Research instruments

1. Nursing records. Obstetric and demographic information on each of the women delivering during the study months was extracted from the nursing Kardex and transferred on to a data collection sheet designed for the purpose.

2. Questionnaires
Postal questionnaire at ten days postnatal   ⎫ sent to all women
Postal questionnaire at one month postnatal   ⎬ agreeing to take
Postal questionnaire at three months postnatal   ⎭ part.

3. Interviews
Interview at ten days postnatal   ⎫ with a sample of the women –
Interview at one month postnatal   ⎬ (approximately one-tenth of the
Interview at three months postnatal   ⎭ cohort).

Ethical committee approval and access

Approval for the project was granted by the Research Ethics Committee of the local Health Board. Both the Director of Nursing Services (Midwifery) and the chairman of the obstetricians' staff committee gave permission for the researcher to have access to the women's nursing Kardexes and to visit the wards daily to ask women to participate in the study. The Directors of Nursing Services in the community and relevant GPs were informed; all agreed to support the study. For those women who lived outside the local Health Board, individual letters were sent to the relevant midwifery and health visiting managers as well as to their GPs.

Exploratory phase of the study

An exploratory phase was undertaken in order to identify those aspects of postnatal care that were of concern to women and to health professionals. This was achieved by means of a series of unstructured interviews with recently delivered women from postnatal support groups, a National Childbirth Trust postnatal support group, members of a well woman centre, midwives and health visitors. Each group was given a short explanation of the research project and asked for their views on the strengths and weaknesses of postnatal care. The views expressed in the first interviews were wide ranging and produced many different insights into postnatal care. By the final interview several common themes had emerged, from the interviews held with the women. Some of these themes were negative, whereas others were positive; they included:

- conflicting advice;
- fragmented and routinized care;
- complaints about the number of and timing of visits;
- appreciation of the support and help provided during the first weeks at home.

The development of the main study questionnaires and interview schedules was based on three sources: the themes that had emerged from the interviews with women, a literature review, and professional concerns about postnatal care. The women also volunteered to participate in pre-testing of the questionnaire prior to a pilot study, and this help with the study was greatly appreciated.

Women who took part in the exploratory phase were also involved in piloting the questionnaires, together with another group of women recruited from postnatal clinics. These women were somewhat different to those who took part in the main study as their babies were older, although all were less than one year old. The women noted any questions that they did not understand or could not complete with the pre-coded answers provided and the time it took to complete the questionnaires. The majority were able to complete the questionnaires in 10–20 minutes, even when dealing with a fractious baby. As a consequence of the pilot study, the wording and layout of some questions were changed and some categories added to the pre-coded questions.

Sample recruitment

The main study sample comprised a cohort of women who gave birth in one Scottish hospital during a summer and a winter month of 1986. Women with live babies below 1500 g birthweight, who were being recruited for another study, were excluded. The purpose of using this kind of cohort was to represent the normal range of women delivering in a regional hospital.

All the women were informed individually on their first postnatal day of the nature and purpose of the study, and that they had the option to refuse to return the questionnaires during each phase of the study. Personal recruitment on an individual basis allowed for the inclusion of women with premature babies, stillbirths and neonatal deaths who had to be approached with particular sensitivity. Of the 675 women who delivered in these months, 30 were not eligible or refused to take part. There was no formal mechanism for recording consent as this was assumed to have been given if the questionnaires were returned.

Every tenth woman approached during the recruitment period in hospital was asked if she would agree to being interviewed at home. Those who did not want to be interviewed or were not present in the ward were replaced by the woman with the next study number. An appointment for the interview was made at this time; all women involved were given telephone numbers to contact if they wanted to change the date or time of the interview or, on reflection, to refuse to participate in this stage of the study.

The questionnaires

The 645 women were sent postal questionnaires at ten days, at one month and at three months after delivery. These questionnaires sought their perceptions of the care provided by midwives, extent of support at home, ability to cope with the baby's demands and household management, as well as access to other maternity services. Most of the questions in all three questionnaires were pre-coded and asked respondents to tick an appropriate box. The response rates to the questionnaires were 83% (536/ 645) at ten days, 80% (520/645) at one month and 76% (493/645) at three months. The open-ended questions were coded after all had been returned. The accuracy of the coding was checked by another researcher on 10% of the questionnaires chosen at random after the coding was complete. The error level of 0.16% was considered to be within acceptable limits.

The interviews

A sub-sample of women (51, 8%) agreed while in hospital to be interviewed at home at the same time intervals at which the questionnaires were posted. A slightly larger proportion of women in the interview group were not employed outside the home during pregnancy compared with the cohort as a whole. This might indicate a greater willingness in this group to be interviewed in the home, as they were more likely to be there during the day.

The semi-structured interview schedules were based on the questionnaires and allowed for greater exploration of those aspects of postnatal care of concern to women. As they were part-coded with space to allow for replies which did not fit pre-coded questions, the women's comments were written down at the time and later transcribed. Although most reports were straightforward, the more complex replies were read back to the interviewee to check if it agreed with what she had said. Thirty-three women (64% of the group) were interviewed on three occasions, and a further 14 were interviewed once or twice. The transcribed material was then analysed in order to identify the main themes emerging and the range of views expressed in relation to each.

FINDINGS

The study generated a substantial volume of findings on many aspects of the care provided by community midwives for women during the postnatal period (Murphy-Black, 1989). Findings on three main topics are discussed in this chapter:

- aspects of care provided by community midwives during the first ten days after delivery (from the questionnaire sent to the 645 women on the tenth postnatal day);
- women's perceptions of the advice given to them by community midwives (from the interviews);
- women's views of the help that they were given by community midwives (from the questionnaire sent at one month after delivery).

First, data on the cohort's characteristics are presented (figures are presented for all 675 women eligible to participate).

Cohort characteristics

The 675 women who gave birth during the study months comprised 1% of the total births in Scotland in 1986. The summer month was slightly busier with 359 deliveries compared with 316 in the winter month. As the study hospital contained the regional special care baby unit, there were some women (7%) who lived outside the city postal limits.

Comparison of the demographic and obstetric data of all the women who gave birth during the study months demonstrated no statistically significant differences between those in the summer and winter months in terms of marital status, socioeconomic group, parity, gestation of pregnancy, or type of delivery. Comparison with the annual deliveries of the hospital showed there were fewer caesarean sections and more forceps deliveries in the study months. The percentage of caesarean sections during the study (12%) is, however, closer to the percentage for all of Scotland (13%) than the hospital annual rate of 16%. Of the 85 caesarean sections, 52 (61%) were emergencies. The rate of illegitimate births in the local Health Board was 21 per 100 live births while in the study sample there were 25% who were unmarried.

As there were nine pairs of twins there was a total of 684 babies. There were no differences between the study months in terms of sex, birthweight or method of feeding the babies. Breast feeding was the method chosen by 339 women (50%) immediately after birth. There were more babies born in the winter month who were admitted to SCBU (10% compared with 5% of the summer babies) but this difference did not reach a significant level ($\chi^2 = 8.819$, df $= 4$, $p = 0.06$). Although there were no significant differences in the Apgar score at one minute, there were significantly more babies in the winter group with an Apgar score of seven or below at five minutes after birth (7% compared with 3%; $\chi^2 = 6.01$, df $= 1$, $p = 0.01$). There were two stillbirths, one in each month and three neonatal deaths, all of which occurred in the summer month. The perinatal mortality rate (7.3 per thousand) was slightly lower than the rate for the Health Board (8.0 per thousand) and all Scotland (10.2 per thousand) for 1986 (Information Services Division, 1988).

Women's reports of care provided by community midwives

The first questionnaire completed by women at ten days after delivery contained a list of possible aspects of care that they could have received from midwives (Table 6.1). This list included physical tasks, most of which were associated with the midwives' screening or monitoring role; and a range of topics concerned with the educational and psychosocial components of care in the postnatal period. The women were asked to indicate which of the aspects listed they had received from midwives and their responses are shown in Table 6.1. The technique of listing items and asking respondents to recall which were relevant in their case is, of course, always open to inaccuracies of original perception and of recall. Data obtained in this study were women's perceptions of their care and these may or may not have been identical to midwives' perceptions of the care that they had delivered to these women. Some indication of the accuracy of women's perceptions is evidenced by the 13% who indicated that the midwife checked their operation scar, as 13% had in fact had a caesarean section and one additional woman had a tubal ligation. Although attention to an operation scar may be more important to women than other aspects of care, it seems reasonable to assume that the women's reports were accurate, particularly as the majority (90%, 484) had completed the questionnaire within two days of the midwives finishing their visits.

Looking at physical aspects of care first, the findings show that nearly every woman reported that the midwives examined their abdomen (to check fundal height) and examined the baby. Over 80% reported that the midwife had taken the women's temperature (86%) and the baby's temperature (83%), and over 70% said their perineum had been examined (76%) and that blood had been taken from the baby (72%); 62% said their breasts had been examined. Other aspects of physical care were much less frequently reported, for example, removing stitches (17%) and taking blood pressure (13%). The educational aspect of care reported most frequently was discussion of feeding the baby (92%). Other aspects were reported less frequently: cleaning the cord was reported by 47% of respondents; discussion of baby bathing and nappy changing by 23% each, although less than 4% were actually shown the last two tasks. Psychosocial aspects of care featured prominently in that 90% of women said the

Table 6.1 Aspects of midwives' care reported by women (*n* = 536)

Aspects of care	Once or more		Never	Not answered
	No.	*%*	*No.*	*No.*
Examined abdomen	520	97	7	9
Examined baby	495	92	20	21
Discussed feeding baby	491	92	31	14
Discussed mother	485	90	41	10
Took mother's temperature	462	86	27	47
Let mother talk about herself	458	85	64	14
Took baby's temperature	443	83	72	21
Examined perineum	407	76	118	11
Took blood from baby	388	72	118	39
Examined breasts	330	62	192	14
Showed how to clean the cord	254	47	245	37
Discussed family planning	145	27	364	27
Discussed baby bathing	128	23	372	36
Discussed nappy changing	121	23	381	34
Removed stitches	93	17	321	122
Took blood pressure	69	13	419	48
Checked operation scar	68	13	287	181
Helped with feeding baby	27	5	463	46
Showed how to change a nappy	20	4	467	49
Showed how to make a bottle feed	19	4	460	54
Showed how to bath a baby	5	1	484	47

Source: complied by the author.

midwives discussed their health and 85% said that they were given the opportunity to talk about themselves. Family planning, however, had been discussed with only 27% of women.

Women's perceptions of their care were analysed by a number of variables. Analysis by parity, and by delivery (comparing spontaneous deliveries with instrumental and caesarean deliveries) showed no statistically significant differences in the incidence of physical monitoring, educational or psychosocial aspects of care reported by the women. Differences did emerge, however, when perceptions of care were analysed by time of discharge from hospital and by method of feeding.

Time of discharge from hospital by care given. Analysis of care by time of discharge from hospital, reported by women, is shown in Table

6.2. Findings show that women discharged early (up to and including the fourth day) were more likely than those discharged later to report that tasks were undertaken or issues discussed. Using the χ^2 test of significance, physical tasks reported significantly more frequently by those discharged

Table 6.2 Aspects of midwives' care reported by women discharged early and late from hospital

	Discharged early (n = 315)		Discharged late (n = 221)		
	No.	%	No.	%	
Examined abdomen	321	(99)	206	(93)	**
Examined baby	304	(96)	190	(86)	***
Discussed feeding baby	290	(92)	199	(90)	ns
Discussed mother	288	(91)	195	(88)	ns
Took mother's temperature	279	(89)	182	(82)	**
Let mother talk about herself	268	(85)	168	(76)	ns
Took baby's temperature	280	(89)	163	(74)	***
Examined perineum	260	(82)	146	(66)	***
Took blood from baby	293	(93)	94	(42)	***
Examined breasts	210	(67)	118	(53)	**
Showed how to clean the cord	166	(53)	87	(39)	*
Discussed family planning	88	(23)	57	(26)	ns
Discussed baby bathing	70	(22)	58	(26)	ns
Discussed nappy changing	67	(21)	54	(24)	ns
Removed stitches	82	(26)	10	(4)	***
Took blood pressure	42	(13)	27	(12)	ns
Checked operation scar	4	(2)	64	(29)	@@@
Helped with feeding baby	15	(5)	12	(5)	ns
Showed how to change a nappy	7	(2)	13	(6)	@
Showed how to make a bottle feed	6	(2)	13	(6)	@
Showed how to bath a baby	2	(1)	3	(1)	ns

Levels of significance:

*	$p < 0.05, > 0.01$	⎫	
**	$p < 0.01, > 0.001$	⎬	Reported more frequently by those discharged early
***	$p < 0.001$	⎭	

@	$p < 0.05, > 0.01$	⎫	
@@@	$p < 0.001$	⎬	Reported less frequently by those discharged early

Source: compiled by the author.

early were 'examination of the abdomen' ($p = 0.005$), 'examination of the breasts' ($p = 0.002$) and 'examination of the perineum' ($p = 0.001$); 'removal of stitches' ($p = 0.001$) and 'taking the mother's temperature' ($p = 0.01$). 'Letting the mothers talk', 'discussion about the mother', 'family planning' and 'taking the blood pressure' were each reported more frequently by the early discharge group but not at statistically significant levels. The only issue reported less frequently by the early discharge group was the 'checking of the operation scar'.

Findings for care involving the baby showed that the women who were discharged early reported the following more frequently: 'examination of the baby' ($p = 0.0002$); 'taking the temperature' ($p = 0.0001$); 'taking blood' ($p = 0.0001$) 'cleaning the umbilical cord' ($p = 0.02$) and, but not at a statistically significant level, 'discussing feeding the baby'. A number of issues concerning baby care were reported less frequently by the women discharged early: these included 'demonstrating nappy changing' ($p = 0.05$) and 'making a bottle feed' ($p = 0.03$). 'Discussion and demonstration of baby bathing', 'help with feeding baby' and discussing 'nappy changing' were also reported less frequently but not at significantly different levels. This group of women were no more likely to have had these tasks demonstrated to them by hospital midwives than those women who were discharged later, in fact the opposite is more likely to have been the case. It might therefore have been expected that community midwives would have paid particular attention to demonstrating these aspects of care to the early discharge group, but findings show that this was not the case.

Method of feeding by care given. Although the issue of infant feeding is explored in greater depth elsewhere (Murphy-Black, 1989), those findings relating to method of feeding by care given by the midwives are included in this chapter. Feeding was classified as bottle feeding, complete breast feeding or partial breast feeding. Partial breast feeders were those women who were breast feeding their babies and gave additional feeds of milk, water or juice.

The 21 issues listed previously were analysed by feeding method for the 534 mothers who had given details (Table 6.3). There were no statistically significant differences in the percentage of the two breast feeding groups who reported the following: 'examination of the breasts', 'examination of the baby' and 'help with feeding the baby'. The bottle feeders, however, reported these activities less frequently, at a level that was statistically significant. Compared with the complete breast feeders and the bottle feeders, a greater percentage of the partial breast feeders reported 'help with feeding the baby' and being 'shown how to make a bottle feed', at a statistically significant level. There were no differences between the three groups in the other issues from the original list which were not concerned with feeding.

Table 6.3 Methods of feeding by aspects of midwives' care reported by women

Method	Complete breast feeding (n = 198)		Partial breast feeding (n = 67)		Bottle fed only (n = 269)		
	No.	%	No.	%	No.	%	
Examined breasts	132	67	45	67	153	57	*
Examined baby	193	98	64	96	239	89	**
Let mother talk	184	93	64	96	210	78	***
Talked about feed	187	94	65	97	239	89	ns
Helped feed the baby	10	5	8	12	9	3	@@@
Showed making a bottle feed	2	1	6	9	11	5	@@

Levels of significance:
* $p < 0.05, > 0.01$ ⎫
** $p < 0.01, > 0.001$ ⎬ Reported less frequently by bottle feeders
*** $p < 0.001$ ⎭

@@ $p < 0.05, > 0.01$ ⎫
@@@ $p < 0.001$ ⎬ Reported more frequently by partial breast feeders
Source: compiled by the author.

The finding that the majority of partial breast feeders reported midwives talking to them about feeding is to be welcomed. However, the issue of feeding does not appear to have been a major factor for the midwives, as 88% of the partial breast feeders did not report actually receiving help. The number of partial breast feeders who were shown how to make a bottle feed could be viewed in two ways: either the midwife realized that these mothers were not shown how to make a bottle feed in hospital because they did not need to do so while they were there, but once back at home they needed this skill; or that it became a self-fulfilling prophecy in that the women were shown how to bottle feed 'in case' they needed to and then they changed to bottle feeding because they had learnt how to do so.

Midwives advice: findings from interveiw study

The women who were interviewed were asked to comment about any advice that they may have been given by the midwives. The responses were varied, and ranged from complaints about conflicting advice, through indifference to appreciation of the advice that they had received. Conflicting advice, which has been the focus of attention in other studies (Filshie *et al.*, 1981; Maternity Services Advisory Committee, 1985; Ball, 1987; Farleys, 1988; Williams, 1988; Porter and Macintyre, 1989), was only concerned with feeding or related issues. Some of the conflict arose from the midwife giving advice in a situation in which the mother did not see a problem:

> The midwife said try feeds every four hours – she had been sleeping for five hours and in the hospital they told me to leave her five hours. When I tried four hours she consumed so much – well her stomach wasn't used to it, she was up all night howling – didn't get any peace until 5 a.m. The next day I decided to do my own thing and that was the only night I've really had to be up with her.

So why did you feed her 4-hourly?

> Well the midwife said and I was under the impression that every newborn needs 4-hourly feeds. But she's a big baby 10 lb born and OK, she lost when we came home, 9 lb 10 oz she was then but now she's 10 lb again. Even with 5-hourly feeds I've had to wake her the majority of time for a feed. (W21)

In the next examples, the midwives are responding to a problem:

> My baby was not passing wind easily so one said give him gripe water and the other said don't so I was mixed up what to do. (W27)

But advice is ignored when it doesn't work:

> She advised me to feed him every three hours, 15 minutes on each side when the baby was not settled. That didn't work so I ignored it. All the midwives have different ways of doing things, they give opposing advice about leaving the baby crying. One said give a bottle; the other one said never give a bottle. The baby won't take a bottle anyway. (S7)

These quotes indicate that the midwives who visited these particular women made no attempt to help them find the cause of the unsettled baby or suggest what they might do about the crying. It was perhaps fortunate that the baby solved the conflicting advice about the bottle, but it is regrettable that the 'midwives have different ways of doing things' could not be translated into a series of options which midwives could have presented to the woman.

Ball (1987) noted that conflicting advice had a marked effect on the woman's self-image in relation to feeding her baby, and argues that women need to gain confidence which has to be built up by praise and encouragement. Anxious mothers, taking on a new skill, will seek advice from anyone available. Conflicting advice, especially from midwives or other professional staff, is confusing. Women may conclude that the fault is theirs and that they have failed in a key aspect of caring for their babies. Inch (1982) maintained that more women in fact give up breast feeding as a result of destroyed confidence and sore nipples than insufficient milk.

Not all advice was conflicting, however, and much of it was greatly appreciated by the women as the following comments illustrate:

It was good – in fact fantastic. She explained much more about the Milton and with the cot, he could of suffocated with the pillow – and I did ken from the last (baby) but you forget how stupid you can get. I hadna' thought it. It is the wee things that hadna' occurred to me. (S25)

I found it very helpful – everything I asked – she helped me. I tried all her wee things, the things she said and they worked. She asked me things and found that I knew how he worked and that it was going well. (W16)

Mothers' assessment of help given by midwives

The second questionnaire, sent to women a month after the birth, included an open ended question which asked if they thought that there was any way they could have had more help from the midwives who came to see them. The majority (60%) of the 520 women who returned the questionnaires made no comment; 26% said that the midwives could not have given them any more help, while others commented on the quality of the help they gave (see Table 6.4).

Those women who did answer the question were most likely to make a general positive comment, for instance:

I find the midwives very helpful in the things that they have done and if I wanted to know anything they told me, they were very good. (456)

I thought the aftercare was excellent and very reassuring. (501)

Some of the general comments, however, were negative in tone:

I saw three different midwives. The first who called was unable to answer some of my queries – she advised me that if she did not call the following day she would ensure that her colleague who called would have answers. The colleague who called the following day knew nothing about this. She also gave information on other matters which in some respects was directly contradictory to what had been said the previous day by the first midwife. The third midwife who called was very helpful. (389)

Table 6.4 Number of women who gave examples of additional help they could have had from the midwives

No response	314	(61%)
No further help wanted	137	(26%)
Comment(s) made about help wanted	69	(13%)
Total	520	(100%)

Details of comment(s) made	*(n = 69)* * No.
Positive statement about amount/quality of help	44
Visits at inconvenient times or rushed	15
Negative statement, wanted more help not specified	10
Lack of information/explanation/demonstration of care	9
Positive statement about midwives/midwives' advice	7
Poor communication/didn't listen	5
Wanted baby care undertaken	5
Other	5
Would have liked visits after 10 days	4
Wanted midwife present at feed	2

* Some of these 69 women made more than one comment.
Source: compiled by the author.

Other comments referred to specific aspects of postnatal care; some were positive, others negative. Lack of physical care was a source of complaint from some women. In this example, the strength of feeling seems entirely justified:

> The midwife who came to see me was hopeless. She sat and watched (the TV) while I tried to find out if my stitches had turned septic but to no avail. (285)

Other women had clear expectations of physical care to be provided by the midwives. One said:

> Weigh the baby instead of bringing the baby back to the hospital twice, just for a weight check on the seventh and tenth day following caesarean section, especially when I could hardly walk straight and had difficulty going up stairs . . .
> Bath the baby for me at least once when I'm still not mobilizing well . . .

Three different midwives came to see me and baby but none
of them checked our temperatures. My baby was never checked
thoroughly apart from looking at the umbilical cord only. (626)

Perhaps the second woman did not appreciate the midwife's role today,
namely to give advice and support combined with monitoring the condition
of woman and baby. If midwives feel they do not have the time to bath or
weigh babies or that their time should not be spent on these tasks, perhaps
this should be made clear, either through antenatal classes or in the course
of explaining their role at the first home visit. Only five women (1%)
recorded that the midwife had shown them how to bath their babies (Table
6.1, page 133). Another study reported that 95% of the women left
hospital knowing how to bath a baby (Williams, 1988) so community
midwives might feel that baby bathing is not part of their educational role.

Other examples of educational help which midwives could have given
the woman demonstrate the need to build up the confidence of the new
mother:

They didn't explain about his cord or how to clean it. (239)

More information on breast feeding would have been helpful. (340)

More general reassurance that some day the baby would settle down,
that all babies cry a lot and you are not alone in not coping. (433)

As with each aspect of care considered, however, the positive comments
outnumbered the critical ones:

I thought they were very helpful and good at giving advice about any
of my questions about baby, myself and feeding. (527)

The psychosocial aspects of care provided by midwives are possibly the
most difficult to define, plan for and carry out. The diversity of the women's
needs demonstrated in the following examples shows both the demanding
nature of the community midwife's job and the impact that a single
midwife can make on a woman during a very sensitive period of her life:

Some advice on heating my house without electricity which I'm £400
in arrears, heating my home for my last child of 16 months. (362)

I think it would generally be helpful for midwives to remind mothers
how difficult it is looking after another human being 24 hours a
day. Because this is not stressed (no doubt for fear of encouraging
depression) I think women who are having problems (i.e. probably
99.9% of women) feel inadequate because everyone else seems to
be finding it easy, or at least can cope. A bit more public honesty

about the demands placed on mothers might: (a) increase male understanding of how difficult motherhood is; (b) improve women's feelings about their ability to cope and increase their self-confidence; (c) give increased status to motherhood, e.g. it is comparable to nursing a bed-bound adult 24 hours a day caring for all that adult's needs; (d) prevent people entering parenthood unaware of the difficulties – particularly young people. (117)

The midwife who came to see me and my baby wasn't at all nice. She shouted the first day she came as my doorbell wasn't working. My mother had to tell her to be quiet. She didn't really talk about how I felt, she seemed to do her job and then leave. I got the impression that she was tired of her job. I guess if she had come to see me and this was my first baby, I would have burst out crying. She seemed to find fault in everything I had done, I hope no one else has to put up with what I did. When I had my two other children the midwives were great and very helpful. (375)

Appeared in too much of a hurry. (455)

This final statement should stand alone without additional commentary!

I felt that the midwives acted like doctors – they came to see if baby and mum were well – no real help was given. (685)

There were also comments about the timing and patterns of visits, help with feeding, poor communication, the number of midwives who visited, and lack of continuity of care, which are reported elsewhere (Murphy-Black, 1989).

There is a danger that the critical comments reported here will leave a false impression of women's views. The large majority of respondents chose either not to reply to the question or to answer positively. The adverse comments are emphasized, not because community midwives give a bad service, but to encourage all those who try to meet the needs of postnatal women to examine their own practice.

DISCUSSION

Findings from this study on care provided in the community during the postnatal period do not support anecdotal accounts reported elsewhere of midwives ignoring women to concentrate on the babies (*NT News*, 1985). Although there were a small number of comments complaining about the midwives ignoring the women, most of the evidence indicated that care was given to both women and their babies.

There was no difference in the incidence of aspects of care reported by women with previous experience of childbearing and by those who had become a mother for the first time. Moreover, there were no differences in this respect between those who had operative or instrumental deliveries and those who had a spontaneous delivery. The women discharged before the first day were more likely than those discharged later to report that the midwives undertook physical care; some aspects of this care is dictated by the length of time since delivery or the age of the baby. For many years the Midwives' Rules have not only stated the physical care and/or monitoring to be carried out by the community midwives but have also specified the action to be taken in the event of detecting a deviation from the normal (Central Midwives Board, 1962; Central Midwives Board for Scotland, 1965). As discussed earlier in the chapter some of these Rules have been in existence since the days when puerperal fever was common and frequently a cause of death. The midwife had to take the woman's temperature twice a day for the first three days and once a day until the tenth day. A rise in temperature above 100 °F had to be notified to the Medical Officer of Health (Central Midwives Board for Scotland, 1965). Puerperal fever is now rare and the more recent version of the Midwives' Rules (United Kingdom Central Council, 1986) reflects the decrease in this postnatal complication in that midwives are now expected to judge what care is needed and give it when appropriate. Findings from this study indicate, however, that there are certain physical tasks, such as temperature taking, which are undertaken for nearly all postnatal women irrespective of need. Eighty-six per cent of women in the study reported that their temperature was taken, compared with only 13% who reported blood pressure recording. If midwives can assess which women should have their blood pressure recorded, they should be able to assess those who should have their tempreature taken and not do it because it is routine.

Women who were discharged early were less likely than those discharged later to report that the midwives discussed or demonstrated aspects of baby care (e.g. feeding, bathing, nappy changing). However, these are the women who have had less time in hospital to learn these skills. As there are no differences in the reports from multiparous compared with primiparous women, it would appear that midwives do not base their decision making on the women's previous experience. Although psychosocial and educational aspects of the midwives' role are recognized as important, they were never stated in the Midwives' Rules as clearly as the physical aspects of care and perhaps this explains why these aspects of care are not undertaken as frequently.

The aspects of care which were reported by nearly all the women are in fact mainly physical (such as examination and temperature taking), although discussion about feeding the baby and the woman herself were reported by over 90% of mothers. Other aspects of care, which were only reported by a small number of women, do not appear to be selected according to the mother's needs. For instance, helping with feeding the baby was reported by only 5% of mothers. Breast feeding is a matter of concern in that the proportion of women who start to breast feed is small but also that those who do start, abandon it very quickly. The OPCS surveys of 1985, for example, showed a reduction of breast feeders from 48% to 29% in Scotland and 65% to 40% in England and Wales between birth and six weeks (Martin and White, 1988). Findings from this study showed that 50% of women intended to breast feed in the first 24 hours and by a month 44% were breast feeding.

Community midwives need a number of skills to meet the physical, educational and psychosocial needs of postnatal women. Two themes of particular importance emerged from this study. These two themes are time and assessment; they are evident in both the questionnaire and interview material included in this chapter and in the findings presented in the full report on the project (Murphy-Black, 1989). It was clear that the midwives were pressed for time. In many of the comments about conflicting advice it was also clear that midwives did not assess the needs of the women. If individual midwives have the opportunity to assess women's needs, it may be possible to offer a more efficient and appropriate service to those for whom help is really needed. There were some midwives who did identify women who had problems feeding their babies, such as those who combined breast with bottle feeds, but only a small proportion of this small group actually reported receiving help. All members of this group of women could be helped further if they were identified as needing help.

Some of the women in the study reported conflicting advice, with the midwives often contradicting that given by another midwife the day before. This problem could also be reduced if midwives were able to base their advice on that given previously by colleagues. It is possible to present women with a series of options and then encourage them to try different methods of feeding or coping with a crying baby without being dogmatic and implying that the advice given before was wrong. Identifying those women with feeding problems and not giving conflicting advice both require assessment of the needs of individual women. It has been demonstrated in another study that given the appropriate setting and support, community midwives do develop new skills that are needed in the community (Davies and Evans, 1991).

Hospital midwives are constantly viewed by others while they work. On the whole community midwives work alone, with no other professional to monitor the reactions of women to the care they give. Research projects, such as this and others which examine quality assurance issues have one aim, to improve the care of women and babies. It is not done in the spirit of criticism of the often hard pressed community midwives. It is worth noting that the community midwives who visited the women participating in this project were under particular stress as the number of available beds in the hospital postnatal wards had been reduced.

ACKNOWLEDGEMENTS

The Nursing Research Unit is funded by the Chief Scientist Office of the Scottish Office Home and Health Department. This chapter is part of a study undertaken as part of the Core Programme of research, directed by Dr Alison Tierney. The views and conclusions are those of the author and do not reflect those of the funding body.

A copy of the full report *Postnatal care at home: a descriptive study of mothers' needs and the maternity services* may be obtained from the Nursing Research Unit, University of Edinburgh, 12 Buccleuch Place, Edinburgh EH8 9LW (cost £4.00, cheques to be made payable to University of Edinburgh). The questionnaires and interview schedules are published separately as an appendix (cost £2.00, cheques to be made payable to University of Edinburgh).

REFERENCES

Amos, A., Jones, L. and Martin, C. (1988) *Maternity services in Lothian: a report on a survey of users' opinions.* Department of Community Medicine and Research Unit in Health and Behavioural Change, University of Edinburgh.

Askham, J. and Barbour, R.S. (1987) The role and responsibilities of the midwife in Scotland. *Health Bulletin*, **45**(3), 153–9.

Ball, J. (1984) Adaptations to motherhood. *Nursing*, **2**(21), 623–4.

Ball, J. (1987) *Reaction to motherhood: the role of postnatal care.* Cambridge University Press, Cambridge.

Barnett, Z. (1984) Yesterday, today and tomorrow in postnatal care: the 1984 Dame Rosalind Paget Memorial Lecture. *Midwives Chronicle and Nursing Notes*, **97**(1162), 358–64.

Bent, E.A. (1982) The growth development of midwifery. In P. Allan and M. Jolley (eds) *Nursing, midwifery and health visiting since 1900.* Faber & Faber, London.

Boyd, C. and Sellars, L. (1982) *The British way of birth.* Pan Books, London.

Campbell, J.M. (1923) *The training of midwives.* Ministry of Health reports on public health and medical subjects, No. 21. HMSO, London.

Campbell, J.M. (1924) *Maternal mortality.* Ministry of Health reports on public health and medical subjects, No. 25. HMSO, London.

Campbell, J.M. (1927) *The protection of motherhood.* Ministry of Health reports on public health and medical subjects, No. 48. HMSO, London.

Central Midwives Board (1962) *Handbook incorporating the Rules of the Central Midwives Board*, 25th edn. William Clowes & Sons, London.

Central Midwives Board (1980) *Handbook incorporating the Rules of the Central Midwives Board*, 1st edn. Hymns Ancient and Modern, Suffolk.

Central Midwives Board for Scotland (1944) *Rules framed for the Central Midwives Board for Scotland.* George Robb & Co., Edinburgh.

Central Midwives Board for Scotland (1965) *Rules framed for the Central Midwives Board for Scotland.* Oliver & Boyd, Edinburgh.

Davies, J. and Evans, F. (1991) The Newcastle community midwifery care project. In S. Robinson and A.M. Thomson (eds) *Midwives, research and childbirth*, Vol. 2. Chapman & Hall, London.

Department of Health and Social Security (1970) Standing Maternity and Midwifery Advisory Committee. *Domiciliary midwifery and maternity bed needs* (Chairman: J. Peel). HMSO, London.

Department of Health and Social Security (1988) *Hospital in-patient enquiry: maternity tables 1982–1985*. HMSO, London.

Farleys Report (1988) *Is having babies the end of life as we know it?* Crookes Healthcare, Nottingham.

Filshie, S., Williams, J., Senior, O.E., Osbourn, M., Symonds, E.M. and Backett, E.M. (1981) Postnatal care in hospitals – time for a change. *International Journal of Nursing Studies*, **18**, 93–5.

Flint, C. (1991) Continuity of care provided by a team of midwives – the Know Your Midwife Scheme. In S. Robinson and A.M. Thomson (eds) *Midwives, research and childbirth*, Vol. 2. Chapman & Hall, London.

Inch, S. (1982) *Birthrights: a parents' guide to modern childbirth*. Hutchinson, London.

Information Services Division, Common Services Agency for the Scottish Health Service (1970) *Scottish health statistics*. HMSO, Edinburgh.

Information Services Division, Common Services Agency for the Scottish Health Service (1980) *Scottish health statistics*. HMSO, Edinburgh.

Information Services Division, Common Services Agency for the Scottish Health Service (1988) *Scottish health statistics*. HMSO, Edinburgh.

Jacoby, A. (1988) Mothers' views about information and advice in pregnancy and childbirth: findings from a national study. *Midwifery*, **4**, 104–110.

Laryea, M. (1989) Midwives and mothers' perceptions of motherhood. In S. Robinson and A.M. Thomson (eds) *Midwives, research and childbirth*, Vol. 1. Chapman & Hall, London.

Lewis, P. (1987) The discharge of mothers by midwives. *Midwives Chronicle and Nursing Notes*, **100**(1188), 16–18.

Martin, J. and White, A. (1988) *Present day practice in infant feeding: third report of a working party of the Panel on Child Nutrition*. HMSO, London.

Maternity Services Advisory Committee for England and Wales (1985) *Maternity care in action*, Parts I, II and III. HMSO, London.

Mugford, M., Somchiwong, M. and Waterhouse, I.L. (1986) Treatment of umbilical cords: a randomised controlled trial to assess the effect of treatment methods on the work of midwives. *Midwifery*, **2**, 177–86.

Murphy-Black, T. (1989) *Postnatal care at home: a descriptive study of mothers' needs and the maternity services*. Nursing Research Unit Report, University of Edinburgh.

NT News (1985) Mothers can feel ignored in baby oriented postnatal care. *Nursing Times*, **81**(28), 10.

Porter, M. and Macintyre, S. (1989) Psychosocial effectiveness of antenatal and postnatal care. In S. Robinson and A.M. Thomson (eds) *Midwives, research and childbirth*, Vol. 1. Chapman & Hall, London.

Rider, A. (1985) Midwifery after birth. *Midwives Chronicle and Nursing Notes*, **97**(1161), October Supplement.

Robinson, S. (1985) Midwives, obstetricians and general practitioners: the need for role clarification. *Midwifery*, **1**(2), 102–13.

Robinson, S. (1990) Maintaining the independence of the midwifery profession: a continuing struggle. In J. Garcia, R. Kilpatrick and M. Richards (eds) *The politics of maternity care*. Oxford University Press, Oxford.

Robinson, S., Golden, J. and Bradley, S. (1982) The role of the midwife in the provision of antenatal care. In M. Enkin and I. Chalmers (eds) *Effectiveness and satisfaction in antenatal care*. Spastics International Medical Publications/William Heinemann, London.

Robinson, S., Golden, J. and Bradley, S. (1983) *A study of the role and responsibilities of the Midwife*. NRU Report No. 1. Nursing Research Unit, King's College, London.

Royal College of Midwives (1987) *Towards a Healthy Nation: a policy for the maternity services*. RCM, London.

Seel, S. (1987) A mutual trust. *Nursing Times, Community Outlook*, **83**(March), 8–9.

Sleep, J. (1991) Perineal care – a series of randomized controlled trials. In S. Robinson and A.M. Thomson (eds) *Midwives, research and childbirth*, Vol. 2. Chapman & Hall, London.

Social Services Committee (1980) Second report from the Social Services Committee Session 1979–80. *Perinatal and neonatal mortality* (Chairman: Mrs R. Short). HMSO, London.

Theobald, G.W. (1959) Home on the second day: the Bradford experiment, the combined maternity scheme. *British Medical Journal*, **2**, 1364–7.

Thomson, A.M. (1989) Why don't women breast feed? In S. Robinson and A.M. Thomson (eds) *Midwives, research and childbirth*, Vol. 1. Chapman & Hall, London.

United Kingdom Central Council for Nursing, Midwifery and Health Visiting (1986) *Handbook of Midwives' Rules*. UKCC, London.

Walker, A. (1954) Midwife services. In J. Munro Kerr, R.W. Johnstone and M.H. Phillips (eds) *Historical review of British obstetrics and gynaecology (1800–1850)*. Livingstone, Edinburgh and London.

Williams, S. (1988) *Maternity survey*. Ayrshire and Arran Health Board.

Wood, A. (1963) The development of the midwifery services in Great Britain. *International Journal of Nursing Studies*, **1**, 51–8.

Woollett, A. and Dosanjh-Matwala, N. (1990) Postnatal care: the attitudes and experiences of Asian women in east London. *Midwifery*, **6**(4), 178–84.

tocol was submitted to, and approved by, a hospital ethics com-
The instruments used were Stein's Daily Scoring System (Stein,
nd interviews with a sub sample of the study participants. In the
g sections Stein's Daily Scoring System is described first, followed
process of recruitment, data collection and data analysis.

Stein's Daily Scoring System

Daily Scoring System (SDSS), shown in Figure 7.1, was developed
cally to measure the 'maternity blues' (Stein, 1980), and has subse-
y been used in other studies of mood changes in the puerperium
Stein, 1982). The SDSS investigates the presence/absence of 13
on symptoms and, for nine of them their intensity, if present. The
ident is asked to indicate whether the symptoms headache, feeling
le, difficulty concentrating, forgetfulness and confusion (labelled
in Figure 7.1) are present by recording 'yes'. For the symptoms
ssion, weeping, anxiety, tension, restlessness, exhaustion, dream-
d anorexia (labelled A–E and G–I in Figure 7.1) the respondent
tes which of between three and four statements most accurately de-
s how they feel that day. For this study another symptom, sleepless-
(labelled F in Figure 7.1), was added to the group where intensity
be indicated. A score is computed by adding the numbers by the
ments in A–E and G–I and for the other symptoms a response of
scores one point. In Stein's study the range of scores was 0–26 and a
of eight or more was considered to indicate a significant mood swing.
he symptom 'sleeplessness' was not part of the original SDSS the
s achieved in the F category were analysed separately.
he split half reliability was 0.75 and the score correlates significantly
the score on the General Health Questionnaire ($r = 0.8$). The General
th Questionnaire (Goldberg, 1972) is a well-validated screening instru-
which provides a quick and reliable way of identifying patients with
niatric symptoms.
ata from the SDSS was used to investigate the incidence and manifes-
ns of the maternity blues, and to investigate whether a similar reaction
e maternity blues had occurred in the surgical patients after operation.

Recruitment of participants

sample size for the two groups (postnatal women and postoperative
ents) had to be large enough to enable comparisons to be made but
ageable within the time and resource constraints of the study. Poten-
participants were recruited from the postnatal wards of a Consultant
t, and gynaecological, general and orthopaedic surgical wards.

CHAPTER SEVEN

The maternity blues in postpartum women and postoperative patients

Valerie Levy

This chapter describes a study that explored various aspects of the maternity blues and the extent to which a similar syndrome is experienced by
patients after surgery. The impetus for the study arose when I experienced
a blues-like reaction a few days after surgery and it occurred to me that the
'third day blues' may not be confined to puerperal women. This idea was
reinforced by the nursing staff on the ward who said that dysphoric reactions were common after surgery. I was however unable to find any
research evidence that the third day blues could occur after surgery as well
as after childbirth – the literature was almost silent on this topic. I was
sufficiently intrigued to investigate further; hence this study.

The study was not difficult to set up; indeed, if it had been I would not
have undertaken it, as it had to be done in addition to my work as a
midwifery tutor. Nor was it expensive. The total cost probably came to
under £100. I did apply for a small grant from the locally organized
research committee but was unsuccessful. The committee thought it was a
worthwhile subject of study, but asked me to take advice on the research
protocol from a doctor before reapplying. It often seems difficult for a
midwife or nurse to convince committees such as these, in which medical
staff are usually in a majority, of the validity of her (or his) proposed
research. Since the cost was minimal I decided not to proceed further with
the grant application. Furthermore, I had already sought advice from
several people – doctors and others – and their help is gratefully acknowledged at the end of this chapter.

BACKGROUND

The 'maternity blues' refers to the brief period of emotional lability affecting approximately 60% of women (e.g. Pitt, 1973) in the first week of the
puerperium. Neither the cause nor the precise nature of the maternity
blues has yet been determined. It would appear reasonable to relate the

blues to the hormonal upheavals occurring in the early puerperium but, so far, attempts have failed to demonstrate conclusively an association between the levels of various hormones and the blues (Nott *et al.*, 1976).

Is the maternity blues a normal occurence? The blues must certainly be differentiated from postnatal depression and puerperal psychosis, which are pathological and potentially dangerous conditions. Paykel *et al.* (1980) state that the blues is a transient, self-limiting condition with no known serious psychiatric after effects, and so common as to be considered normal. Stein (1982) in an excellent review of the maternity blues quotes Kraupl-Taylor (1980) who suggests that whether a condition is deemed to be an illness depends on the degree of therapeutic concern it arouses, and the maternity blues fails to elicit such feelings. Indeed, Bourne (1975) writes that many midwives and doctors consider an attack of the blues is almost essential to relieve tension after delivery. Stein (1982) also quotes from Scadding (1967) who defines an illness as 'a specified common set of characteristics by which living organisms differ from the norm of the species in such a way as to place them at a biological disadvantage'. Since the incidence of the blues is fairly consistently reported at around 50% to 60% of newly delivered women (Robin, 1962; Pitt, 1973) and has been noted worldwide, that is, in the UK, the USA, Africa (Harris, 1981), the West Indies (Davidson, 1972) and Japan (Morsbach *et al.*, 1983) the blues cannot be said to be an abnormal condition and in this sense cannot be regarded as pathological.

It may, however, be argued that the blues does indeed place the mother (and her baby) at a biological disadvantage; Sheehan (1981) emphasizes that the early weeks of the puerperium constitute a crisis for the primipara as her role changes, and Lesh (1978) suggests that the blues are an additional source of anxiety for mothers, placing them under mental stress when they need all their resources to care for their babies and to learn new skills. Furthermore, Cox *et al.* (1982) found that in seven out of 16 women experiencing a severe attack of the blues, the dysphoria persisted to develop into postnatal depression lasting several months. Cox and colleagues comment that the blues is therefore not necessarily trivial or fleeting, but may be an important predictor of postnatal depression.

The maternity blues would, therefore, appear to be a normal occurence, but severe episodes may render the mother temporarily incapable of caring for her baby and may be a predictor of postnatal depression.

The maternity blues is an ill-defined condition. Most descriptions of the blues emphasize its dysphoric elements and crying is cited as being the predominant feature of the blues (Yalom *et al.*, 1968; Pitt, 1973; Oakley and Chamberlain, 1981). Crying episodes are not necessarily associated with depression, however (Yalom *et al.*, 1968), but may be triggered by a heightened sensitivity to many factors (Robin, 1962; Pitt, 1973). Mood is labile and may feature euphoria as well as dysphoria (Kendell *et al.*, 1981;

Stein, 1982). Insomnia and nightmares are somet 1982). The woman may feel that she is confused a 1968), and may also feel tired, worried, restless Stein, 1982).

A hitherto common assumption in these and have been that the blues is unique to the pue however, particularly those working on surgical their patients often become tearful a few days aft to this study) I asked them, several nurses said were a reaction to general anaesthesia and a few were also mothers or midwives) thought the dysph maternity blues. One sister, working on a female warned her patients to expect a bout of tears and after the operation 'just like after having a baby'.

Raphael (1974) found that a condition similar may follow hysterectomy. Her study involved 100 p of age, undergoing hysterectomy for non-malignar these women experienced postoperative blues on th The blues were characterized by crying, sadness and '

There is some evidence that the blues may be ex types of surgery. Lindemann (1941), in his study of p surgical operations, refers to Cobb *et al.* (1938), who postoperative psychoses, consisting mainly of altered 'such as is often seen in the so-called symptomatic p cious anaemia or the puerperal states'.

The study reported in this chapter adds to the sma on 'blues' after surgery, as well as providing infor experiences of the maternity blues. The latter findi of implications for midwives and these are discussed i the chapter.

AIMS AND METHODS

The aims of the study were to:

1. investigate the incidence and manifestation of the
2. establish whether a reaction similar to the materni enced by postoperative patients;
3. elicit comments from postnatal women and post experiencing the blues regarding the factors preci tress, and their perceived needs during this time.

The study was undertaken in one hospital and entailed o tion about the blues from women on maternity wards (and female patients on surgical wards ($n = 91$). Before sta

Figure 7.1 Stein's daily scoring system.

Number . . . . Date . . . . .

In the first part of this questionnaire there are several groups of statements. Please circle the number of the one statement that most accurately describes how you have felt today. If there are two or more statements in a group that describe how you feel please circle the highest one. Thank you for your help.

A 0. I do not feel depressed today
  1. I feel a little depressed today
  2. I feel quite depressed today
  3. I feel so depressed it is quite painful

B 0. I do not feel like crying
  1. I feel as though I could cry, but I have not actually cried
  2. I have shed a few tears today
  3. I have cried for several minutes, today but for less than half an hour
  4. I have cried for more than half an hour

C 0. I feel no more anxious or worried than usual
  1. At times today I have felt anxious and worried
  2. At times today I have left very anxious and worried
  3. At times today I have been in a state of panic

D 0. I feel calm and relaxed
  1. I feel somewhat tense
  2. I feel very tense

E 0. I feel no more restless than usual
  1. I feel a little restless
  2. I feel very restless and find it difficult to settle to anything

F 0. I slept well last night
  1. I slept fairly well last night
  2. I did not sleep very well last night
  3. I hardly slept at all last night

G 0. I don't feel any more tired than usual
  1. I have less energy than usual
  2. I feel exhausted for most of the day

H 0. Last night I did not dream
  1. Last night I had a dream
  2. Last night a dream woke me from my sleep

I 0. My appetite is the same as usual
  1. My appetite is not so good as usual
  2. My appetite is worse today
  3. I have no appetite today

Lastly, please answer YES or NO to the following: Today, have you experienced:

L Headache . . . . .
M Feeling irritable . . . . .
N Difficulty concentrating . . . . .
P Forgetfulness . . . .
Q Confusion . . . .

Source: Stein 1980, amended by the author.

Postnatal women. Women in the maternity group were approached on their first postnatal day and invited to participate in the study. Verbal and written explanations of the study were given to each woman individually. Every woman who delivered was invited to participate except for those whose baby had died or was seriously ill. Recruitment continued until the required number (61) of women had agreed to participate.

Postoperative patients. In the surgical groups, women and men who had undergone various types of surgical operations were approached on the first postoperative day and invited to take part in the study. Terminally ill patients were not included as it was thought unreasonable to concern them with questionnaires at such a time. Women undergoing termination of pregnancy were also excluded as their responses were likely to have been influenced by extraneous psychological factors. All respondents were aged between 16 and 50 years in order to facilitate comparisons with the maternity group. Apart from these exclusions, every postoperative patient in the study wards was invited to participate until a sufficient number had been recruited ($n = 91$).

The study wards all carry out both major and minor surgery within their specialities. There is, however, no clear distinction between major and minor surgery. For the purposes of this study, patients discharged home within 48 hours of surgery were assessed as having had minor surgery and those remaining longer than 48 hours, major surgery. Numbers in each group invited to participate and agreeing to do so were as shown in Table 7.1.

Data collection

Administration of Stein's Daily Scoring System questionnaire (SDSS). The SDSS was administered to each respondent every day from the second to the sixth (inclusive) postnatal or postoperative day.

The respondents were asked:

1. to circle the number of the statement which most accurately described
   · how he or she had felt during the day;
2. to complete the SDSS during the evening, preferably at the same time each day, in order to provide an opportunity to review the events of the day and to minimize the effects of circadian rhythms;
3. not to discuss their responses with anyone.

Verbal instructions were reinforced by written instructions at the beginning of each SDSS.

Collection of the SDSSs and gathering of comments. The SDSSs were collected from inpatients each morning by myself and new ques-

Table 7.1 Number in each group invited to participate and agreeing to do so

Group	Invited to participate	Agreed to participate
Female major surgical	29	29
Female minor surgical	31	30
Male major surgical	18	18
Male minor surgical	14	14
Total	92	91

Source: compiled by the author.

tionnaires issued for later completion. This personal contact provided an opportunity to gather information about the recalled feelings of the respondent regarding the dysphoria. By means of a semi-structured interview schedule, respondents who had experienced dysphoria the previous day (as assessed by quick scrutiny of the current SDSS) were invited to comment about any aspect of their distress they thought appropriate, for instance, what they thought had precipitated the dysphoria, who they had wanted with them at the time, and how they thought they could best have been helped. Only those who indicated they had experienced dysphoria were interviewed.

Constraints of time and money prevented me from visiting respondents who had been transferred home and therefore only hospital inpatients were asked to provide comments.

Respondents transferred home before the sixth day were given a supply of SDSSs and stamped addressed envelopes, and asked to return the completed forms by post.

SDSS response rates

Some respondents did not return a complete set of questionnaires. The numbers in each group who did so, and upon which the analysis is based are shown in Table 7.2 (page 154).

It was not possible to discover the reasons for the incompleteness or non-return of the questionnaires. This implies a possible source of bias as the non-compliant individuals may have experienced a severe episode of the blues that prevented them from complying, or alternatively may not have experienced dysphoria and thought it not worthwhile to return the questionnaires.

Table 7.2 Questionnaire response rates

Group	Agreed to participate	Returned all questionnaires
Postnatal women	61	42 (69%)
Female major surgical (FS major)	29	28 (96%)
Female minor surgical (FS minor)	30	22 (73%)
Male major surgical (MS major)	18	16 (89%)
Male minor surgical (MS minor)	14	9 (64%)
Total	152	117 (77%)

Source: compiled by the author.

Data analysis

Diagnosis and incidence of the blues. The blues was assessed as having occurred when 8 points or more was scored on the SDSS on one or more days. As noted earlier, a score of 8 or more signifies, according to Stein (1980), that 'the blues' has occurred. Scores from the insomnia category were analysed separately and did not contribute to the diagnosis of the blues, as insomnia had not been included as an item in the original instrument.

Manifestation of the blues. Stein (1982) discusses the uncertainty regarding the manifestion of the maternity blues; for instance it is not clear whether confusion is part of the syndrome. There appears to be agreement, however, that tearfulness is the predominant feature of the blues (Yalom *et al.*, 1968). Crying was therefore taken to be the central symptom and correlations were sought between crying and the other 12 items included in the SDSS.

The total individual symptom score was calculated in each respondent for days 2 to 6 inclusive. Each symptom score was then correlated with the crying score. Pearson's correlation coefficient was calculated to establish the degree of linear relationship between crying and each of the other variables. The *t* statistic was then calculated from the value of the sample correlation coefficient and the number of XY pairs in order to give the probability value.

Comparison of the blues between the groups of respondents.
The manifestations of the blues were then compared between the maternity and surgical groups. The data were not normally distributed and

so the Mann-Whitney test was used to evaluate the difference between symptom score distributions in the surgical groups compared with those in the maternity group. Probability values were then calculated from the standard normal distribution.

Data processing. The processing was done by myself using my personal BBC B microcomputer. At first, I could find no suitable commercially produced statistics program and had to write my own (which lacked something in sophistication, to say the least). Now there are many commercially produced, 'user friendly' programs available which can be used on personal computers.

Analysis of comments. The comments made by those respondents who had experienced dysphoria were examined for major themes. This produced eight major categories and each comment was then allocated to one of these.

FINDINGS

The study population

Table 7.3 (page 156) shows the age range and type of delivery of the postnatal women and the age range and type of operation of the four groups of postoperative patients. The majority of the postnatal women had a normal delivery (30/42). Hysterectomy was the commonest operation among the female major surgical group (11/28). Overall the operations undergone by the surgical patients encompassed a very wide range of conditions.

Incidence of the blues

Table 7.4 (page 157) shows the number of respondents in each group experiencing the blues (i.e. a score of 8 or more on the SDSS). The figures indicate that postoperative women are as likely to experience the blues as postnatal women. Although the number of postoperative men in the sample is small, the figures provide an indication that dysphoria may also occur in this group.

Timing of the blues. There appears to be important differences between the postpartum and postoperative groups in the timing of the blues; this is shown in Figure 7.2. Postpartum dysphoria peaked on days 3 and 4, whereas postoperative dysphoria tended to be worse immediately after the operation and progressively diminished. This finding is consistent with those of Pitt (1973), Stein (1980) and more recently Kendell *et al.* (1984).

Table 7.3 Study groups: age and type of delivery/operation

Maternity (*n* = 42)	Examination under
Age: mean 27, range 18 to 40,	anaesthetic 2
SD6	Change intrauterine
Modes of delivery:	contraceptive device 1
Normal 30	Lengthening ERCB 1
Instrumental 7	Menisectomy 2
Caesarean section 5	Internal fixation of elbow 1
—	Fixing fractured finger 1
Surgical operations:	Excision bursa 1
Female surgical major (*n* = 28)	
Age: mean 39, range 17 to 50,	**Male surgical major (*n* = 16)**
SD10	**Age: mean 29, range 19 to 43,**
Hysterectomy, ovaries	**SD9**
conserved 8	Appendicectomy 3
Hysterectomy and	Hemicolectomy 1
oopherectomy 3	Evacuation haematoma after
Pelvic floor repair 1	amputation leg 1
Appendicectomy 2	Tendon graft finger 1
Fixing fractured condyle of	Replacement tibial screws 1
humerus 1	Repair shoulder dislocation 1
Femoral varus osteotomy 1	Bone graft tibia 1
Lumbar discectomy 2	Removal patella wires 1
Lumbar sacral fusion 1	Laminectomy 1
Menisectomy and arthroscopy 1	Internal fixation tibia and
Exploration septic arthritis of	fibula 2
knee 1	Removal Richard's screw 1
Removal of hip plate 1	Lumbar sacral fusion 1
Removal cervical rib 2	Insertion nail into femur 1
Bilateral Kellars operation 1	**Male surgical minor (*n* = 9)**
Pinning femur 1	**Age: mean 28, range 17 to 43,**
Total hip replacement 1	**SD9**
Arthrodesis of foot 1	Abscess gluteal cleft 1
Female surgical minor (*n* = 22)	Arthroscopy 2
Age: mean 35, range 16 to 45,	Removal elbow wires 1
SD10	Removal elbow nodules 2
Evacuation retained products 4	Internal fixing fractured
Dilation and curettage 6	malleolus 1
Tubal ligation 2	Drainage axillary abscess 1
Laparoscopy 1	Excision pilonidal sinus 1

Source: compiled by the author.

Table 7.4 Incidence of 'blues' in each study group

Group	Number experiencing blues	
	No.	*%*
Maternity ($n = 42$)	25	60
Female surgical major ($n = 28$)	19	68
Female surgical minor ($n = 22$)	13	59
Male surgical major ($n = 16$)	5	31
Male surgical minor ($n = 9$)	0	0

Source: compiled by the author.

Figure 7.2 Timing of the blues.

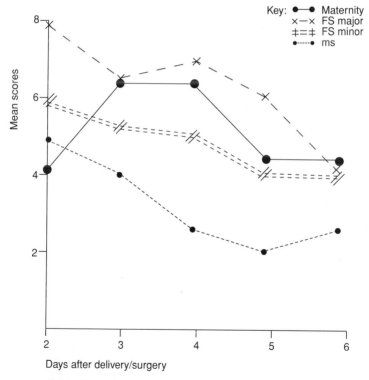

Source: compiled by the author.

Kendell *et al.* found that mood changes after caesarean section peaked on the fifth day in a similar fashion to those following vaginal delivery, but found no peaking following hysterectomy: instead, hysterectomy mood change ratings fell progressively from day 2 onwards.

Manifestations of the blues

Three main points emerge from Figure 7.3 which shows the pattern of scores for each symptom in the study groups over the two to six day period.

First the postnatal group scores show that crying, depression, loss of appetite, irritability and dreaming peak at the fourth day, with anxiety, tension, headache, loss of concentration, restlessnes, insomnia, tiredness and confusion peaking at the third or second day. Secondly, the scores for the groups of postoperative patients also peak, although the pattern is often different to that for the postnatal women. Thirdly, for most of the symptoms, the female patients (particularly those who had major surgery) recorded higher scores than male patients.

Correlation of individual symptoms with crying

Table 7.5 (page 164) shows the correlation of individual symptoms with crying for each of the study groups. In the postnatal group the symptom scores correlating most significantly with the crying scores were found to be depression, tension, anxiety, restlessness, lack of concentration, confusion and tiredness. In the female major surgical group the symptom scores correlating most significantly with the crying scores were found to be depression, tension, anxiety, lack of concentration, tiredness, anorexia, forgetfulness and insomnia. In the female minor surgical group, the symptom scores correlating most significantly with the crying scores were tension and depression. None of the men undergoing minor surgery said that he had cried, and so the symptom scores were correlated with the crying scores in only the major surgical group. In the male major surgical group the only symptom score correlating significantly with the crying scores was depression.

Comments made by participants who had experienced the blues

The comments made by participants whose SDSS scores indicated that they had experienced the blues fell into eight main categories. All of the comments made in each of these categories are included and are quoted almost verbatim. The respondent's group and number of days following delivery or operation is noted after each quote.

Ann Cyzewski

1. Often no convincing reason could be given for crying:

No particular reason. I felt it building up all day. I cried all day and all night. (Maternity, day 3)

I couldn't understand why I was crying; I'm not a tearful sort of person. There was no reason for my tears. (FS Major, day 3)

There was no particular reason for my tears. (FS Major, day 4)

No reason. Crying didn't worry me – I've had it before after operations. (FS Major, day 4)

I cried for no special reason, I just felt fed up and wanted to be mobile. The next day I cried before lunch, just feeling sorry for myself. (FS Major, day 5)

Figure 7.3 Patterns of symptoms in different groups of patients: (a) depression; (b) anxiety; (c) crying; (d) tension; (e) anorexia; (f) headache; (g) irritability; (h) concentration; (i) restlessness; (j) insomnia; (k) tiredness; (l) dreaming; (m) forgetfulness; (n) confusion.

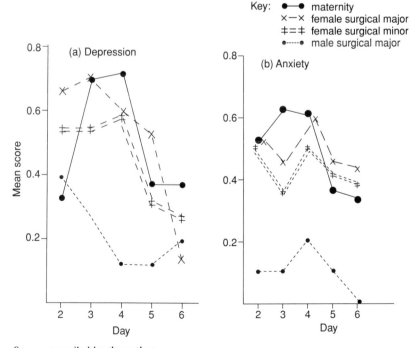

Source: compiled by the author.

Figure 7.3 *Continued*

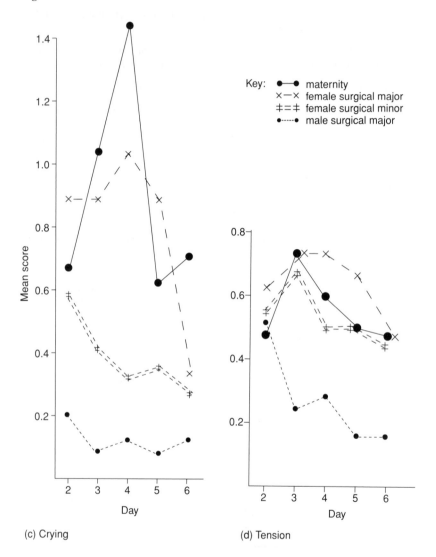

Key:
●—● maternity
×—× female surgical major
‡=‡ female surgical minor
•····• male surgical major

(c) Crying

(d) Tension

Figure 7.3 *Continued*

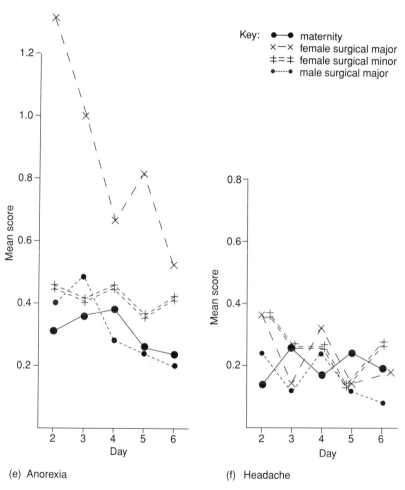

(e) Anorexia   (f) Headache

Source: compiled by the author.

Figure 7.3 *Continued*

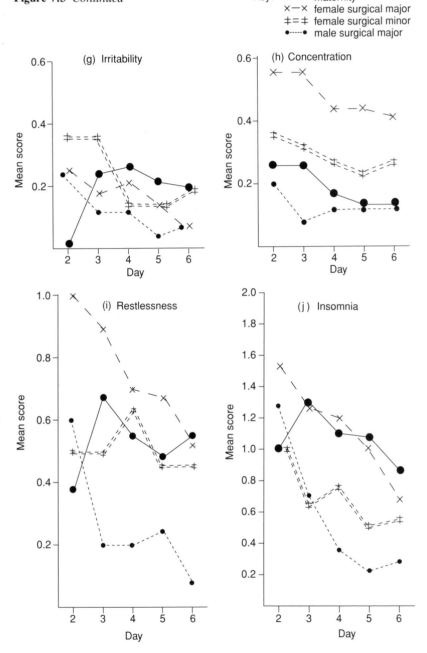

Figure 7.3 *Continued*

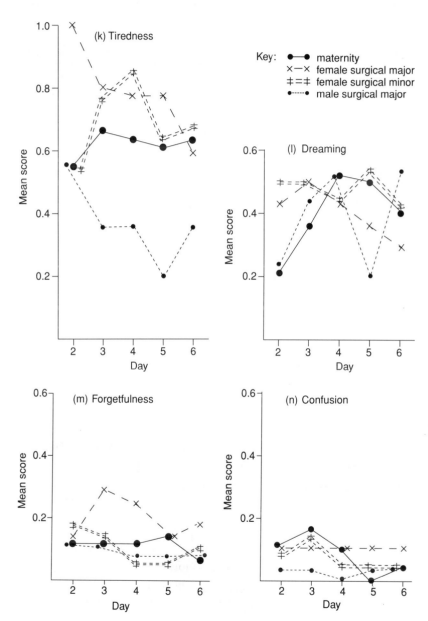

Source: compiled by the author.

Table 7.5 Correlation of individual symptoms, with crying in the study groups

	Pearsons correlations			
Symptom	Postnatal	FS major	FS minor	MS major
Depression	0.713[a]	0.626[a]	0.555[b]	0.650[b]
Tension	0.645[a]	0.591[a]	0.610[b]	0.010NS
Anxiety	0.583[a]	0.591[a]	0.466[c]	0.467[c]
Lack concentration	0.431[b]	0.566[b]	−0.091NS	−0.106NS
Restlessness	0.423[b]	0.433[a]	0.220NS	0.236NS
Confusion	0.397[b]	0.446[a]	0.385[c]	−0.176NS
Tiredness	0.394[b]	0.566[b]	0.206NS	0.106NS
Irritability	0.390[c]	0.205NS	0.150NS	0.328NS
Anorexia	0.331[c]	0.580[b]	0.390[c]	0.131NS
Forgetfulness	0.318[c]	0.586[b]	0.500[c]	−0.134NS
Insomnia	0.260[c]	0.504[b]	0.048NS	0.424[c]
Headache	0.059NS	0.343[c]	−0.042NS	0.285NS
Dreaming[d]	0.017NS	0.072NS	0.234NS	0.199NS

[a] <0.0006;
[b] <0.005;
[c] <0.05;
NS Not significant.
[d] The night **before** the crying.
Source: complied by the author.

2. On other occasions respondents mentioned physical causes that may have precipitated their tears:

> Everything was building up – my stitches were sore, I hadn't had my bowels open, my breasts were sore and my milk was going straight through the baby. Also I have thrombophlebitis. (Maternity, day 3)

> I was feeling tearful anyway first thing in the morning, and then I had to wait all day to be got out of bed. I had a corset put on early, and it was very uncomfortable. (FS Major, day 4)

> Just generally fed up and depressed. I'll probably have to go for another operation and I'm worried about that too. (MS Major, day 3)

The catheter not coming out was the last straw. My father has just been admitted to hospital and I'm worried about him. (FS Major, day 3)

3. Some cried because they felt tired:

It hits you at night – I couldn't cope, too tired. I can cope with one thing, but not all this and the baby too. The nurses (*sic*) took the baby into the nursery – wonderful, made all the difference. (Maternity, day 3)

I was tired, it's difficult to sleep in hospital. (Maternity, day 3)

I had 12 visitors in the afternoon – I couldn't cope with that. They kept picking up the baby and upsetting her. (Maternity, day 3)

I felt tearful, cold, shaking. I just wanted to sleep, I didn't want anyone with me. There was nothing anyone could have done. (Maternity, day 4)

I was transferred to a convalescent hospital later on, the transfer arrangements were awful, and I was very upset and tearful by the time I arrived. I was also exhausted by the long, uncomfortable journey. I was still crying the next day. (FS Major, day 5)

4. Others cried at visiting times, or because they missed their families and were homesick:

I was thinking of my other child. A magazine article reminded me. (Maternity, day 1)

I don't think I would have cried if my husband hadn't been there. (Maternity, day 4)

I was missing my husband, I cried when he visited. I just wanted my husband to talk to, this helped a lot. (Maternity, day 3)

I had a sleepless night, and cried when my daughter came. I missed my family. (Maternity, day 4)

I cried at visiting time – no particular reasons. (FS Major, day 2) (The same comment was made by another surgical patient on her sixth day.)

A comment made by a man who took part in the pilot study is worthy of inclusion here.

I just burst into tears when my wife and family visited – I was so embarrassed. My wife was upset and my son and his wife had to go and wait in the waiting room. I've never done such a thing before, we couldn't figure out what was going on or why I should be crying. (Prostatectomy, day 4)

5. Some women cried because of pleasant events:

The nice things people were saying to me in letters and when they visited made me cry. (FS Major, day 2)

I cried at a telegram from my husband overseas with the Navy. (Maternity, day 3)

No particular reason. When the priest offered me communion it made me cry. (FS Major, day 3)

6. Some women in the maternity group cried because they were worried about their babies:

I had to leave the baby behind in SCBU. I was surprised to cry – I thought the tears happened on the third day. (day 5)

My baby is on SCBU, and has a feeding problem. (day 4)

I didn't think the baby was getting enough milk. I was upset by different advice. (day 3)

Three women cried because (they said) their babies were jaundiced and had to have phototherapy (days 4, 5, 6).

7. None of the respondents felt the midwives or nurses could have helped them during their distress:

I didn't want anyone – nurses (*sic*) or family. I told the nurses to go away, I felt stupid. They tried to help but I didn't want anyone. (Maternity, day 4)

I didn't want anyone, just wanted to be left in peace. (Maternity, day 3)

I wanted my husband with me, but there wasn't anything anyone could do to help me. (Maternity, day 3)

I didn't want anyone with me, but it might have been different if I had known the nurses (*sic*) on duty. (Maternity, day 3)

I didn't want anyone with me. (FS Major, day 3)

I was better by myself, no-one could have helped. (FS Major, day 2) (The same comment was made by another surgical patient on day 2.)

I preferred to be on my own. I phoned my sister – a familiar voice helped. (FS Major, day 4)

I wanted to be on my own. Then my mum visited and I cried again, but I was glad my mum was there. (FS Major, day 5)

I just wanted to be left alone. (FS Major, day 4)

Another surgical patient made the same comment.

I felt tearful first thing in the morning but wanted to be by myself. (FS Major, day 5)

8. Two women experienced violent dreams which upset them:

I felt numb. I woke up during the night, crying, after weird dreams. In the dream, my home turned into a field, someone stole my baby's clothes and I told my husband to go off with another woman. (Maternity, day 3)

Last night I had violent dreams; someone put a bomb under my skirt, and I was blown up into the sky. I was bombing everyone in sight. (Maternity, day 4)

One woman who had had a ruptured tubal pregnancy had also experienced a particularly vivid nightmare a few days after the event. Unfortunately she failed to complete the questionnaires properly and so was not included in the study, but her dream is described here:

I had a terrible nightmare, I walked into a room and there was a row of dolls there, they suddenly came to life and screamed 'kill her, kill her'. (day 4)

DISCUSSION

This study has shown that the dysphoria called the maternity blues, which is so commonly associated with the puerperium, is not unique to this situation. A similar type of dysphoria appears to occur postoperatively in women and to a lesser extent in men. There was no significant difference in the symptom pattern between postpartum and postoperative women; indeed, after major surgery there was slightly more dysphoria than after childbirth (Table 7.4, page 157). The manifestations of the dysphoria are also similar, particularly between the female groups, as evidenced by the correlations between crying and other symptom scores (Table 7.5, page 164).

The only important difference between postpartum dysphoria and postoperative dysphoria appears to be in the timing (Figure 7.2, page 157). In this study it was found that postpartum dysphoria showed peaking on days 3 and 4, whereas postoperative dysphoria tended to be worse immediately after the operation and progressively diminished. As noted earlier this finding is consistent with those of Pitt (1973), Stein (1980) and more recently Kendell *et al.* (1984).

However, looking at individual symptoms in patients undergoing a wider spectrum of surgical operations, this present study shows that several symptoms peak in a similar way to the postpartum group (Figure 7.3, pages 159–63) and, furthermore, many postoperative patients indicated by their comments that their dysphoria occurred suddenly and unexpectedly at or around the third or fourth postoperative day. Many of the symptoms correlating significantly with crying in the postpartum group show similar peaking or non-peaking patterns throughout the groups (Figure 7.3). In his study of 37 postpartum patients, Stein (1980) found the peaking symptoms to be depression, crying, irritability, restlessness, dreaming and headache, whereas exhaustion, poor concentration and anorexia started at a relatively high level and declined throughout the rest of the week. This present study has identified symptom patterns similar in many respects to those described by Stein.

Some symptom patterns may perhaps be partially explained by the general physical discomfort experienced in the early postoperative days, particularly following major surgery, or alternatively by ward procedures. For example, postoperative insomnia scores start at a high level and then decline throughout the rest of the week, whereas postpartum insomnia scores peak on the third day (Figure 7.3). This possibly reflects the local policy of 'rooming in' the woman with her baby from the second or third night onwards, thus making it more difficult for her to obtain a good night's sleep.

Of interest are the differences between men and women regarding postoperative mood changes. The differences seem to be those of degree; mood changes appear to occur in men in a similar fashion to those in the female groups, but at a reduced level (Figure 7.3). This may represent a genuinely lower level of mood changes in men after operations, or it may indicate a greater reluctance in men to admit to such depressive feelings. Blumenthal (1975), measuring depressive symptomology in the general population, gave a point prevalence (as measured by the Zung scale – a 20-item scale measuring symptoms of depressive illness (Zung, 1965)) – of 32 per 100 for women and 12 per 100 for men. She points out that this could be due to differences in feelings of depression, or else differences in response styles between men and women.

It has long been known that both the postpartum and postoperative periods are times at which the risk of a major psychosis are increased (Stengel *et al.*, 1958). During both of these times women were found to be more at risk than men. This finding may have some relevance to the observation in this present study that postoperative dysphoria is more common in women than in men.

The comments elicited from respondents who had experienced the blues are remarkably similar throughout the groups. Often, no convincing reason could be given for the dysphoria; several women had been taken by surprise by their tears. Some women could partially, but not completely, explain the reason for their distress. Perceived setbacks in recovery, or problems with their babies, triggered the tears that were not far off anyway. Happy events could have the same effect; this accords with findings (Yalom *et al.*, 1968) that puerperal women cried for numerous reasons other than sadness. Other women felt they could fully explain the reasons for their tears. Several respondents said they cried because they were tired. It has long been recognized that wards are often noisy at night, and patients who desperately need to sleep are unable to do so. Laryea (1984a) points out that women may find it difficult to sleep in a postnatal ward with several other occupants. (When else in his or her adult life would an individual consent to sleep in a room with several strangers?) Ball (1987) advocates a flexible approach to 'rooming in' policies and recommends that babies should be removed to the nursery when necessary to allow the woman a good night's sleep.

Hospital wards are usually busy areas; surgical and postnatal wards do not always provide the tranquillity desired by many postoperative patients and postnatal women. Laryea (1984b) comments that, because of their fast pace, it is difficult to achieve the relaxed atmosphere that should prevail in postnatal wards. Instead of allowing the woman to concentrate exclusively upon her baby and herself, in many cases we (both as professionals and members of the public) impose upon her various intrusions and concerns. For example, unrestricted visiting was a cause of considerable stress to one postnatal woman in this study. Many maternity units have adapted rooms in delivery suites to facilitate a more 'homely' atmosphere; perhaps consideration needs to be given in the design of postnatal wards to provide surroundings more conducive to the tranquility and privacy desired by many newly delivered women.

The embarrassment felt by patients experiencing the blues may have been reduced if they had been warned beforehand. The importance of giving relevant information to preoperative patients is well documented; for example, Hayward (1975) found that giving relevant preoperative information reduced postoperative pain, and Boore (1978) found that preoperative teaching of surgical patients reduced postoperative stress. Prior knowledge of the condition may be helpful in assisting patients to accept the dysphoria for what it is – a temporary distrubance of mood that is not likely to last for long.

Several respondents said they preferred to be alone during their distress; none had wanted nurses or midwives with them (but one respondent commented that it might have been different had she known the staff on duty). Some would have liked close members of their family with them; indeed, the arrival of such people often coincided with the onset of crying. This may be alarming to 'visitors', who may arrive to floods of tears from their relatives and it would seem reasonable to warn them of the possibility of postnatal or postoperative dysphoria. Newly delivered women and their families are often aware that the blues may occur a few days after childbirth, but postoperative dysphoria is not so well recognized and may cause considerable distress to the relatives as well as the patient. It may be helpful, therefore, to warn patients undergoing surgery and their relatives, of the possibility of postoperative dysphoria.

Several women reported violent dreams. Gentil and Lader (1978) found that anxious patients tend to experience terrifying dreams; the dreams reported in this present study may indeed be an indication of intense anxiety but this would require further study. In the meantime, anxious patients should be forewarned of the possibility of frightening, upsetting dreams a few nights after delivery or surgery, and night staff aware that newly delivered women or postoperative patients may experience nightmares.

To summarize, respondents in the postpartum and major surgical groups made very similar comments regarding the blues, which further suggests that a condition very similar to the maternity blues is also experienced following surgery. During these periods the crying threshold appears to be lower than usual; often, no reason can be given to account for the tears but frequently a precipitating factor can be identified which may be rectifiable, such as tiredness or discomfort.

The cause of the blues remains uncertain, despite extensive biochemical investigation. An underlying assumption of these investigations is that the blues is a condition peculiar to the early puerperium, and that biochemical changes occurring after childbirth are therefore likely to be responsible. If the blues is not unique to the puerperium, however, it is unlikely that the large drop in sex hormones is responsible. Indeed, Nott et al. (1976) showed no difference between blues and non-blues cases regarding their levels of sex hormones. If biochemical changes are responsible for this dysphoria, then these changes should be present both postoperatively and postpartum.

Cortisol is known to rise in pregnancy and postoperatively and has been implicated in mood changes. Starkman et al. (1981) found that a blues-like syndrome frequently occurs in patients with Cushing's disease. If postoperative dysphoria is precipitated by an increased output of cortisol then it could be expected that major surgery, which causes greater adrenal stress, would result in a higher incidence of dysphoria than minor surgery, and this has been found to be the case in this study.

Endorphins have also been implicated in mood changes (Koob and Bloom, 1983). Beta-endorphin levels increase during periods of stress, such as surgery (Cohen et al., 1981; Mirrales et al., 1983) and during pregnancy and labour (Thomas et al., 1982). However, Newnham et al. (1984) found no correlation between the postpartum blues and beta-endorphin levels at delivery or 24 hours after delivery, or with the rate of fall of beta-endorphin levels in the 24 hours after delivery. Whatever the precise cause of the postpartum and postoperative blues, it is possible that the dysphoria is a reaction to a period of acute stress. Similar periods of dysphoria have been noted following other stressful events; Yalom *et al.* (1968) mention the similarity of the postpartum blues to the 'end phenomenon' – a dysphoric reaction noted after periods of intense paratroop training (Basowitz *et al.*, 1955), and Brudel (1984) found that men present at their wives' deliveries often developed a blues-like reaction in the early postnatal period.

CONCLUSION

This was an exploratory study, and no attempt was made to control several important variables such as the type of operation, delivery, medication, or the length of stay in hospital, all of which would have been likely to have affected the findings to some extent. Furthermore, the study is small and no firm conclusions may be reached regarding patterns of dysphoria (particularly in men) following surgery; a more extensive study is needed that also takes into account the variables mentioned above. Nevertheless, the results of this study have shown that the transient dysphoria commonly seen in the early puerperium, and known as the postpartum, maternity, or third day blues, is also experienced by women and to some extent, men a few days after surgery. Therefore in the search for the cause of the maternity blues, it may be helpful to study the same parameters in postoperative dysphoria. As indicated in the discussion section of this chapter, there is much however that midwives can do to alleviate the distress that may be caused by the postpartum blues.

If I were to repeat this study, besides controlling factors mentioned in the discussion (such as the type of delivery or surgery), I would place more emphasis upon the interviews with respondents regarding their dysphoria, particularly those who had experienced intense dysphoria. The time I was able to allocate to these interviews was constrained by the needs of my 'real' work as a tutor; it is difficult and frustrating to carry out an interview in any depth when one knows one is expected in the classroom in 15 minutes and the respondent is going home later that morning . . . I am sure I missed a wealth of information that would have contributed enormously to the richness of the data. In a future study, given no constraints of time or money, I would follow up a sample of respondents by visiting them at home. Home interviews feature prominently in subsequent research that I have undertaken, and revealed a much more satisfactory depth of detail.

Research – where does one stop? One study leads to another; unexpected findings appear which beg further enquiry. One such phenomenon from the blues study was the number of puerperal women whose dysphoria, instead of peaking round about the third day, persisted throughout the week. Could this be predictive of postnatal depression? I have recently completed a study to suggest factors predictive of postnatal depression that may be identifiable by midwives. This second study has been funded by the Iolanthe Trust and the Cornwall and Isles of Scilly Health Authority and is supervised by Exeter University and Cornwall College.

ACKNOWLEDGEMENTS

In setting up this study one of my main problems had lain in finding expert advice within reasonable travelling distance. Good sources of advice were available, however, it was just a question of asking around. Eventually I found my way to the Principal of Cornwall College of Further and Higher Education, Mr L. Piper. My special thanks are due to him, not only for his good advice but also for his interest and enthusiasm which gave me much needed encouragement. Research is often a lonely occupation and it is easy to become dispirited and out of touch. It is wonderful how a few words of encouragement, or interest, can stimulate flagging enthusiasm and restore reality. Dr Nigel Powell provided help and advice with statistics; for which I am very grateful. My thanks to Dr G. Stein, Consultant Psychiatrist, who developed the SDSS and gave me much good advice. My thanks also to Dr S. Bhanji, Consultant Psychiatrist, Mrs S. Bose, Senior Midwifery Tutor, Mrs P. Kitch, Librarian, the nursing and midwifery staff at Treliske, City and Redruth Hospitals, and the postnatal women and postoperative patients who took part in the study.

REFERENCES

Ball, J.A. (1987) *Reactions to motherhood: the role of postnatal care.* Cambridge University Press, Cambridge.

Basowitz, H., Persky, H., Korchin, H. and Grinker, R. (1955) *Anxiety and stress.* McGraw-Hill, New York.

Blumenthal, M.D. (1975) Measuring depressive symptomology in a general population. *Archives of General Psychiatry*, 32, Aug, 971–8.

Boore, J. (1978) *Prescription for recovery.* Royal College of Nursing, London.

Bourne, G. (1975) *Pregnancy.* Pan Books, London.

Brudel, L.F. (1984) Paternity blues and the father-child relationship. In J.D. Call, E. Galenson and R.L. Tyson (eds) *Frontiers of infant psychology*, Vol. 2. Basic Books, New York.

Cobb, S. and McDermott, N.T. (1938) *Medical Clinics of North America*, 22, 569–76.

Cohen, M., Pickar, D., Dubois, M., Roth, Y., Naber, D. and Bunney, W. (1981) Surgical stress and endorphins (letter). *Lancet*, 1, 213–14.

Cox, J.L., Connor, Y. and Kendell, R.E. (1982) Prospective study of the psychiatric disorders of childbirth. *British Journal of Psychiatry*, **140**, 111–17.

Davidson, J. (1972) Postpartum mood changes in Jamaican women. *British Journal of Psychiatry*, **121**, 659–63.

Gentil, M. and Lader, M. (1978) Dream content and daytime attitudes in anxious and calm women. *Psychological Medicine*, **8**(2), 297–304.

Goldberg, D.P. (1972) *The detection of psychiatric illness by questionnaire.* Oxford University Press, London.

Harris, B. (1981) Maternity blues in East African clinic attenders. *Archives of General Psychiatry*, **38**, 1293–5.

Hayward, J. (1975) *Information – a prescription against pain.* Royal College of Nursing, London.

Kane, F., Harman W., Keeler, M. and Ewing, J. (1968) *British Journal of Psychiatry*, **114**, 99–102.

Kendell, R.E., McGuire, R.J., Connor, Y. and Cox, J.L. (1981) Mood changes in the first 3 weeks after childbirth. *Journal of Affective Disorders*, **3**, 317–26.

Kendell, R.E., Mackenzie, W.E., West, C., McGuire, R.J. and Cox, J.L. (1984) Day to day mood changes after childbirth – further data. *British Journal of Psychiatry*, **145**, 620–25.

Koob, G.F. and Bloom, F.E. (1983) Behavioural effects of opioid peptides. *British Medical Bulletin*, **39**, 89–94.

Kraupl-Taylor, F. (1980) The concepts of disease. *Psychological Medicine*, **10**, 419–24.

Laryea, M.G. (1984a) *Postnatal care – the midwife's role.* Churchill Livingstone, Edinburgh.

Laryea, M.G. (1984b) Postnatal Care – the Midwife's Role. Churchill Livingstone, Edinburgh.

Lesh, A. (1978) Postpartum depression. *Current Practice in Obstetric and Gynecological Nursing*, **2**, 52–64.

Lindemann, E. (1941) Observations of psychiatric sequelae to surgical operations in women. *American Journal of Psychiatry*, **98**, 132–9.

Mirrales, F., Olaso, M., Fuentes, T., Lopez, F., Laorden, M. and Puig, M. (1983) Presurgical stress and plasma endorphin levels. *Anaesthiology*, **59**, 367–8.

Morsbach, G., Sawaragi, I., Riddell, C. and Carswell, A. (1983) The occurrence of maternity blues in Scottish and Japanese mothers. *Journal of Reproductive and Infant Psychology*, **1**, 29–35.

Newnham, J.P., Dennett, P.M., Ferron, S.A., Tomlon, S., Legg, C., Bourne, G.L. and Rees L.H. (1984) A study of the relationship between circulating β-endorphin-like immunoreactivity and postpartum blues. *Clinical Endocrinology*, **20**, 169–77.

Nott, P., Franklin, M., Armitage, C. and Gelder, M. (1976) Hormonal changes and mood in the puerperium. *British Journal of Psychiatry*, **128**, 379–83.

Oakley, A. and Chamberlain, G. (1981) Medical and social factors in postpartum depression. *Journal of Obstetrics and Gynaecology*, **1**, 182–7.

Paykel, E., Emms, E., Fletcher, J. and Rassaly, E. (1980) Life events and social support in puerperal depression. *British Journal of Psychiatry*, **136**, 339–46.

Pitt, B. (1973) Maternity blues. *British Journal of Psychiatry*, **122**, 431–3.

Raphael, B. (1974) Parameters of health outcome following hysterectomy. *Bulletin of the Post Graduate Committee in Medicine, Sydney*. Dec, 214–19.

Robin, A. (1962) Psychological changes of normal parturition. *Psychiatric Quarterly*, **36**, 129–50.

Scadding, G.H. (1967) Diagnosis, the clinician and the computer. *Lancet*, **2**, 877–82.

Sheehan, F. (1981) Assessing postpartum adjustment. *Journal of Obstetric, Gynecological and Neonatal Nursing*, **10**(1), 19–32.

Starkman, M.N., Schteingart, D.E. and Schork, M. (1981) Depressed mood and other psychiatric manifestations of Cushing's syndrome: relationship to hormone levels. *Psychosomatic Medicine*, **3**(1), 3–18.

Stein, G. (1980) The pattern of mental change and body weight change in the first postpartum week. *Journal of Psychosomatic Research*, **24**(3–4), 165–71.

Stein, G. (1982) The maternity blues. In I. Brockington and R. Kumar (eds) *Motherhood and mental illness*. Academic Press, London.

Stengel, E., Zeitlyn, B.B. and Rayner, E.H. (1958) Postoperative psychosis. *Journal of Mental Science*, **104**, 389–402.

Thomas, T.A., Fletcher, J.E. and Hill, R.G. (1982) Influence of medication, pain and progress in labour on plasma beta-endorphin-like immuno-reactivity. *British Journal of Anaesthesia*, **54**, 401.

Yalom, I., Lunde, D., Moos, R. and Hamburg, D. (1968) Postpartum blues syndrome. *Archives of General Psychiatry*, **18**, 16–27.

Zung, W. (1965) A self-rating depression scale. *Archives of General Psychiatry*, **12**, 63–70.

CHAPTER EIGHT

Retention in midwifery: findings from a longitudinal study of midwives' careers

Sarah Robinson and Heather Owen

A longitudinal study documenting the careers of midwives has been in progress at the Nursing Research Unit of Kings College, London University, for more than a decade. Two large cohorts of midwives have been followed up at regular intervals since they qualified; one group in 1979, the other in 1983. The study had two main aims: first, to ascertain whether extending post-registration midwifery education from 12 to 18 months was accompanied by an increase in the proportion of newly qualified midwives who felt adequately prepared to practise as a midwife, in the proportion who intended to do so, and the extent to which these intentions were subsequently translated into practice; second, to obtain information on various aspects of life as a midwife, particularly those that may be relevant to retention. Three phases of data collection have been completed to date: Phase 1 at the time that each cohort qualified; Phase 2 in 1986 and 1987 and Phase 3 in 1989. Further phases of data collection are planned.

The research is of importance for three reasons. **First**, it provided an answer to the questions posed above concerning the effect of lengthening the post-registration midwifery course. **Second**, it has produced findings on a wide range of midwives' experiences after qualifying that are relevant to an understanding of careers in the midwifery profession whatever the educational route to registration. **Third**, it demonstrates the value of longitudinal as opposed to cross-sectional designs in gaining an understanding of the development of careers over time.

A substantial volume of findings have been generated in the course of the project and have been made available in a number of reports and papers (Golden, 1980; Robinson, 1986a, 1986b, 1986c; Robinson and Owen, 1989; Owen and Robinson, 1990, 1992; Robinson *et al.*, 1992; Robinson, 1993). This chapter presents some of the findings for each of the project's two main aims. The first section looks at issues that the study has explored concerning the education and subsequent careers of midwives.

The rationale for using a longitudinal design and the methods employed at each of the three phases are described, and this is followed by presentation and discussion of a seclection of findings. At the time that Phase 1 for the 1979 cohort was undertaken, the term 'midwifery training' was used rather than 'midwifery education'. This was reflected in the wording of the questionnaires developed at the time and so is retained in the presentation and discussion of findings in this chapter.

BACKGROUND TO THE STUDY

The background to the study was longstanding concern about attrition from the midwifery profession. This concern had two main foci: first, the relationship to retention of different educational routes to registration as a midwife; second, the extent to which subsequent attrition was related to dissatisfaction with various aspects of life as a midwife. In order to examine these issues, the study took the form shown in Figure 8.1.

In Phase 1 views held about the adequacy of training and career intentions expressed at qualification by a cohort of midwives who had taken an 18 month course were compared with the views and intentions expressed by a cohort who had taken a 12 month course. In Phases 2 and 3 information was obtained from members of both cohorts about the careers they had subsequently followed, together with their experiences and views of many aspects of life as a midwife, particularly those identified as relevant to retention. This section provides a brief background to the main issues researched in the project to date.

Figure 8.1 Structure of Midwives' Career Patterns Project

Phase 1 (a) 1979: Questionnaires sent to midwives qualifying after a 12 month course
      (b) 1983: Questionnaires sent to midwives qualifying after an 18 month course

Phase 2 (a) 1986: Questionnaires sent to all members of both cohorts
      (b) 1987: Questionnaires sent to all those who responded in 1986 and who had practised midwifery

Phase 3 1989: Questionnaires sent to all phase 2(a) respondents

---

Source: compiled by the author.

Educational routes to registration

In relation to attrition two main issues emerge from the history of training courses leading to registration as a midwife:

- first, the extent to which nurses have taken midwifery training in order to enhance a nursing career rather than to practise as a midwife;
- second, whether those who wish to qualify as midwives should first qualify as nurses.

The history of these two interrelated issues, from the start of this century onwards, has been the subject of a number of extensive reviews. Attempts to reduce the numbers of nurses taking post-registration midwifery training for reasons other than wishing to practise as a midwife, have been reviewed by Bent (1982), Robinson (1986a, 1991) and by Mander (1989). The history of midwifery courses for non-nurses and the arguments advocated both for and against their desirability, have been reviewed by Radford and Thompson (1988 and Chapter 10 in this volume). As these references are widely available, a review of the history of first level midwifery education is not included here, but the main points are outlined in order to provide a context for the design and findings of this study.

The problem of nurses taking midwifery training but not intending to practise midwifery has been in evidence ever since the examination and registration procedures for midwives were established in the early years of this century. This situation would not necessarily be problematic, apart from the waste of training facilities entailed, if sufficient midwives remained to staff the service adequately. Since the Second World War, however, the professional and statutory bodies for midwifery have maintained that there are insufficient midwives in post (e.g. Central Midwives Board, 1957; Ministry of Health, 1959; Royal College of Midwives, 1964; Central Midwives Board, 1983).

Although changes made in the length and structure of training since 1902 have been concerned primarily with developments in maternity care, they have also been aimed at deterring nurses from qualifying for a profession in which they do not intend to practise. The training was initially of three months duration for both nurses and non-nurses; it was extended to four months for nurses and six months for non-nurses in 1916 and to six months and one year respectively in 1926. However, lengthening the training did not deter nurses from training for reasons other than wishing to practise midwifery, in fact they represented an ever increasing proportion of those qualifying. Another attempt at resolving the problem was made in 1938 when the training was divided into two periods, the first being spent in hospital and the second mainly in the community. It was hoped that Part 1 would be regarded as sufficient for nursing posts that required a midwifery qualification and for entry into health visitor training; however, this division of training not only failed to reduce the numbers who took both parts and then did not practise, but also led to dissatisfaction with the training itself. The loss of midwives after training continued after the Second World War but, as noted, was also accompanied by a shortage of midwives that has persisted until the present time. Findings from two post-war studies that examined attrition showed that a substantial proportion of those qualifying as midwives did not practise midwifery or did so for a short time only (Ministry of Health *et al.*, 1949; Ramsden and Radwanski, 1963).

Against this background of continuing attrition from the profession and concern about staffing levels, the extent to which student midwives felt sufficiently confident to practise was accorded considerable importance during the 1970s. In 1968 the two-part training was finally replaced by the single period course, but in subsequent years, staff at midwifery training schools maintained that 12 months was insufficient time to cover the syllabus adequately and in particular to develop confidence in clinical skills (Central Midwives Board, 1977). The Board consequently decided to extend training to 18 months for State Registered Nurses and to three years for those without nursing qualifications; the new course was introduced in September 1981. As Stewart (1981) commented, it was hoped that the extension of time would be 'used to develop clinical skills and to give opportunities for the midwife to become confident and wish to practise as a midwife'. The newly qualified midwife's confidence in her clinical competence was regarded as an essential factor in subsequent decisions as whether to practise midwifery. We took the view, however, that if any conclusions were to be drawn as to whether the extended training did have the desired effect on midwives' confidence and career intentions, then data on these issues had first to be obtained from midwives who had taken a 12 month course, in order that a comparison could subsequently be made. This was the aim of Phase 1 of the project.

Turning now to the issue of non-nurse midwifery education, then the proportion of midwives in training and in practice who are not qualified nurses has shown a steady decline, particularly since the Second World War (see Chapter 10 in this volume). Some of the committees that investigated the maternity services in general and/or the midwifery services in particular did not address this question at all (e.g. Ministry of Health, 1959). Others counselled against direct entry, either because they took the view that nursing was an essential pre-requisite for midwifery (e.g. Ministry of Health, 1929; Royal College of Obstetricians and Gynaecologists, 1944) or promotion prospects for direct entrants were so poor that it was unfair to encourage this portal of entry to the profession (Ministry of Health *et al.*, 1949). More recent committees recommended a common foundation training followed by specialization in midwifery or in the various branches of nursing (Department of Health and Social Security, 1972; United Kingdom Central Council, 1986). Renewed interest in non-nurse midwifery education was expressed in the late 1970s and 1980s among the profession itself. This had a threefold impetus: the need for midwives who could meet the growing demand of women for less medically dominated childbirth, namely, midwives who could practise with autonomy and who had not first been socialized into a nursing role; the associated recognition that midwifery is a separate profession from nursing and as such required separate educational programmes; and a range of workforce considerations (these points are amplified in Chapter 10 of this volume).

Aspects of life as a midwife

The relationship to retention of extending post-registration midwifery training from 12 to 18 months provided the original impetus for the project. From the outset, however, it was recognized that a range of aspects of life as a midwife might have a bearing on retention, irrespective of original career intentions, and consequently were explored in Phases 2 and 3. These aspects were identified from earlier research in the Unit on the role of the midwife, from an ongoing literature review and from pilot studies for the current project; they comprised the following:

- the division of responsibility between midwives and medical staff for normal maternity care;
- opportunities for individual midwives to pursue their own professional development;
- conditions of service;
- the practicalities of combining family commitments with work as a midwife and its effect on career progression.

Data on each of these topics were of relevance not only to the question of retention, but also provided much needed information on the extent to which the maternity services were fully utilizing midwives' skills in the 1980s and on the quality of the professional environment in which midwives were practising. Each is briefly discussed in turn, together with relevant research, in order to provide a framework for the questions asked in Phases 2 and 3.

The division of responsibility between midwives and medical staff. Midwives in Britain are qualified to provide care on their own responsibility throughout pregnancy, labour and the puerperium and to recognize those signs of abnormality that require referral to medical staff. A continuing theme in the more recent history of midwifery, however, is the extent to which these responsibilities have been eroded by the increasing involvement of medical staff in this process. This in turn has been identified as a source of dissatisfaction and a possible reason for leaving;

consequently it was explored in the course of this study. The trend was identified as early as 1947 by the Working Party on Midwives (Ministry of Health *et al.*, 1949). It was not until the early 1970s, however, that it became a major issue of concern.

The incidence of obstetric interventions, which had begun to rise in the 1960s, climbed sharply in the 1970s (Butler and Bonham, 1963; Chalmers and Richards, 1977; Chamberlain *et al.*, 1978; Government Statistical Service, 1980). This meant an increase in the proportion of women in labour in whose care medical staff participated and who were not managed entirely by midwives. At the same time an increasing number of units developed policies for the 'active management' of labour which staff were required to follow; these included, for example, the frequency of vaginal examinations, when to rupture membranes, and the length of time to be allowed for the second stage of labour. Medical staff became increasingly involved in the antenatal care of women with normal pregnancies, and many midwives' clinics were closed down. This was partly due to the delegation of care to community staff, and to the view that hospital visits should be for the purpose of assessment by the obstetrician. Childbirth became characterized by the philosophy that 'labour is only normal in retrospect' (Percival, 1970): a philosophy which overshadowed the role of the midwife in caring for women who experienced a normal pregnancy, labour, and puerperium.

Midwives became increasingly concerned about the erosion of their role by the medicalization of childbirth (e.g. Royal College of Midwives, 1977; Brain, 1979; Barnett, 1979). No information existed, however, on the overall extent to which the midwife's role was being eroded, and whether this varied in different practice settings. A national survey of midwives, obstetricians, general practitioners, and health visitors was undertaken by the first author of this chapter and colleagues, with funding from the Department of Health and Social Security (Robinson *et al.*, 1983; Robinson, 1985a, 1985b, 1985c, 1989a), in order to provide this information. The survey found that although midwives were responsible for much of the care provided for childbearing women, many were not able to exercise their clinical judgement in decision making about the management of that care. In the antenatal period, less than 5% of hospital midwives and less than a third of community midwives took responsibility for assessing the course of pregnancy; the majority worked in clinics in which either medical staff examined women or did so after the midwife had already examined them. A substantial majority of midwives worked in labour wards in which certain decisions that are basic to the management of labour were either made by medical staff or determined by unit policy. Over 80% of those who took part in the survey worked in units in which medical staff also examined normal postnatal women and made the decision as to when they and their babies were fit to go home.

The end of the 1970s was in many ways a turning point for the profession, with the recognition that certain trends in the health services over the past two decades had undermined various aspects of their contribution to maternity care. The 1980s witnessed a response to this situation, with many midwives involved in setting up schemes which made full use of their knowledge and skills, and enabled them to provide continuity of care from early pregnancy to the end of the postnatal period (see Robinson, 1990, for a review of these developments).

Despite these developments and research that showed that midwives achieve as good perinatal outcomes as medical staff and higher levels of client satisfaction (Robinson, 1989b), the under use of midwifery skills continued to be a cause for concern. Subsequent research (e.g. Department of Health and Social Security, 1984; Garforth and Garcia, 1987, 1989; Garcia and Garforth, 1989, 1991), has shown that midwives' responsibilities for clinical assessment and decision making concerning the management of care continue to be restricted in much the same way as our earlier study demonstrated (Robinson *et al.*, 1983). Various official publications appeared on the subject (e.g. Central Midwives Board for Scotland *et al.*, 1983) recommending that the maternity services be organized in a way that enabled midwives to practise with the level of responsibility for which they are qualified. This study provided an opportunity to examine the extent to which this was the case in a wide variety of posts and practice settings, together with the midwives' satisfaction with their experience and their views on the effect, if any, that satisfaction in this respect might have on retention.

Continuing professional development. The second area of life as a midwife, identified as relevant to retention, was opportunities for continuing education and other aspects of professional development. The importance attached to the provision that health service professions make for the continuing education and development of their members have featured in a number of publications from government departments and professional organizations. Two of the most recent examples are the UKCC's document on the *Post-registration education and practice project* (United Kingdom Central Council, 1990) and the English National Board's Framework for *Continuing education and training* (English National Board, 1990).

In these two documents, as in many others that have addressed the subject, it is taken as a given that continuing professional education of health practitioners enhances both the quality of care that they deliver and their own career development. It is maintained that the latter contributes to job satisfaction and this in turn has a positive effect on retention. In midwifery, a growing range of post-basic and in-service opportunities are available. Post-basic qualifications include the Post-Graduate Certificate in Education for Adults (Midwifery), which has replaced the Midwife Teachers' Diploma, the Diploma in Professional Studies (Midwifery), which has replaced the Advanced Diploma in Midwifery, National Board courses relevant to midwifery practice and education, a variety of nationally recognized courses such as diplomas in counselling and certificates in antenatal education and degrees at bachelor, masters and doctoral level. In addition to statutory refresher courses, in-service courses on a range of topics relevant to midwifery are offered by university departments, the Royal College of Midwives, organizations such as MIDIRS, maternity units, individual health authorities, and NHS trusts. Up dating courses for those who are returning after a break are available in some areas and a recent innovation is the production of a distance learning programme for midwives who have been out of practice for a while (South Bank University, 1992).

Research published to date on opportunities for midwives to continue their professional development is relatively scant. Consequently little is known about midwives' perceptions of their own continuing education needs, how many have attended courses, factors that facilitate or militate against doing so, and what effect, if any, continuing education has on patient care and individual careers. Research that has been undertaken shows that a high proportion of midwives regard continuing education as important (Maclean, 1980; Clarke and Rees, 1989), that a number of factors militate against course attendance (Sugarman, 1988; McCrea, 1989) and that clinical updating is the topic specified most frequently when respondents are asked about their preferences for the content of future courses (Maclean, 1980; Parnaby, 1987; Clarke and Rees, 1989).

An area neglected until relatively recently is the continuing education needs of practitioners who are not working for reasons such as childcare or a period of unemployment. Recognizing the potential importance that opportunities for continuing education may have on encouraging a return to work, the Department of Health (1988) has recommended the implementation of 'keeping in touch' schemes. Views of non-working midwives, recently explored in a small scale interview study by Midgely (1993), showed that nearly all would be interested in a 'keep in touch' programme for midwives. Finally, research on aspects of professional development for midwives, such as mentorship and career guidance, is notable by its absence, although a number of unpublished studies are recorded in the Midwifery Research Database (Renfrew and Simmons, 1991).

The paucity of empirical studies on professional development for midwives is echoed in nursing also, as demonstrated by a recent comprehensive review of the literature by Barriball and colleagues (1992). In view of the foregoing, several questions on continuing professional development in midwifery and its relationship to retention were included in this study.

Conditions of service. Reports from the 1940s onwards have shown that dissatisfaction with conditions of service have tended to head the list of reasons why nurses and midwives leave the health service (e.g. RCN, 1942, 1964; Ministry of Health *et al.*, 1947; Royal Commission on the Health Service, 1978; Martin and MacKean, 1988; Price Waterhouse, 1988; Buchan and Stock, 1990). It is outside the scope of this chapter to review the wide body of literature on the subject, suffice it to say that pay, shortage of staff and unsocial and inflexible hours have featured most prominently.

Given the importance of conditions of service in relation to retention, a number of questions on the subject were included in Phases 2 and 3 of the study. At Phase 3, several additional questions were included on the Clinical Grading Review, since its implementation was accompanied by much adverse publicity on the effect it might have on retention.

Combining working as a midwife with family responsibilities. The fourth area of life as a midwife investigated in the project focused on combining work with family responsibilities and its relationship to retention. In the health services over the last few years increasing attention has focused on strategies to encourage and enable women to combine work with caring for a family. Women who leave to have children and do not return, represent a loss to the profession of the skills and experience gained since qualification and a reduction in the total workforce if they are not replaced. This is of particular concern to those health service professions comprised primarily of women, such as midwifery and nursing. Strategies for retention have focused on keeping in touch about developments in nursing and midwifery and job opportunities, combined with 'return to nursing' courses when employment is resumed (Laurent, 1989; Standring, 1989) flexible hours (O'Byrne, 1989), job sharing (Lathlean, 1987), and childcare facilities (Hurst *et al.*, 1990). Flexible hours, in particular, have been shown to be of prime importance to women returners in many spheres of work (Martin and Roberts, 1984). In relation to nurses and midwives, Hockey (1975) found flexible hours to be the single most important incentive cited for attacting staff back and Moores *et al.* (1983) showed that lack of flexible working hours was the main obstacle preventing the return of a large pool of qualified staff keen to resume a career.

Breaks in employment for childcare affects individual career development as well as the overall composition of the workforce. Studies of women in many occupations have shown that breaks in employment are often associated with lack of career progress (Joshi, 1989) and in some cases with downward mobility (Dex, 1990). Whether through choice or necessity a return to work is often to a part-time post, and these tend to be concentrated in lower grades. The Women and Employment Study illustrates this, showing that 37% of women had returned to a lower occupational level following childbirth, and that this was strongly associated with returning part time (Martin and Roberts, 1984). Various studies have demonstrated that the majority of nurses and midwives take part-time posts on returning from a period of childcare (e.g. Hockey, 1975). As in other occupations, however, part-time posts in nursing and midwifery are concentrated in lower grades (Corby, 1991; Equal Opportunities Commission, 1991). A number of studies have shown that despite the increasing proportion of nurses and midwives who are women with children; they make slower career progress than either men or women without children (e.g. Hutt, 1985; Davies and Rosser, 1986; Equal Opportunities Commission, 1991).

In view of the major influence that family responsibilities may have on retention in midwifery, various questions on the subject were included at all three phases of this study.

AIMS, DESIGN AND METHODS

Having considered the range of issues with which the project has been concerned, this section discusses the aims of each of the three phases and the methods that were adopted.

Phase 1 – two cross-sectional surveys

Phase 1 aimed to establish whether extending midwifery training from 12 to 18 months led to the hoped-for increase in the proportion of midwives who qualified feeling adequately prepared to practise midwifery and in the proportion who intended to do so. It was not originally undertaken as the first phase of a longitudinal panel study, but rather as two cross-sectional surveys, designed to produce comparable data about the two cohorts. A national survey by questionnaire was the method of choice for Phase 1 for several reasons. Large numbers were needed to determine whether significant differences existed between the two cohorts in relation to views about training and career intentions. A national sample was required in order to militate against biases that might result from only including particular catchment areas of students and types of training school. Questionnaires were the only feasible method of data collection given the numbers involved and the geographical dispersion of the two cohorts.

A pilot study was undertaken in 1978. A questionnaire covering reasons for training, career intentions and views about various aspects of the course was developed and tested by means of interviews with a group of midwives qualifying in the early part of the year, and then by postal versions sent to a larger group qualifying later that year. The revised questionnaire was then sent to 932 midwives who qualified in 1979 after a 12 month course, representing a quarter of those qualifying that year; lists of those qualifying in 1978 and in 1979 were made available by the then Central Midwives' Board. Then the same questionnaire was sent to 931 midwives who qualified in 1983 after an 18 month course, also representing a quarter of the year's qualifiers; lists were made available by the English National Board. Following the initial questionnaire and one reminder letter, response rates of 84% (782) and 89% (828) were achieved for the two cohorts respectively. Phase 1 was regarded as a completed study after the questionnaire was sent to the 1983 cohort at qualification and findings were made available (Golden, 1980; Robinson 1986a, 1986b, 1986c, 1991).

Phases 2 and 3 – advantages of a longitudinal panel design

From the early 1980s onwards concern had been growing about attrition from the nursing and midwifery workforce, and it was thought that information about the post-qualification experiences of the two cohorts of midwives might usefully contribute to an understanding of factors associated with attrition that would be relevant to all midwives, whatever their route to registration. At the same time information would be provided as to whether those who had taken the 18 month course had been more likely to stay than those who had taken the 12 month course. Consequently two further phases were undertaken; Phase 2 in 1986 and 1987 and Phase 3 in 1989.

The fact that contact had been established with the cohorts at the time that they qualified provided an excellent opportunity to undertake a longitudinal panel study, i.e. one in which the same individuals are questioned on more than one occasion. Such a study had a number of advantages when compared with the option of undertaking a new cross-sectional study to explore the problem of attrition with a different group of midwives. Before describing the methods used, some of the advantages of longitudinal panel studies are discussed, as well as the particular problems that they entail.

Change at the individual level. Firstly, longitudinal panel studies allow for analysis of events and change over time at the **individual** level as well as at the **aggregate** level. Thus having documented midwives' career intentions at qualification, information at later stages in their careers would indicate whether intentions were put into practice, reasons advanced for changes in plans, and the extent to which midwives moved between midwifery and other occupations and had breaks in employment.

Inaccuracy of recall. Secondly, longitudinal panel studies mitigate against inaccuracy of recall. In a cross-sectional study midwives who have been qualified for several years can be asked about their intentions at qualification, but their answers may be affected by inaccurate recall over time or by *post hoc* rationalization of a work history that for some reason did not accord with original intentions. A longitudinal design makes it possible to explore whether attrition occurs as a consequence of the intended role of midwifery in people's career plans, or whether it is in response to working conditions.

Responding to new events. Thirdly, longitudinal studies can also document responses to new events. For example, the period between Phase 2 (1986) and Phase 3 (1989) of the project saw the introduction of the Clinical Grading Review. Consequently a question on gradings awarded under the review and the effect that it might have on career intentions was included at Phase 3.

As well as advantages, however, longitudinal studies also pose considerable methodological problems, in particular those of attrition at successive phases of data collection and complexity of data analysis. Attrition at each stage is a major problem since those who do respond may differ markedly from those who do not, so leading to increasing loss of representativeness (Douglas and Bloomfield, 1973; Hoinville *et al.*, 1978; Goldstein, 1979; Cohen and Manion, 1980; Waterton and Lievesley, 1986). Attrition may be due to loss of interest in the study or failure to maintain records of change of address. The overriding task of the longitudinal panel researcher is to get as high a proportion of the group in question recruited into the study at the outset and to maintain interest and high response rates thereafter.

The complexity of longitudinal data, particularly those concerned with life events, is often underestimated, with the result that data may remain under explored (Marsh and Gershuny, 1991). Specific problems are also encountered such as censoring (i.e. events being incomplete at the start and/or end of the study period) and time varying explanatory variables such as marriage (Allison, 1984; Uncles, 1988; Marsh and Gershuny, 1991). However, recent years have seen substantial developments in the methods of longitudinal data analysis available for the quantitative or qualitative study of individuals over time. Whereas in 1973 Carr-Hill and Macdonald commented that 'adequate tools (conceptual and computational) for the handling of sociological life-histories are unavailable', some 18 years later Dex was able to report that 'life and work history analyses have been an area of social science where substantial and exciting developments have taken place, particularly over the last two decades' (Dex, 1991).

Attrition of subjects and complexity of data analysis, together with high initial costs and problems in maintaining continuity of personnel and comparability of research items over time, has meant that most studies of health service careers have been conducted using cross-sectional designs and longitudinal studies are few and far between. Exceptions in nursing and midwifery include follow-up studies of graduates from nursing degree courses (see Brooking *et al.*, 1989; Winson, 1993, for reviews), some of the studies undertaken by the Institute of Manpower Studies (e.g. Waite *et al.*, 1989) and Mander's study of midwives (Chapter 9 in this volume). Lack of longitudinal studies of careers is not confined to nursing and midwifery however. In a review of the literature on motivation for career development, Law and Ward (1981) draw attention to the paucity of studies which have examined the relationship between career choices and subsequent work patterns, noting that those which do exist are primarily in the field of school leavers' aspirations and subsequent careers.

Phases 2 and 3 – aims and methods

Returning now to our study, the aims of Phase 2 were to re-establish contact with all members of the two cohorts and to obtain information on:

1. career paths since qualification, both in and out of midwifery;
2. experience of midwifery posts in relation to the four areas identified as particularly relevant to retention, and discussed in the background section of this chapter namely:
   - division of responsibility with medical staff,
   - opportunities for continuing professional development,
   - views on conditions of service,
   - combining work with family commitments;
3. reasons for leaving midwifery, future career intentions and views as to what would encourage retention.

The original plan of sending a questionnaire covering these topics to each member of the cohort proved not to be feasible because of the length entailed in providing for all possible sequences of posts and activities since qualification. Even though recipients were directed to skip questions not applicable to them, the overall effect was of a dauntingly long questionnaire that would have militated against a high response rate. Consequently a different strategy was adopted. All cohort members were sent a short questionnaire in which they were asked to complete a career chart of numbered lines showing details of posts held and other specified activities since qualification, to recall their career intentions at qualification and to provide some biographical details. If they had not practised midwifery they were asked to say why this had been the case. A four page summary of findings from Phase 1 was included in the hope that this feedback would enhance midwives' interest in and commitment to a study in which most of them had already taken part.

Those who returned the first questionnaire and indicated that they had practised as midwives were then sent a second questionnaire, tailored to fit the particular career they had followed, as indicated by their completed career chart. This comprised blocks of questions for each of the kinds of posts that could have been held, and each individual's questionnaire was made up of the blocks of questions applicable to the particular posts that they had held. Questions were also included on educational qualifications and opportunities, why midwives leave the profession, views on what factors might encourage them to return, and future career intentions. Anticipating the possibility of undertaking a long-term follow-up study, i.e. Phase 3, a form was enclosed with each of the second questionnaires, asking if the respondent would be willing to take part in a longitudinal study and, if so, to keep us up to date with changes of address.

Both questionnaires were developed and tested by means of first discussing each question with a small group of midwives on a one-to-one basis, then sending amended versions by post to a second group, and finally sending a revised version, also by post, to a third group. Each group of midwives included some who were practising midwifery, some who had practised but were not doing so at the time of the pilot study and some who had never practised. In order to assess the likely response rates a reminder letter and a duplicate questionnaire were sent to non-respondents four weeks after the initial mailing, and a second reminder some three weeks later.

Although the response rates at Phase 1 were very high for a postal survey (84% for the 1979 cohort and 89% for the 1983) the task of re-establishing contact with members of these two cohorts, some seven and three years later respectively, was somewhat daunting. The first strategy was to locate them on the UKCC database. Working within the guidelines of the Data Protection Act, all but a few members of the two cohorts were traced by this means. If the address on the database was the same as that we had at Phase 1, we sent the first questionnaire to that address; if it was different, the UKCC did not give us the new address but forwarded it to the midwife on our behalf. Each midwife was asked to provide us with their current address so that the second questionnaire could be mailed direct from the Unit; all but a handful did so.

Rather than send reminders to the same address for non-respondents, these were first checked against mailing lists held by the Royal College of Midwives and the Health Visitors Association. If the address was the same, a reminder letter and another copy of the questionnaire was sent from the Unit; if it was different then the reminder was forwarded on our behalf. Further reminders and questionnaires were then sent to every possible address held for each non-respondent. Finally those who had responded were asked if they could help us trace members of their set who had not done so. Response rates achieved are shown in Table 8.1.

The main aims of Phase 3 of the study were similar to those of Phase 2 in that they included obtaining information about careers followed, and views and personal experiences in relation to midwifery. As noted earlier,

Table 8.1 Response rates at Phases 1, 2 and 3 of the Midwives' Careers Project

	1979 cohort	*1983 cohort*
Phase 1 1979/1983		
Number in cohort	932	931
Number returning the questionnaire at qualification	782	828
Phase 1 response rate	84%	89%
Phase 2(a) 1986		
Number sent Phase 2(a) questionnaire	932	931
Number returning questionnaire	536	629
Response rate as proportion of cohort	58%	68%
	(536/932)	(629/931)
Number returning a Phase 1 and a Phase 2 questionnaire	490	581
Response rates proportion of Phase 1 respondents who returned a Phase 2 questionnaire	63%	70%
	(490/782)	(581/828)
Phase 2(b) 1987		
Number who had practised midwifery by 1986 and sent a Phase 2(b) questionnaire	394	524
Number returning questionnaire	319	431
Response rate as proportion of number sent	87%	82%
	(319/394)	(431/524)
Phase 3 1989		
Number who had practised midwifery by 1986 and sent a Phase 3(a) questionnaire	394	524
Number returning questionnaire	288	407
Response rate as proportion of number sent	73%	78%
	(288/394)	(407/524)
Number who had not practised midwifery by 1986 and sent a Phase 3(b) questionnaire	96	57
Number returning questionnaire	80	38
Response rate as proportion of number sent	83%	67%
	(80/96)	(38/57)

Source: compiled by the authors.

one of the advantages of a longitudinal panel study is the opportunity to explore experiences and views about new events with people for whom a substantial database already exists. Consequently the Phase 3 questionnaire included questions on gradings awarded under the Clinical Grading Review and its effects, if any, on intentions to stay in, to leave or to return to the profession. Moreover, by 1989 when Phase 3 of the study was undertaken, increasing attention was focusing on the problem of combining health service work with family commitments and keeping in touch with professional developments while taking a break from full-time employment. The subject had been included in the Phase 2 questionnaires, but not in the depth that was now felt to be warranted. Consequently in the Phase 3 questionnaire, respondents were asked about their experiences in this respect for the whole period since qualification.

In order to keep the questionnaire to a manageable length and maximize chances of high response rates, however, it was not feasible to include questions on these two new areas (Clinical Grading Review and combining work and family) as well as retain all the Phase 2 questions on aspects of midwifery posts; consequently the latter were reduced in number. The questionnaire for those known to have practised midwifery between qualification and 1986 differed slightly from the one sent to those known not to have practised midwifery by this time.

A short summary of the Phase 2 findings was enclosed with both questionnaires. As in Phase 2 it was hoped that feedback of this kind would increase interest and commitment. Both the Phase 3 questionnaires were developed and tested with a group of midwives; as in Phase 2 they represented a range of levels of involvement in the profession. By Phase 3, it seemed a waste of time and money to send questionnaires to those who had not responded at Phase 2. Consequently questionnaires were sent to Phase 2 responders only, using the address currently held in 1989. Addresses of non-respondents were checked against those held on the UKCC database and, as at Phase 2, reminder letters and duplicate questionnaires were sent out twice. Response rates achieved are shown in Table 8.1 (page 189).

Response rates and representativeness of the data

Every effort was made to maximize response rates at Phases 2 and 3 of this longitudinal study. Strategies described included the following:

- developing and testing questionnaires with a pilot group to ensure that they were valid, reliable and of acceptable length;
- checking reliability of addresses;
- enclosing short feedback reports to maintain interest;
- sending reminder letters and duplicate questionnaires to every known address;

- asking those who had responded if they could help us to contact members of their set who had not done so.

Response rates for longitudinal studies can be presented as a proportion of the total cohort eligible to reply or as a proportion of those responding at previous phases. Both of these are shown for this project in Table 8.1 and demonstrate that high response rates were obtained at each phase. It is important to consider, however, how representative the respondents were at each phase. The very high response rates achieved for Phase 1 (84% and 89% for the two cohorts respectively) means that confidence can be placed in findings concerning midwives' views and intentions at the time of qualification.

In the course of tracing the whereabouts of the two groups of midwives at Phase 2 (1986), we obtained as much information about each individual as possible. In particular, information from the UKCC indicated whether they had ever notified an intention to practise midwifery, and this subsequently enabled us to assess whether respondents differed markedly from non-respondents. Information about respondents from the returned questionnaires combined with information about non-respondents from the UKCC database showed that respondents were much more likely than non-respondents to have practised midwifery: 87% compared with 57% in 1979 and 90% compared with 49% in 1983. The practisers among the respondents did, in fact, represent a substantial majority of the practisers in the cohort as a whole: 66% of the 1979 practisers (435/660) and 79% of the 1983 practisers (568/715). Consequently, Phase 2 findings concerning experiences of practising as a midwife can be viewed with confidence. However, those who had not practised midwifery were under represented among the respondents: 37% of the 1979 non-practisers (100/271) and 30% of the 1983 non-practisers (61/201). At Phase 3 we did not have the time or resources to ascertain whether non-respondents had practised midwifery in the period between 1986 and 1989. The response rates at Phase 3 are, however, sufficiently high for confidence to be placed in the findings.

Data handling and analysis

The Phase 1 questionnaires were coded and inputted by Unit staff as were the career charts from the Phases 2 and 3 questionnaires. The other Phase 2 and 3 questions were coded and inputted by temporary staff recruited for the purpose. Analysis of longitudinal data is potentially very complex and as described previously these data often remain under analysed. To some extent this was the case with this project and this was for two reasons: first, the main research questions could be answered by relatively simple techniques; namely:

- assessing whether the proportion of each cohort expressing a particular intention or holding a midwifery post at specified times differed significantly;
- linking answers given at one phase with those at another in order, for example, to assess the extent to which intentions were put into practice;
- providing descriptive information about experiences as a midwife.

Secondly, this study of midwives' careers was the first longitudinal study undertaken at the Unit and at the time that it was carried out we had not developed the statistical and computing expertise necessary for more complex analysis. This expertise has subsequently been developed in the course of our current longitudinal studies of careers of registered general nurses, registered mental nurses, and nursing graduates. In due course, therefore, the substantial database that we now hold on midwives' careers could be subjected to more complex analysis; this in turn can then be linked to subsequent phases of data collection.

Three aspects of the analytic procedures that were used are relevant to the findings presented in this chapter and so are described here.

Career path summaries. Completed career charts revealed an immense diversity not only in the posts held and activities pursued since qualification, but also in the order in which they were undertaken. A coding procedure was therefore devised to group these diverse career paths into broader categories which could form the basis of subsequent analyses. First, current posts or activities were grouped into the following eight categories:

1. midwifery;
2. nursing;
3. health visitors course/health visiting;
4. health care related post, other than midwifery, nursing or health visiting;
5. non-health care related post;
6. full-time study;
7. unemployment;
8. maternity leave and/or caring for children.

Secondly, all possible combinations of posts and activities leading up to the one currently held was allocated a separate code. Those currently practising midwifery, for example, included:

- continuous practice as a midwife since qualification;
- practised midwifery, unemployed, on maternity leave, now practising midwifery;
- practised midwifery, practised nursing, now practising midwifery;

- practised nursing, took other employment, went on maternity leave, now practising midwifery.

Examples of respondents currently practising nursing included:

- practised midwifery, now nursing;
- nursing since qualified as a midwife, never practised midwifery.

Using this system, the 1979 data revealed 151 different combinations and the 1983 data 86 combinations for the period between qualification and Phase 2 and between qualification and Phase 3. Thirdly, these combinations were grouped into various broader categories which were then used for subsequent analysis.

Other aspects of career paths were also summarized in order to compare the two cohorts; these included:

- the total number of months spent in midwifery practice since qualification;
- the type of midwifery career followed (i.e. practice, teaching and/or management);
- the highest grade reached;
- the number of posts held;
- the proportion of midwifery practice spent in full-time employment and the proportion in part-time employment.

One of the aims of the study was to compare the career paths of those who qualified in 1979 after a 12 month course with those who qualified in 1983 after an 18 month course. By November 1986 (the cut off point for the career chart in Phase 2), the former group had been qualified for seven years and the latter for three. In order to provide comparable data on the two groups, a summary of the careers followed by the 1979 respondents up until November 1982 (i.e. three years after qualification) was also coded and inputted into the database. By March 1989, the 1979 group had been qualified for ten years and the 1983 group for six. Again, in order to compare the progress of the two groups, the careers of the 1979 respondents were summarized as at 1985, as well as at 1989, thus providing a summary of careers followed by both groups over a six year period since qualification.

Units of analysis. Four different units of analysis were used in the exploration of data and presentation of findings. The most frequent was the individual midwife; the other three were 'post', 'period of clinical experience' and 'period of absence from midwifery'. In Phase 2 of the project each midwife was sent a separate set of questions for **each** midwifery post that she had held. Experiences and views often varied considerably from post to post and so it would have been meaningless to have worked out an average for each respondent, of (for example) the rating given in each post for satisfaction with support from senior staff. Figures are presented therefore for 'post' and not for 'person'. The set of questions for each post contained questions about the main aspects of care which the post might have entailed, namely antenatal care, care in labour and delivery, postnatal care and special care. Two issues were relevant to selecting the appropriate unit of analysis for these data. First, a midwife may have worked in, for example, the antenatal clinic in one post, but not in another and so post was not an appropriate unit of analysis. Secondly, experiences of the provision of care often varied from one post to another; for instance, in the antenatal clinic in one post a midwife was responsible for the abdominal examination whereas in another post this procedure was usually performed by medical staff. It was not possible to 'average' out this experience and so findings on care are presented by 'period of clinical experience'. In Phase 3 respondents were asked several questions about each period of absence that they had had from midwifery for childcare purposes. As with periods of clinical experience, events varied from one period of absence to another and so could not be 'averaged' out for each individual. Findings on this subject are therefore presented by period of absence and not by individual midwife.

Statistical analysis. The test for significant differences between proportions (Armitage, 1971) was used when comparing the two cohorts in terms of career intentions and subsequent retention.

FINDINGS

Findings presented in this chapter include those relating to the main research questions and those that demonstrate the strength of a longitudinal panel design in documenting careers over time; they are as follows:

1. comparison of career intentions and careers followed by the two cohorts;
2. career events over time;
3. some aspects of four areas of life as a midwife, relevant to retention;
4. views and experiences in relation to retention.

Phase 1 findings on reasons for wishing to qualify as a midwife, career intentions at the beginning and at the end of training, and views about the course and its adequacy as a preparation for practice have been widely disseminated elsewhere (Golden, 1980; Robinson, 1986a, 1986b, 1986c, 1991). In this chapter therefore, only the Phase 1 findings relating to career intentions at qualification are included since they were subsequently linked to data collected at Phases 2 and 3.

In tables that follow the totals vary according to the phase(s) at which the data were collected, the sub-group(s) in question, and the unit of analysis (see previous section on data analysis). To aid clarity, the phase from which data are drawn is indicated in the table headings.

Career intentions and careers followed; comparison of those who took an 18 month course with those who took a 12 month course

Career intentions at qualification. Members of the two cohorts were asked to state their career intentions in relation to practising midwifery at the time that they qualified. Newly qualified midwives may intend to work as a midwife for a short time in order to consolidate their training before moving to another area of work. Intending to work as a midwife does not therefore necessarily entail making a career in midwifery. A contribution to the profession is made, however, by all those who put their training into practice, albeit that this may be as a short-term commitment rather than as a career. We were interested in the proportion of newly qualified midwives coming into both these categories and in whether or not the two cohorts differed in this respect.

The range of possibilities in relation to practising midwifery, shown in Table 8.2 (page 196), was developed during the course of the project's pilot study. The first three possibilities indicate an intention to practise as a midwife, even if only for a short time, and have been subtotalled within the table to show the overall proportion of respondents who expressed an intention to practise. Similarly, the fourth and fifth possibilities have also been subtotalled within the table to show the overall proportion of midwives who did not express an intention to practise.

The largest proportion of respondents in both cohorts expressed uncertainty as to whether they would practise midwifery for a short time only or for a career. The subtotals for those who intend to practise midwifery having qualified, show that this is the case for a substantial majority of both cohorts, with the figure for the 1983 cohort representing an increase of 12% over that for the 1979 qualifiers (85% compared with 73% $p < 0.00001$).

Turning now to those who intended to make a career in midwifery, then 7% more of the 1983 cohort than of the 1979 cohort came into this category; 24% compared with 17% ($0.001 < p < 0.005$). However, 24% is still very much a minority of the total number of midwives qualifying. Phase 1 of this longitudinal study therefore demonstrated that extending the midwifery course from 12 to 18 months was not associated with the hoped-for increase in the proportion of midwives who reached the end of the course with a definite intention to make a career in midwifery. Moreover, when asked why they had taken midwifery training, the reasons

Table 8.2 Career intentions after qualifying as a midwife: 1979 and 1983 cohorts (Phase 1 data)

Career intentions in relation to practising as a midwife	*1979 cohort*		*1983 cohort*	
	%	No.	%	No.
Intending to make a career in midwifery	17	136	24	199
Intending to practise midwifery but not sure whether for a short time or for a career	40	310	49	403
Intending to practise for some time as a midwife, but not to make midwifery a career	16	127	12	102
Total expressing an intention to practise	**73**	**573**	**85**	**704**
Not sure whether want to practise at all as a midwife	15	115	7	58
Not intending to practise midwifery after qualifying	12	91	6	46
Total not expressing an intention to practise	**26**	**206**	**13**	**104**
No answer	—	3	2	20
Total	100	782	100	828

Source: compiled by the authors.

given most frequently by both cohorts were to broaden experience and improve career prospects.

Careers followed after qualification. Findings from Phases 2 and 3 of the project showed the extent to which the two cohorts differed in the proportion who practised midwifery in the years after qualification. Using the coding system for summarizing careers over comparable periods of time (see page 192) each respondent was allocated to one of the categories shown in Tables 8.3 and 8.4.

The findings for Phase 2 (Table 8.3) show that three years after qualification 8% more of the 1983 qualifiers were practising midwifery than of their 1979 counterparts ($p < 0.025$). Similar proportions of both cohorts were on maternity leave having practised midwifery (11% and 13%) or

Table 8.3 1979 and 1983 cohorts: Career summary three years after qualifying (Phase 2 data)

Career summary	1979 cohort in 1982		1983 cohort in 1986	
	%	*No.*	*%*	*No.*
1. Practising midwifery having done so continuously since qualifying	29	142	37	214
2. Practising midwifery having only had breaks for maternity leave	6	28	21	56
3. Practising midwifery having had breaks for maternity leave and/or other occupations	14	67	10	57
Total practising midwifery	**48**	**237**	**56**	**237**
4. On maternity leave having only practised midwifery	7	34	10	57
5. On maternity leave having practised midwifery and other occupations	4	22	3	19
Total on maternity leave who had practised midwifery	**11**	**56**	**13**	**78**
6. In other occupation having practised midwifery	19	95	20	119
Total who had practised midwifery	**79**	**388**	**90**	**524**
7. Never practised midwifery	21	102	10	57
Total	100	490	100	581

Source: compiled by the authors.

were in other occupations or activities having practised midwifery (19% and 20%). Twenty-one per cent of the 1979 qualifiers had never practised midwifery compared with 10% of the 1983; this difference is primarily a reflection of the fact that the 1979 non-practisers were more likely to have returned a questionnaire than the 1983 non-practisers (see page 191).

The data from Phase 3 of the study demonstrated a continuation of this

Table 8.4 1979 and 1983 cohorts: Career summary six years after qualifying (Phase 3 data)

Career summary	1979 cohort in 1985				1983 cohort in 1989			
	Practised after qualifying		Not practised after qualifying		Practised after qualifying		Not practised after qualifying	
	%	No.	%	No.	%	No.	%	No.
1. Practising midwifery having done so continuously since qualification	23	65			27	109		
2. Practising midwifery having only had breaks for maternity leave	12	36			17	71		
3. Practising midwifery having had breaks for:								
a) other occupations	12	35			4	18		
b) other occupations and maternity leave	6	16			7	29		2
Total in midwifery practice	**53**	**152**			**56**	**227**		
4. On maternity leave having only practised midwifery	8	23			12	50		
5. On maternity leave having practised midwifery and had breaks for other occupations:	9	25			7	29		1

Total on maternity leave	*17*	*48*			*19*	*79*		
6. In another occupation having practised midwifery	30	85	100	80	24	97	3	1
7. Never practised midwifery	1	3			1	4	87	33
8. Incomplete information							3	1
Total	100	288	100	80	100	407	100	38

Source: compiled by the authors.

trend and this is shown in Table 8.4 (page 198). As described on page 190 those who had not practised midwifery by Phase 2 (1986) were sent a slightly different questionnaire in Phase 3 to those who had done so, and so figures are shown separately for these two groups.

Figures in the first and third columns show that the two cohorts differed little in terms of the proportion who were practising midwifery six years after qualification (53% and 56%), the proportion to have done so continuously (23% and 27%) and the proportion on maternity leave having practised as midwives (17% and 19%). Information in the career charts showed that 80 members of the 1979 cohort had not practised midwifery between qualification and 1985. By Phase 2 (1986), 57 members of the 1983 cohort had not practised midwifery since qualifying, and figures in column 4 of Table 8.4 show that of the 38 who returned a questionnaire in Phase 3 (1989) only four had subsequently practised as midwives. This cohort therefore differed little from their 1979 counterparts in the proportion who took up midwifery having **not** done so in the early years after qualification. The Phase 2 and 3 findings, combined with those for intentions at qualification, demonstrated that extending training from 12 to 18 months made little difference to retention levels in the profession. These findings were widely reported at the time and contributed to the decision to introduce pre-registration midwifery training (Radford and Thompson, 1988; Kent and Maggs, 1992).

The role of a longitudinal panel design in exploring career events over time

The findings described in the previous section provide information on the proportion of each cohort who expressed an intention to practise midwifery or otherwise, and on the proportion who were in practice three and six years later. The strength of a longitudinal panel study, such as this one, is that it permits analysis of change at the individual level as well as at the aggregate level. As the same individuals have been questioned on three occasions, the data can be analysed to show the extent to which individual intentions were subsequently translated into practice, and on the extent to which those who were practising midwifery three years after qualification were also doing so four years later, i.e. the extent to which people moved in and out of the profession.

Translating career intentions into practice. Table 8.2 (page 196) showed respondents' career intentions in relation to practising midwifery at the time that they qualified. Table 8.5 (page 202) shows the extent to which career intentions at the time of qualification were translated into practice by those who responded at Phase 2 and Phase 3. Before discussing the findings the table format requires a brief explanation. Along the top are the five categories for intentions in relation to practising midwifery, first shown in Table 8.2. The categories down the side are further groupings of the career summary groups shown in Tables 8.3 (page 197) and 8.4 (page 198). Thus the three categories that entail having worked in midwifery **only** and not in other employment are grouped together (i.e. practising midwifery continuously, practising midwifery with breaks only for maternity leave, and on maternity leave having only practised midwifery). Similarly the four categories that relate to working in midwifery **and** in other occupations are also grouped together (i.e. practising midwifery having had breaks for other occupations, practising midwifery having had breaks for other occupations and maternity leave, on maternity leave having practised midwifery and other occupations, and in another occupation having practised midwifery). The other category, never worked as a midwife, remains unchanged. For the 1979 cohort, (the top half of the table) career intentions expressed at qualification by subsequent events are shown for three years and seven years after qualification (the 1986 Phase 2 data) and ten years after qualification (the 1989 Phase 3 data). The bottom half of the table shows career intentions expressed at qualification by the 1983 cohort by subsequent events three years later (the 1986 Phase 2 data) and six years later (the 1989 Phase 3 data).

Taking the 1979 cohort first, then the findings show that three-quarters of those who had intended to make a career in midwifery had only practised as midwives in the first three years after qualifying. Although not shown in the table, two-thirds of this group had in fact practised continuously and one-third had taken breaks for maternity leave. The proportion who subsequently worked in other occupations as well, inceases from 20% three years after qualification to 38% by ten years on. Those who had not intended to practise midwifery were equally likely to have fulfilled their intentions in the first three years in that 74% had not practised at all, and this proportion remained similar at seven and ten years hence also.

Just over half of those who had been uncertain at qualification as to whether they would practise midwifery for a short time or make it a career had in fact only practised midwifery (four-fifths of whom had done so continuously), and had not worked in any other occupation. By seven and ten years, however, this proportion had dropped to approximately a third, with a concomitant increase in those who had spent time in other occupations. Of those who had intended to practise for a short time, a third had worked only as midwives for the first three years after qualification whereas the majority had moved on to other occupations. However, these proportions remained constant over the seven and ten year period as well. Findings for those ·who had been uncertain as to whether they would practise midwifery at all after qualifying showed that over half had not

Table 8.5 1979 and 1983 cohorts: career intentions at qualification by practised midwifery in subsequent years (Phases 1, 2 and 3 data)

Career summary	1. Make a career in midwifery			2. Practise midwifery but not sure whether for a short time or for a career			3. Practise midwifery for a short time, but not to make it a career			4. Not sure whether want to practise midwifery at all			5. Not to practise midwifery at all		
	3 yrs after qualification %	7 yrs %	10 yrs %	3 yrs after qualification %	7 yrs %	10 yrs %	3 yrs after qualification %	7 yrs %	10 yrs %	3 yrs after qualification %	7 yrs %	10 yrs %	3 yrs after qualification %	7 yrs %	10 yrs %
							1979 COHORT								
Worked only as midwives (with or without breaks for maternity leave)	75	63	56	54	39	31	36	32	34	7	3	4	2	0	0
Worked as midwives and in other occupations (with or without breaks for maternity leave)	20	32	38	41	58	65	58	61	57	37	43	35	24	29	23
Never worked as a midwife	4	5	6	5	4	4	6	5	7	56	53	60	74	71	77
Total number of respondents in group	(88)	(88)	(71)	(191)	(191)	(133)	(79)	(79)	(61)	(73)	(73)	(55)	(58)	(58)	(47)

1983 COHORT

	3 yrs after qualification	6 yrs after qualification	3 yrs after qualification	6 yrs after qualification	3 yrs after qualification	6 yrs after qualification	3 yrs after qualification	6 yrs after qualification	3 yrs after qualification	6 yrs after qualification
Worked only as midwives (with or without breaks for maternity leave)	80	74	62	53	40	37	9	5	0	4
Worked as midwives and in other occupations (with or without breaks for maternity leave)	19	25	37	46	57	63	27	36	28	24
Never worked as a midwife	1	1	2	1	3	—	64	59	72	70
Total number of respondents in group	(145)	(116)	(296)	(234)	(61)	(41)	(33)	(22)	(32)	(23)

Source: compiled by the authors.

done so, and most of those who had done so had also spent time in other occupations.

The findings for each of the five corresponding groups for the 1983 cohort over the three and six year period after qualification demonstrate the same pattern as that described for the 1979 cohort, albeit with some small percentage differences. Two main trends emerge from these data: first, the majority of respondents put their original career intentions into practice; second, those most likely to do so are those whose plans were the most definite in relation to midwifery, i.e. to make it a career or not to practise at all.

Recollecting career intentions. As noted on page 185 of this chapter, one of the advantages of longitudinal panel studies is that respondents can be asked about intentions and decisions at or near the time that they occur. Findings in this respect are therefore not subject to inaccuracy of recall over time, or to a possible *post hoc* rationalization of events that may not have accorded with original intentions. Data from the midwives' careers project provide an interesting demonstration of this point. In Phase 2 (1986) all respondents were asked to recollect their career intentions at the time that they qualified. In fact just under half (48%) of the 1979 cohort and just over half (55%) of their 1983 counterparts gave the same answer as that given in the questionnaire they had completed at qualification. The degree of concordance varied, according to the intentions expressed, as shown in Table 8.6. Those most likely to express the same intention on both occasions (shown in bold figures) were those who intended to make a career in midwifery and those who intended not to practise midwifery at all. The other three groups were less likely to have accurately recollected their original intentions. Further analyses, not included in this chapter, showed that the majority of those who had done what they intended to do gave the same answer, whereas the majority of those who had not done so, gave a different answer.

Moving in and out of midwifery. Tables 8.3 and 8.4 (pages 197 and 198) compared the two cohorts in terms of the proportion of respondents in each of the main career summary categories at three and at six years after qualification. For each cohort further analysis of data shows the extent to which individuals in a particular career summary category at one point in time had moved to another at a subsequent point. Career summaries were made for the 1979 cohort at three, six and seven years after qualification. Table 8.7 (page 206) shows career summaries at three years by those at seven years, and indicates that overall there seems to be little movement between midwifery and other occupations.

Thus of the 142 midwives who had been in continuous practice in the first three years after qualification, just over half (57%) had continued

Table 8.6 1979 and 1983 cohorts: career intentions after qualifying as a midwife by career intentions after qualifying as recollected in 1986 (Phases 1 and 2 data)

Career intentions after qualifying as recollected in 1986	Career intentions expressed at time of qualification									
	1. Make a career in midwifery		2. Practise midwifery but not sure whether for a career or short time only		3. Practise midwifery for a short time but not to make it a career		4. Not sure whether want to practise midwifery at all		5. Not to practise midwifery at all	
	1979 %	1983 %	1979 %	1983 %	1979 %	1983 %	1979 %	1983 %	1979 %	1983 %
1. Make a career in midwifery	**69**	**79**	30	28	19	21	8	3	2	3
2. Practise midwifery but not sure whether for a career or short time only	19	16	**44**	**51**	29	37	12	3	9	3
3. Practise midwifery for a short time but not to make it a career	8	3	17	17	**35**	**44**	12	33	7	19
4. Not sure whether want to practise midwifery at all	2	1	5	2	9	—	**27**	**18**	10	9
5. Not to practise midwifery at all	—	—	4	2	8	3	40	42	**73**	**66**
Total number in group	100 (88)	100 (145)	100 (191)	100 (296)	100 (79)	100 (61)	100 (73)	100 (33)	100 (58)	100 (32)

Source: compiled by the authors.

Table **8.7** 1979 cohort: Career summary three years after qualifying by career summary seven years after qualifying (Phase 2 data)

Career summary seven years after qualifying	Career summary three years after qualifying						
	Midwifery only			Midwifery plus other occupations			
	1. Practising midwifery having done so continuously since qualifying %	2. Practising midwifery having only had breaks for maternity leave %	3. On maternity leave having only practised midwifery %	4. Practising midwifery having had maternity leave and/or breaks for other occupations %	5. On maternity leave having practised midwifery and other occupations %	6. In other occupation or activity having practised midwifery %	7. Never practised midwifery %
Midwifery only							
1. Practising midwifery having done so continuously since qualifying	57	—	—	—	—	—	—
2. Practising midwifery having only had breaks for maternity leave	13	79	38	—	—	—	—
3. On maternity leave having only practised midwifery	8	—	27	—	—	—	—
Midwifery plus other occupations							
4. Practising midwifery having had breaks for maternity leave and/or other occupations	7	4	12	72	18	16	5
5. On maternity leave having practised midwifery and other occupations	—	—	—	12	36	16	1
6. In other occupation or activity having practised midwifery	14	18	24	16	46	68	1
7. Never practised midwifery	—	—	—	—	—	—	93
8. Total number in category	142	28	34	67	22	95	102

Source: Compiled by the authors.

with no break over the next four. Most of the others in this group had continued to practise midwifery, but had had breaks for maternity leave or other posts. Only 14% had left for another occupation. Just over three-quarters of those who had breaks for maternity leave only in the first three years were practising midwifery at the seven year point. During these four years they may have had further breaks for maternity leave, but they had not spent time in other occupations. Of those who were on maternity leave three years after qualification, having only practised midwifery, 65% had only held midwifery employment during the next four years and had not held posts in other occupations. In summary the majority of respondents whose employment career had **only** involved midwifery in the first three years after qualifying had worked only in midwifery during the next four; only 24% (48/204) had spent time in other occupations.

Turning to the group of respondents in Category 4, i.e. those who were practising midwifery three years after qualifying having had breaks for other occupations (and in some cases for maternity leave as well), then the majority (72%) were practising midwifery at the end of the seven year period. Other findings, not included in this chapter, have shown that this category of midwives had been identified as the most mobile in their first three years, but also the second most likely to reach a sister's post in midwifery (Robinson *et al.*, 1992). This early experience in other occupations does not appear for this group to be associated with a move out of midwifery. The same is not the case, however, for respondents in Categories 5, 6 and 7. Of those on maternity leave who had had other occupational experience in their first three years (Category 5), 36% were on maternity leave at seven years, 46% were in another occupation, and only 18% had returned to midwifery. Two-thirds of those who had practised midwifery after qualifying but were in other occupations at the end of the three year period (Category 6) were still in other occupations some four years later. It was possible that within this time they had practised midwifery for a while and left again; further analyses, not included here, showed that this was not the case for most members of this category. Of the 102 respondents who had not practised midwifery at all in the first three years after qualification (Category 7), 93% had still not done so in the following four. This form of analysis was also pursued with the Phase 3 data obtained in 1989. By this time the 1979 cohort had been qualified for ten years, and an analysis of their career summaries at seven years (from Phase 2) by those at ten years (Phase 3) showed the same pattern as in Table 8.7 – i.e. one of little movement back into midwifery. The same analysis was performed with data from the 1983 cohort; in this case career summaries at three years after qualification (Phase 2 data) cross tabulated by career summaries at six years (Phase 3 data). These two sets of findings are not included here because of constraints of space, but are available in Robinson *et al.* (1992). Suffice it to say that they demonstrate the same trend as shown in Table 8.7, namely one of little movement in and out of midwifery.

The main finding to emerge from the career summaries of respondents is that employment experience in the early years after qualification seems to 'set the scene' for that in subsequent years, as far as retention in midwifery is concerned. Midwives may leave for other employment shortly after qualifying because that was what they always intended to do, or they may leave because of dissatisfaction with midwifery or attractions of other employment. In either case the findings from this longitudinal study suggest that most will not return. The occupations most likely to be pursued by those respondents who had also spent some time in midwifery practice were found to be nursing, followed by health visiting and this was also the case for those who had never practised midwifery.

Aspects of life as a midwife

Four main aspects of life as a midwife identified as particularly relevant to retention were studied in the course of the project:

- professional responsibilities – in particular in relation to those of medical staff;
- professional development, in particular opportunities for continuing education;
- conditions of service;
- combining childcare with work as a midwife.

Together these data provided a wealth of information about the way in which midwives' skills and knowledge are deployed in the health service and the extent to which that service affords midwives satisfying work conditions and opportunities for professional development. The detailed findings are outside the main focus of this chapter, but are available in Owen and Robinson (1992), Robinson *et al.* (1992) and Robinson (1993). In this section, the main points are summarized in order to provide a context for respondents' views on factors relevant to retention, and the latter is the subject of the final section of findings.

Division of responsibility between midwives and medical staff. The topics explored and the questions used in relation to professional responsibilities were the same as that used in the earlier study undertaken by the first author and colleagues, which focused specifically on the role of the midwife (Robinson *et al.*, 1983; Robinson, 1985a, 1985b, 1985c, 1989a). The topics were:

- responsibility for abdominal examinations when women visited antenatal clinics;

- proportion of women examined by a doctor on admission to the labour ward;
- decision making for various procedures in the management of labour and delivery in hospital;
- the frequency with which postnatal women were examined by a doctor;
- who made the decision on fitness for discharge home.

Respondents were asked to indicate whether or not they had been involved in antenatal care, care during labour and delivery, postnatal care or special care in respect of **each** midwifery post that they had held. They were then asked various questions about each aspect of care in which they had been involved. The phrase 'period of clinical experience' was used to describe all experience in each clinical area undertaken in the course of a post.

Antenatal care. Responsibility for decision making about the course of pregnancy focuses on the abdominal examination, as it is when this is undertaken and results of other routine investigations are known (e.g. level of blood pressure, urinalysis) that the overall assessment is made of the well-being of the woman and fetus. Responsibility for the abdominal examination in clinics in which respondents worked in their first and in their subsequent midwifery posts is shown in Table 8.8 (page 210).

Findings for the 1979 respondents indicate that the abdominal examination was carried out by the midwife only in a mere 2% of the periods of antenatal experience undertaken in the course of first posts. This is consistent with the findings of our 1979 survey which demonstrated that only 5% of midwives worked in consultant antenatal clinics in which they alone carried out the abdominal examination (Robinson *et al.*, 1983; Robinson, 1985a, 1985c, 1989a). Findings on first posts held by the 1983 respondents show that the proportion of periods of antenatal experience in which the midwife alone carried out the abdominal examination rose to 8%, and findings on subsequent posts show that the proportion rose to 16% and 19% for the 1979 and 1983 respondents respectively. It seems, therefore, that there has been an increase in the likelihood that midwives will be able to take sole responsibility for the abdominal examination in the years since our earlier study was undertaken, but the proportion is still small.

The most likely situation to occur, however, was that the abdominal examination was carried out by medical staff alone or they repeated it after it had been carried out by a midwife; a total of 67% and 56% for first posts (held by the 1979 and 1983 qualifiers respectively) and 40% and 39% for subsequent posts. Moreover in a further fifth of the periods of antenatal experience, the situation varied, depending on the clinic and/or doctor with whom the midwife was working.

Care of women during labour and delivery. Two questions were

Table 8.8 Division of responsibility between midwives and medical staff for abdominal examination (Phase 2 data)

Division of responsibility between midwives and medical staff for abdominal examination	Periods of antenatal clinic experience in which situation applied			
	In first posts held by		In subsequent posts held by	
	1979 cohort, %	1983 cohort, %	1979 cohort, %	1983 cohort, %
Usually carried out by midwife only	2	8	16	19
Usually carried out by doctor only	11	16	14	15
Carried out by midwife but usually repeated by doctor	56	40	26	24
Carried out by doctor at one visit and by midwife at next alternately	4	2	12	9
Varied depending in which clinic and/or with which doctor working	18	18	23	19
Other	7	14	6	12
No answer	2	1	2	1
Total	100 (164)	100 (247)	100 (239)	100 (192)

Source: compiled by the authors.

asked about the division of responsibility between midwives and medical staff for the care of women during labour and delivery in hospital: first, responsibility for examination of women on admission to the labour ward; second, responsibility for decision making about key aspects of care. Table 8.9 shows that in the majority of periods of labour ward experience women were only examined by a doctor on admission if this was requested by a midwife. Routine examination by medical staff occurred in a fifth or less of these periods of experience, and was more likely to involve some rather than all of the women admitted.

The extent to which midwives were responsible for making decisions about key aspects of the care of women during labour and delivery in hospital was examined in relation to the following: when to carry out vaginal examinations; when to rupture membranes; whether to use a continuous monitoring machine; whether to accelerate labour with a syn-

Table 8.9 Division of responsibility between midwives and medical staff for examination of women on admission to the labour ward (Phase 2 data)

Usual practice for examination of women on admission to labour ward	*Periods of labour ward experience in which situation applied*			
	In first posts held by		*In subsequent posts held by*	
	1979 cohort, %	*1983 cohort, %*	*1979 cohort, %*	*1983 cohort, %*
All women are examined by a midwife on admission and **not** by a doctor unless requested by a midwife	78	79	76	81
Some women were examined by a doctor on admission	15	13	13	10
All women were examined by a doctor on admission	5	4	4	4
Other	2	3	4	2
No answer	—	—	4	4
Total	100 (260)	100 (357)	100 (418)	100 (300)

Source: compiled by the authors.

tocinon infusion; and whether to do an episiotomy. Respondents were asked whether the decision was made by a midwife, by a doctor, or determined by a unit policy. The decision for which midwives were most likely to be responsible was whether to do an episiotomy; this was the case in approximately 90% of periods of labour ward experience undertaken by respondents. Deciding when to rupture membranes was the midwife's responsibility in approximately two-thirds of periods of labour ward experience, and this proportion fell to just over 50% for deciding whether to use a continuous monitoring machine. The decision as to when to carry out vaginal examinations was made by the midwife in just over half the periods of experience undertaken in the course of first posts. In those instances in which decisions about vaginal examinations, rupturing membranes and using a continuous monitoring machine were **not** made by midwives, they were more likely to be the subject of a unit policy than an individual doctor's decision. Accelerating labour with a syntocinon infusion was usually decided upon by a doctor and particularly when the respondent was in a first post.

These findings are very similar to those obtained in our earlier research (Robinson *et al.*, 1983) and so it seems that midwives' responsibilities for decision making in labour did not increase substantially during the course of the 1980s. The main difference was an increase in the likelihood that midwives would make the decision as to whether a continuous monitoring machine should be used (37% of respondents in the 1979 study and just over 50% of periods of experience in this study).

Postnatal care. Two questions were asked about the division of responsibility between midwives and medical staff for care of normal women during that part of the postnatal period spent in hospital: first, frequency of examination by medical staff; second, responsibility for deciding whether women were fit to be discharged home. Findings in Table 8.10 show that many midwives were working in situations in which medical staff also examined women routinely and in some instances on a daily basis. (Figures are shown only for those periods of postnatal experience that were based in hospital.) As well as being qualified to assess the health of the postnatal woman, midwives are also qualified to decide on their own

Table 8.10 Frequency with which normal women are examined by a doctor in the postnatal period (Phase 2 data)

Frequency with which normal women are examined by a doctor in the postnatal period	Periods of postnatal experience in which situation applied			
	In first posts held by		In subsequent posts held by	
	1979 cohort, %	1983 cohort, %	1979 cohort, %	1983 cohort, %
Not unless referred by a midwife	45	54	49	48
Routinely once or twice during their stay	40	35	35	36
Daily	12	7	9	7
Other situation	2	4	6	8
Total	100	100	100	100
	(250)	(359)	(302)	(232)

Source: compiled by the authors.

responsibility when she is fit to be discharged home. In the majority of periods of postnatal experience undertaken by respondents, however, this decision was made jointly by midwives **and** medical staff, and not by the midwife alone.

Division of responsibility and satisfaction. Findings on division of responsibility between midwives and medical staff for normal maternity care during the years 1979 to 1986, show a very similar picture to the one that emerged from our 1979 national survey of the profession, namely that many midwives work in settings in which medical staff are involved in decisions which midwives are qualified to make on their own responsibility. In relation to each period of clinical experience that they had undertaken midwives were asked how satisfied they were with the division of responsibility between themselves and medical staff. Findings for both the 1979 and the 1983 cohorts show that midwives were most likely to be satisfied when they are able to make decisions on their own responsibility and least likely to be satisfied when these were made by medical staff (details in Robinson *et al.*, 1992). Data on the extent to which medical involvement in normal maternity care was cited as a reason for leaving midwifery were obtained at Phases 2 and 3 and are discussed in the final section along with other findings on reasons for leaving.

Continuing professional development. Respondents were asked about several aspects of continuing professional development; findings for those relating to opportunities for in-service education and satisfaction with support and feedback from senior colleagues are included in this chapter.

Opportunities for in-service education. In Phase 2 all participants were asked whether, since qualifying as midwives, they had attended any in-service courses relevant to midwifery. These courses were defined as those organized by the respondent's hospital or employing authority, but which received no nationally recognized certificate; statutory refresher courses were specifically excluded. Less than half had in fact attended an in-service course; 41% of both cohorts. Comparison with other studies shows that this is a larger proportion than that found by McCrea (1989) but smaller than those found by Sugarman (1988) and Clarke and Rees (1989). All respondents were asked if they felt there was a need for greater provision of in-service courses for midwives, whether or not they themselves had attended a course. Over 70% of those respondents who had attended in-service courses and over 70% of those who had **not** done so perceived a need for greater provision of such courses. This finding indicates the importance attached to continuing education by midwives and supports those of other studies (Maclean, 1980; McCrea, 1989; Clarke and Rees, 1989).

Respondents who had attended in-service courses were asked to specify the main topics of each course attended and all respondents were asked to specify the topics that they would like to see addressed at future courses. Findings revealed some interesting differences between the frequency of topics of courses taken and those desired in future. Management courses had been taken by just over a third of each group but desired in future by less than 10%. Very few respondents had attended courses concerned with clinical updating (8% of the 1979 group and 1% of the 1983); this, however, was the topic listed by far the most frequently as desired in the future, by just over half of both groups of respondents. This accords with findings from other studies in which midwives have been asked what topics they would like included in future courses (Maclean, 1980; Parnaby, 1987; Clarke and Rees, 1989). This is perhaps not surprising given the rapid developments in the management of childbirth and the new policies and procedures with which midwives need to become familiar. Moreover, the research literature on continuing education for nurses similarly reveals an emphasis on clinical practice topics when respondents are asked for their views about future course content (Barriball *et al.* 1992).

Midwives' satisfaction with the provision of in-service education in each midwifery post held since qualification is shown in Table 8.11. A 5 point rating scale was provided (1 = very dissatisfied to 5 = very satisfied) and the option of not applicable, was included when appropriate. A mid point (3) of 'neither satisfied or dissatisfied', was included so that respon-

Table 8.11 Satisfaction with the provision of in-service education (Phase 2 data)

Satisfaction ratings	Posts held by			
	1979 cohort		1983 cohort	
	First, %	Subsq., %	First, %	Subsq., %
Very dissatisfied	14	9	13	13
Fairly dissatisfied	34	25	27	22
Neither satisfied or dissatisfied	18	20	16	16
Fairly satisfied	23	27	30	31
Very satisfied	6	12	9	11
No answer	8	8	5	8
Total number of posts held	319	514	431	379

Source: compiled by the authors.

dents who were not satisfied, were not forced to express dissatisfaction. Although the figures do not reach a majority, they do indicate a substantial degree of dissatisfaction with the provision of in-service education. These figures are consistent with other findings on in-service education from this project; namely less than half of the respondents having attended a course, and 70% saying that there should be greater provision.

Support and feedback for midwives. As the UKCC has recently reiterated, regular feedback on work from senior colleagues is recognized as important for professional development and particularly for newly registered practitioners (United Kingdom Central Council, 1990). Respondents in this study were asked therefore to rate their satisfaction with feedback received during each midwifery post held since qualification (the rating scale was the same as that for provision of in-service education). Although respondents were more likely to be satisfied than dissatisfied with feedback, nonetheless there was a substantial minority of posts for which this was not the case. For 27% of first posts held by the 1979 cohort and 31% held by the 1983, respondents had been 'very' or 'fairly' dissatisfied with feedback, and corresponding figures for subsequent posts were 21% and 22% for the two cohorts respectively.

Conditions of service. Satisfaction with conditions of service, particularly pay, staffing levels and flexible hours has been identified as a major factor in decisions to leave health service work (see page 183) and consequently some information was obtained on this issue at both Phases 2 and 3 of this study.

Satisfaction ratings with conditions. At Phase 2 respondents were asked, in relation to each of the midwifery posts that they had held, about their satisfaction with levels of pay, fitting home and/or social life around hours of work, catering and car parking facilities for staff and the availability of affordable accommodation. Although catering and car parking facilities have not featured predominantly in the literature on conditions of service, pilot work for this study showed that both were the subject of concern to midwives.

As shown in Table 8.12 (page 216) satisfaction was least likely to be expressed with levels of pay, particularly by the 1983 cohort. Satisfaction was most likely to be expressed with fitting social and/or home life around hours of duty. As with other aspects of working conditions, however, the 1983 cohort were less likely to be satisfied than the 1979 cohort.

Views on staffing levels. Adequacy of staffing levels has long been of concern to midwives (see page 177). As these can vary from one clinical area to another, respondents were asked whether, in their opinion, there had been enough midwives on duty to provide care in each of the periods of clinical experience that they had undertaken. Findings show that the postnatal period was the aspect of care most likely to be regarded as short

Table 8.12 Satisfaction with aspects of working conditions (Phase 2 data)

Aspects of working conditions

Satisfaction ratings	Level of pay				Fitting social and/or home life around hours of duty				Catering facilities for staff				Transport facilities to and from work				Car parking facilities			
	Posts held by				Posts held by				Posts held by				Posts held by				Posts held by			
	1979 cohort		1983 cohort		1979 cohort		1983 cohort		1979 cohort		1983 cohort		1979 cohort		1983 cohort		1979 cohort		1983 cohort	
	1st, %	Sbq, %	1st, %	Sbq, %	1st, %	Sbq, %	1st, %	Sbq, %	1st, %	Sbq, %	1st, %	Sbq, %	1st, %	Sbq, %	1st, %	Sbq, %	1st, %	Sbq, %	1st, %	Sbq, %
Very dissatisfied	21	14	37	20	1	3	5	6	11	14	19	20	11	5	14	8	15	20	25	27
Fairly dissatisfied	32	27	39	29	14	12	19	14	19	20	25	25	12	9	7	5	22	17	27	21
Neither satisfied nor dissatisfied	20	17	13	16	19	12	23	14	19	20	16	14	27	23	29	18	9	7	7	9
Fairly satisfied	21	29	10	22	46	42	43	43	34	33	30	25	29	34	25	40	28	30	27	25
Very satisfied	4	12	—	9	15	28	8	19	13	12	8	11	18	24	23	22	25	24	14	14
No answer	1	2	1	4	3	3	2	3	5	2	3	5	2	5	2	7	1	3	1	5
Total number of posts	319	514	431	379	319	514	431	379	319	420	431	322	171	231	214	182	246	387	366	293

Source: compiled by the authors.

Table 8.13 Views on whether there were enough midwives on duty to provide care (Phase 2 data)

Clinical area	Periods of clinical experience for which respondents said that there were not enough midwives on duty to provide care			
	In first posts held by		*In subsequent posts held by*	
	1979 cohort, %	*1983 cohort, %*	*1979 cohort, %*	*1983 cohort, %*
Antenatal clinic	46	50	27	30
	(75/164)	(123/247)	(65/239)	(57/192)
Labour and delivery	39	54	38	45
	(102/260)	(194/357)	(160/418)	(135/300)
Postnatal care	68	80	50	56
	(178/262)	(308/384)	(176/355)	(149/266)
Special and intensive baby care unit	28	26	39	39
	(31/112)	(36/138)	(46/117)	(30/77)

Source: compiled by the authors.

staffed, and particularly so when respondents were in their first post (Table 8.13).

Views on the Clinical Grading Review. One of the advantages of longitudinal studies is that they can respond to new events that may affect people's decisions and, as described earlier, the Clinical Grading Review was such an event in the case of the midwifery profession. We therefore included a question in the 1989 questionnaire that asked respondents about their satisfaction with their grade, and what effect, if any, it had had on their intentions to remain in midwifery. Those not practising as midwives in 1989 were asked what effect, if any, the Clinical Grading Review had had on their intentions with regard to returning to midwifery.

Staff midwives were the group most likely to have been dissatisfied with their grade. Of the Phase 3 respondents, 115 were working as staff midwives; 76% (87) had been given an E grade, and 76% (66) of these said that they should have been given an F grade. Hospital sisters were much less likely to be dissatisfied than staff midwives; most had been given a G grade, with which over three-quarters were satisfied. Similarly, all but three of the community midwives had a G grade, and 71% of these were satisfied. All the midwifery managers, and all but two of the midwifery tutors were satisfied with their grade – usually H for the former and I for the latter.

Respondents who were dissatisfied with their grading were asked what effect, if any, it had had on their intentions to remain in midwifery; half of the 1979 respondents in this category and 59% of their 1983 counterparts mentioned leaving either now or in the future. All respondents were invited to comment on their grading whether or not they were satisfied. Sixty-five per cent of the 1979 cohort and 96% of the 1983 cohort made negative comments about the effects of the Clinical Grading Review on midwifery, even though many of them were satisfied with the grade that they personally had been awarded. In descending order of frequency these comments were lack of recognition of midwives' responsibilities, detrimental/demoralizing effect on the profession, dissatisfaction with grades awarded to colleagues, lack of recognition of the teaching element in midwifery and setting midwife against midwife. Those who were not practising midwifery in 1989 were asked what effect, if any, the Clinical Grading Review had had on their intentions to return. Responses show that the 1983 cohort were much more likely than the 1979 to say it had made a return less likely: 57% compared with 38%. Taken together, the above findings indicate that the implementation of the clinical grading review was not welcomed by midwives.

Combining working as a midwife with family responsibilities. At the time that they qualified as midwives, the majority of both cohorts were single women in their twenties. Just over half were under 25 years, a further third were aged between 25 and 30 years, and only a small proportion (9%) were over 30. Not surprisingly findings from Phase 2 (1986) and Phase 3 (1989) showed a steady increase in the proportion of respondents who were married, had started families and had taken breaks from work for pregnancy and periods of childcare. Members of the two cohorts who were not practising midwifery at the time of Phase 3 were asked to say why this was the case. A wide range of reasons were cited, but the one occurring most frequently was leaving to have a baby and/or look after children (32% of the 1979 respondents and 37% of the 1983). Twenty-nine per cent of the 1979 cohort said that they left because they were unable to find a post with hours which they could combine with family responsibilities. For the 1983 cohort, the percentage to give this reason was smaller (18%); they had only been qualified for six years by this time, not ten like their 1979 counterparts and so were less likely to have reached the point of having a family and planning to return to work.

As outlined on page 183, increasing attention in recent years has focused on breaks that women have in their employment for childcare purposes and on the effect of these on retention and individual career development. To add to knowledge about this event in relation to midwives, the Phase 3 questionnaire included a number of questions about any breaks in employment since qualification from which the respondent had subsequently returned to a midwifery post. Between them the 1979 cohort had taken a total of 129 periods of absence from midwifery; the corresponding figure for the 1983 cohort was 157.

One of the strategies identified as increasing the likelihood of a return to work after a break is continued contact with members of the employing authority during the break (Department of Health, 1988). Consequently in relation to each period of absence in which they had continued to live in the same area, all respondents were asked if their employers had kept in touch with them about returning to paid employment. Almost all respondents had in fact continued to live in the same area. During half of these breaks employers had kept in touch about job opportunities (62/124 for the 1979 cohort and 75/151 for the 1983). In just over half of those breaks in which employers had not kept in touch, respondents said that they would have liked some contact (57% and 59% for the two cohorts respectively).

Employers were much less likely to have provided facilities for midwives to keep in touch about developments in their professional field, than they were to have kept in touch about job opportunities. Findings showed that contact about the former had occurred in only 6% of the periods of absence taken by the 1979 cohort and in 9% of those taken by the 1983. For those periods in which no facilities for keeping in touch had been provided, in just over half (52%) of those taken by the 1979 cohort, respondents said that they would have liked to have had some; the corresponding figure for the 1983 cohort was 64%. In summary this study indicated that the majority of midwives taking a break for childcare wish to keep in touch with professional developments but, up until 1989, little provision in this respect appeared to have been made.

As described on page 184, several studies have shown that those nurses with an unbroken employment record advance up the hierarchy of posts faster than those who have had breaks, particularly those who returned to a part-time post. Findings from this study (Robinson *et al.*, 1992; Robinson, 1993) also show that continuous practice, unbroken by periods of childcare, is associated with faster progress up the hierarchy of midwifery posts.

Reasons for leaving midwifery and views on retention

Findings from this longitudinal study of midwives' careers show that although the majority did practise midwifery for a while, less than half were working as midwives three years after qualification (see Table 8.2, page 196). Midwives most likely to stay were those who had intended to make a career in the profession, although the proportion of this group in practice did decrease over time (see Table 8.5, page 202). All those who had held at least one midwifery post provided information about four main aspects of life as a midwife: level of responsibility for clinical decision making, continuing professional development, conditions of service and combining work with family commitments. The final set of findings in this chapter are concerned first with the extent to which aspects of these four areas were cited as reasons to leave, and secondly with views about the relative importance of these aspects in encouraging retention.

At both Phases 2 and 3, those respondents not in practice were asked why they had left. They were presented with a list of possible reasons that had been identified from the literature, from our earlier work on the role of the midwife (Robinson *et al.*, 1983; Robinson, 1985a, 1985b, 1985c, 1989a) and from the pilot study for this project. They were asked to ring all the reasons that had contributed to their decision to leave, and then to indicate the five of these that had been the most important. Since findings for Phases 2 and 3 were similar; only those for the latter are presented (Table 8.14, page 222).

Looking first at the 1979 cohort then the reason cited most frequently in the first five was leaving to have a baby/look after children, and this was followed by being unable to find a post with hours that could be combined with family responsibilities. The 1983 cohort were as likely as the 1979 to cite the former reason; but less likely to cite the latter; they were younger and so probably less likely to be returning to midwifery after a period of absence for child care. Dissatisfaction with staff shortages was the aspect of conditions of service most likely to be given as a main reason for leaving, and for the 1979 cohort this was closely followed by a dislike of working unsocial hours. Of the professional issues listed, increased involvement of medical staff in normal maternity care was cited the most frequently and for approximately one-fifth of both cohorts was included as one of their five main reasons for leaving. Some respondents had felt strongly enough about personnel issues to cite them as a main reason for leaving, albeit less than one-fifth in each case.

All respondents, those in practice as well as those who had left, were asked for their views on what might encourage midwives to stay in or return to the profession. As in the previous question they were presented with a list of factors that had been developed from the literature, from our earlier work and from the project's pilot study. Respondents were asked to ring all those factors that they felt were relevant and to indicate the five that they felt were the most important. Again the findings were similar for both phases and so the Phase 3 findings only are presented here (Table 8.15, page 224).

Over 80% of both cohorts ringed more flexibility in working hours and crèche facilities. A similar proportion of the 1983 cohort ringed increased levels of pay and better staffing levels; the corresponding figures for the

1979 cohort were slightly lower at 77%. These four factors were also the most likely to be included in respondents' list of the five most important, although the order differed for the two cohorts. The 1979 cohort were equally likely to be concerned about flexible working hours as they were about pay and staffing, and this probably reflects the fact that they personally were more likely than the 1983 cohort to have children of school age. Issues concerned with professional responsibility and development were ringed by a substantial proportion of both cohorts, although these did not reach a majority for inclusion in the five most important factors.

Looking back at the findings obtained on the four aspects of life as a midwife, the study provided evidence that not all midwifery posts enabled midwives to practise with the degree of clinical responsibility for which they were qualified, and not all posts provided midwives with adequate opportunities for personal professional development. Findings also showed that both these factors were a source of dissatisfaction for some respondents. However, neither dissatisfaction with professional responsibilities nor professional development were as likely to be cited as a reason for leaving, or as important for retention, as dissatisfaction with conditions of service or problems in combining family life with work as a midwife.

CONCLUSION

This study adopted a 'broad brush' approach in that information was obtained from a large sample of midwives on a wide range of issues relevant to retention in the profession. In this final section we draw together the main themes from the findings obtained to date and look at future needs in relation to research on careers.

The main findings from the project

Firstly, the original impetus for the study was to ascertain whether extending post-registration midwifery training from 12 to 18 months had any impact on subsequent retention. Findings on intentions at qualification (Table 8.2) and at three and six years subsequently (Tables 8.3 and 8.4) demonstrated that the effect was minimal. This contributed to the decision to introduce pre-registration midwifery education programmes, since merely extending the length of post-registration programmes was not adequately addressing the problem of retention.

Secondly, the study demonstrated the power of a longitudinal panel design in analysing movements and change over time at the individual as well as at the aggregate level. For example we were able to show the extent to which individual intentions were subsequently translated into practice (Table 8.5) the extent to which career intentions were accurately recollected (Table 8.6) and the extent to which individuals moved in and

Table 8.14 Reasons for having left midwifery (Phase 3 data)

Reasons	1979 cohort (n = 133)		1983 cohort (n = 176)	
	% listing reason in 1st five	% listing reason	% listing reason in 1st five	% listing reason
Family				
Left to have a baby/look after children	29	32	31	37
Unable to find a post with hours which I could combine with family responsibilities	28	29	16	18
Conditions of service				
Dissatisfaction with staff shortages	23	30	23	35
Dissatisfaction with level of pay	14	22	12	22
Dislike having to work unsocial hours (evenings, weekends)	20	26	11	22
Dislike having to work night duty for periods of time	15	22	11	20
Lack of reasonably priced accommodation	—	1	1	1
Thought health visiting would provide better hours and pay	12	20	12	16
Thought promotion prospects better in nursing	4	4	2	4
Professional issues				
Dissatisfaction with erosion of midwife's role because of increased involvement of medical staff in normal maternity care	18	26	22	28
Dissatisfied because not able to use my midwifery knowledge/skills fully	14	22	20	27

Dissatisfied with too much technological intervention	11	19	14	18
Dissatisfied with lack of opportunity to provide continuity of care	9	16	18	26
Did not enjoy the work	8	9	4	4
Dissatisfied with standards of patient care in midwifery	14	19	12	16
Dissatisfied with health service generally	10	14	10	15
Lack of appreciation from patients	1	2	3	5
Do not feel confident enough to practise	4	8	8	8
Anxious about ability to work on labour ward	5	10	11	18
Fear of litigation	8	10	8	12
Thought health visiting would provide better job satisfaction	14	20	11	14
Personnel issues				
Put off midwifery by:				
attitude of managers to sisters and staff midwives	19	28	15	22
senior managers out of touch with problems of clinical practice	12	22	13	22
lack of support from colleagues during stressful times at work	13	16	15	23

Source: compiled by the authors.

Table 8.15 Views on factors thought to be important in encouraging midwives to stay in and/or return to midwifery (Phase 3 data)

	1979 cohort (n = 288)		1983 cohort (n = 407)	
	% listing reason in 1st five	*% listing reason*	*% listing reason in 1st five*	*% listing reason*
Family commitments				
More flexibility in working hours to fit round family commitments	63	83	61	82
Crèche facilities	51	83	54	87
Setting up bank schemes	21	51	13	52
Conditions of service				
Increased levels of pay	63	77	68	86
Increased pay for living in high cost areas	8	30	9	34
Better staffing levels	58	77	64	86
Better accommodation facilities provided by health authority	4	19	3	19
Car parking facilities	1	21	1	18
Professional responsibility				
Less involvement of medical staff in decision making in normal maternity care	35	62	40	66
More opportunities to provide continuity of care	31	63	30	66
Less technological intervention in childbirth	14	43	18	45

Professional development

More support for newly qualified midwives from senior staff	37	62	35	67
Better promotion prospects	28	51	30	59
Increased provision of in-service education	17	51	15	58
More refresher courses for updating of skills	27	49	15	45
A management structure that ensures midwifery services are managed by midwives	28	63	23	67

Source: compiled by the authors.

out of midwifery in the years after qualification (Table 8.7). The findings, which are important to an understanding of retention, showed that those most likely to stay were those who wanted to make a career in the profession, and that those who left for other occupations were unlikely to return. Such findings could not have been obtained by means of single or repeated cross-sectional surveys.

Thirdly, the study provided information on four areas that have featured prominently in the literature on the experience of working as a midwife. These included the extent to which midwives are able to deploy their skills in the care of childbearing women; opportunities for aspects of individual professional development, satisfaction with conditions of service and the experience of combining family life with work as a midwife. A mixture of positive and negative experiences were revealed in respect of each of these areas, but all merit further and more detailed investigation.

Fourthly, an attempt was made to identify those factors that seemed most relevant to retention. Certainly the study showed that a definite intention to make a career in midwifery was a good predictor of subsequent retention. Other findings showed that concerns about pay and staffing levels and the availability of flexible hours to combine with family life were more likely to have an adverse effect on retention than inadequate opportunities for deployment of skills and individual professional development (Tables 8.14 and 8.15). Issues of pay, staffing levels and flexible hours can be remedied, if desired, by relatively straight forward policy decisions at national and local level. The question of deployment of skill is a more complex issue to resolve since it involves the interrelationship of the role of midwives with that of medical staff.

It could be that those midwives who are dissatisfied with the interrelationship of their role with that of medical staff leave the profession and indeed this study provided some indication that some midwives turned to health visiting as it offered them a greater degree of autonomy of practice. Such a development might leave enough midwives to staff the service, albeit that they were in the main those who were satisfied with exercising a lesser degree of responsibility than that for which midwives are qualified. This is certainly an area which requires greater depth of investigation than was possible by means of the methods adopted for this study. It will also be of particular importance in the context of the careers of those who have opted specifically to practise midwifery by means of the new pre-registration courses.

Directions for future research

Three phases of data collection have now been completed in the course of this longitudinal study of two cohorts of midwives. The main research questions have now been answered, namely that extending the length of post-registration midwifery training had little effect on retention. There is little point therefore in continuing to try and keep in touch with all members of both cohorts to ask about employment in midwifery, particularly those who have never practised since qualifying. However, as the existing phases of data collection have demonstrated, much information relevant to retention and to the practice of midwifery has been obtained which had no relationship to the type of course followed. The two cohorts include several hundred midwives, many of whom have now reached relatively senior positions in the profession and maintaining contact with them affords an opportunity to monitor experience and views in relation to these issues and to respond to new ones that may arise. Consequently plans are in progress to devise two secondary cohorts from the original ones, which comprise those members who are currently practising midwifery or have recently done so.

As well as providing information of relevance to the midwifery profession, the study described in this chapter has also been of importance methodologically. As noted earlier in this chapter longitudinal studies are few and far between in health service research, largely because of their high initial costs, and the complexity of data collection and analysis that they entail. The experience that we gained in the course of studying midwives' careers over time has been used to develop a substantial programme of Department of Health funded longitudinal studies into the careers of registered general nurses, registered mental nurses and nursing graduates. In due course the programme will also include studies of the careers of Project 2000 diplomates. As far as midwives are concerned the most pressing need now is for a longitudinal study to compare the careers of a cohort selected from those qualifying from pre-registration courses with a cohort of those qualifying at the same time from post-registration courses. A longitudinal comparative study was necessary to evaluate effects of lengthening the post-registration course and the same design is required if any conclusions are to be drawn in due course about the impact on the profession of pre-registration midwifery education.

ACKNOWLEDGEMENTS

We should like to thank the following: the Department of Health for funding the project; Josephine Golden who was responsible for much of the work involved in Phase 1 of the project; Keith Jacka for assistance with computing; Carolyn Dereky for administration of the questionnaire mailings; Gian Brown for typing the manuscript, and all the midwives who completed our questionnaires.

REFERENCES

Allison, P.D. (1984) *Event history analysis: regression for longitudinal event data.* Sage University Paper series on qualitative application in the social sciences. Sage Publications, Beverly Hills and London.

Armitage, P.O. (1971) *Statistical methods in medical research*. Blackwell, Oxford.

Balch, B. (1982) Teacher training for midwives: an investigation of the Midwife Teacher's Diploma course 1975–79 at the Royal College of Midwives, London, with special reference to teaching practice. In *Research and The Midwife Conference Proceedings for 1981*. Nursing Research Unit King's College, London University.

Barnett, Z. (1979) The changing pattern of maternity care and the future role of the midwife. *Midwives Chronicle and Nursing Notes*, **92**(1102), 381–4.

Barriball, K.L., While, A. and Norman, I. (1992) Continuing professional education for qualified nurses: A review of the literature. *Journal of Advanced Nursing*, **17**, 1129–40.

Bent, E.A. (1982) The growth and development of midwifery. In P. Allan and M. Jolley (eds) *Nursing, midwifery and health visiting since 1900*. Faber & Faber, London.

Brain, M. (1979) Observations by a midwife. In *Report of a day conference on the reduction of perinatal mortality and morbidity*. Children's Committee and Department of Health and Social Security, HMSO, London.

Brooking, J., Terrey, C. and Howard, J. (1989) A longitudinal study of nurse graduates from King's College, London University. In J. Wilson-Barnett and S. Robinson (eds) *Directions in nursing research*. Scutari Press, London.

Buchan, J. and Stock, J. (1990) *Midwives' careers and grading. IMS Report 201*. Institute of Manpower Studies, University of Sussex, Brighton.

Butler, N.R. and Bonham, D.G. (1963) *Perinatal mortality*. Churchill Livingstone, Edinburgh.

Carr-Hill, R.A. and Macdonald, D.K.I. (1973) Problems in the analysis of life histories. In P. Halmos (ed.) *Stochastic Processes in Sociology. Sociological Review Monograph No 19*. University of Keele.

Central Midwives Board (1957) *Annual Report of the Board for the Year Ending 31.3.57*. Hymns Ancient & Modern Ltd, Norwich.

Central Midwives Board (1977) *Letter from Board to midwifery training schools, regional and area nursing officers regarding the decision to extend the 12 month training to 18 months*. Central Midwives Board, London.

Central Midwives Board (1983) *Financial report on the work of the Board*. Hymns Ancient & Modern Ltd, Suffolk.

Central Midwives Board for Scotland, Northern Ireland Council for Nurses and Midwives, An Bord Altranais, Central Midwives Board (1983) *The role of the midwife*. Hymns Ancient & Modern Ltd, Suffolk.

Chalmers, I. and Richards, M. (1977) Intervention and causal inference in obstetric practice. In T. Chard and M. Richards (eds) *Benefits and hazards of the new obstetrics*. Spastics International Medical Publications, London.

Chamberlain, G., Philipp, E., Howlett, B. and Master, K. (1978) *British births 1970. Vol. 2 Obstetric care*. William Heinemann, London.

Clarke, J. and Rees, C. (1989) The midwife and continuing education. *Midwives Chronicle and Nursing Notes*, **102**(1220), 288–90.

Cohen, L. and Manion, L. (1980) *Research methods in education*. Croom Helm, London.

Corby, S. (1991) When two halves make total sense. *Health Service Journal*, **101**(5621), 20–21.

Davies, C. and Rosser, J. (1986) *Processes of discrimination: a report on a study of women working in the NHS*. Department of Health and Social Security, London.

Department of Health and Social Security (1972) *Report of the Committee on Nursing*. (Chairman: A. Briggs) HMSO, London.

Department of Health (1988) *The way ahead: Report of the career development project group*. Nursing Division, Department of Health, London.

Department of Health and Social Security (1984) *Study of Hospital-based midwives*. A report by Central Management Services. DHSS, London.

Dex, S. (1990) Occupational mobility over women's lifetime. In G. Payne and P. Abbot (eds) *The social mobility of women: beyond male mobility models*. The Falmer Press, Basingstoke.

Dex, S. (1991) Life and work history analyses. In S. Dex (ed.) *Life and work history analyses: qualitative and quantitative developments*. Sociological Review Mongraph No 37. Routledge, London.

Douglas, J.W.B. and Blomfield, J.M. (1973) The reliability of longitudinal surveys. In J.B. McKinley (ed.) *Research methods in health care: A selection of articles from the Milbank Fund Quarterly*. Prodist, New York.

English National Board (1990) *Framework for continuing professional education and training for nurses, midwives and health visitors*. ENB, London.

Equal Opportunities Commission (1991) *Equality management: women's employment in the NHS*. EOC, Manchester.

Garcia, J. and Garforth, S. (1989) Labour and delivery routines in English consultant maternity units. *Midwifery*, **5**(4), 155–62.

Garcia, J. and Garforth, S. (1991) Midwifery policies and policy-making. In S. Robinson and A.M. Thomson (eds) *Midwives – Research and childbirth. Vol 11*. Chapman & Hall, London.

Garforth, S. and Garcia, J. (1987) Admitting – a weakness or a strength? Routine admission of a woman in labour. *Midwifery*, **3**(2), 10–24.

Garforth, S. and Garcia, J. (1989) Hospital admission practices. In I. Chalmers, M. Enkin and M. Keirse (eds) *Effective care in pregnancy and childbirth*. Oxford University Press, Oxford.

Golden, J. (1980) Midwifery training: The views of newly qualified midwives. *Midwives Chronicle and Nursing Notes*, **93**(1109), 190–94.

Goldstein, H. (1979) *The design and analysis of longitudinal studies; their role in the measurement of change*. Academic Press, London.

Government Statistical Service (1980) *1973–76 Hospital in-patient enquiry – maternity tables Series MB4 No 8*. HMSO, London.

Hockey, L. (1975) *Women in nursing: a descriptive study*. Hodder & Stoughton, London.

Hoinville, G., Jowell, R. *et al.* (1978) *Survey research practice*. Heinemann Educational Books, London.

Hurst, K., Jones, R., Pullyblank, R. and Hickling, D. (1990) Retaining staff through crèche provision. *Nursing Times*, **86**(24), 54–5.

Hutt, R. (1985) *Chief officer career profiles: a study of the backgrounds, training and career experiences of regional and district nursing officers.* Institute of Manpower Studies, University of Sussex, Brighton.

Joshi, H. (ed.) (1989) *The changing population of Britain.* Blackwell Press, Oxford.

Kent, J. and Maggs, C. (1982) *An evaluation of pre-registration midwifery education in England: a research project for the Department of Health. Working Paper 1 – Research design.* Maggs Research Associates, Bath.

Kilty, J.M. and Potter, F.W. (1975) *The Midwife Teacher's Diploma.* Research Project. University of Surrey, Guildford.

Lathlean, J. (1987) *Job sharing a ward sisters post.* Riverside Health Authority, Ashdale Press, Peterborough.

Laurent, C. (1989) Born again nurses. *Nursing Times*, **85**(23), 46–7.

Law, B. and Ward, R. (1981) Is career development motivated? In A. Watts, D. Super and J. Kidd (eds) *Career development in Britain: some contributions to theory and practice.* Hobsons Press, Cambridge.

Maclean, G. (1980) *A study of the educational needs of midwives in Wales and how they may be met.* West Glamorgan Health Authority.

Mander, R. (1989) 'The best laid schemes . . .': An evaluation of the extension of midwifery training in Scotland. *International Journal of Nursing Studies*, **26**(1), 27–41.

Marsh, C. and Gershunny, J. (1991) Handling work history data in standard statistical packages. In S. Dex (ed.) *Life and work history analyses: qualitative and quantitative developments.* Routledge, London.

Martin, J.P. and MacKean, J. (1988) *Can we keep nurses in the health service? A study of nurse retention in two health districts.* Department of Sociology and Social Policy, University of Southampton.

Martin, J. and Roberts, C. (1984) *Women and employment: a lifetime perspective.* Department of Employment/Office of Population Censuses and Surveys, HMSO, London.

McCrea, H. (1989) Motivation for continuing education in midwifery. *Midwifery*, **5**(3), 134–45.

Midgely, C. (1993) Continuing education for non-practising midwives. In A. Thomson and S. Robinson (eds) *Research and the Midwife Conference Proceedings for 1992.* Department of Nursing Studies, University of Manchester.

Ministry of Health (1929) *Report of the Departmental Committee on the training and employment of midwives.* HMSO, London.

Ministry of Health (1959) *Report of the Maternity Services Committee.* HMSO, London.

Ministry of Health, Department of Health for Scotland, Ministry of Labour and National Service (1947) *Report on the Working Party on the recruitment and training of nurses* (Chairman: Sir Robert Wood). HMSO, London.

Ministry of Health, Department of Health for Scotland, Ministry of Labour and National Service (1949) *Report of the Working Party on Midwives* (Chairman: Mrs M. Stocks). HMSO, London.

Moores, B., Singh, B.B. and Tun, A. (1983) An analysis of the factors which impinge on a nurse's decision to enter, stay in, leave or re-enter the nursing profession. *Journal of Advanced Nursing*, **8**, 227–35.

O'Byrne, J. (1989) Working flexi-time. *Nursing Standard*, **3**(38), 16.
Owen, H. and Robinson, S. (1990) Researching midwives' careers. In A.M. Thomson and S. Robinson (eds) *Proceedings for 1989 Research and the Midwife Conference*. Department of Nursing Studies, University at Manchester.
Owen, H. and Robinson, S. (1992) Working as a midwife: opportunities and constraints. In A.M. Thomson and S. Robinson (eds) *Proceedings for 1991, Research and the Midwife Conference*. Department of Nursing Studies, University of Manchester.
Parnaby, C. (1987) Surveying the opinions of midwives regarding the curriculum content of refresher courses. *Midwifery*, **3**(3), 133–42.
Percival, R.C. (1970) Management of normal labour. *The Practitioner*, **1221**, 204.
Price Waterhouse (1988) *Nurse retention and recruitment: a matter of priority*. Price Waterhouse, London.
Radford, N. and Thompson, A. (1988) *Direct entry: a preparation for practice*. University of Surrey, Guildford.
Ramsden, D. and Radwanski, P. (1963) *Some aspects of the work of the midwife*. Dan Mason Nursing Research Committee of the National Florence Nightingale Memorial Committee, London.
Renfrew, M. and Simmons, M. (1991) *MIRIAD: Midwifery Research Database*. National Perinatal Epidemiology Unit, Oxford.
Robinson, K. (1992) The nursing workforce; aspects of inequality. In J. Robinson, S. Gray and R. Elkan (eds) *Policy issues in nursing*. Open University Press, Milton Keynes.
Robinson, S. (1985a) Normal maternity care: whose responsibility? *British Journal of Obstetrics and Gynaecology*, **92**(1), 1–3.
Robinson, S. (1985b) Midwives, obstetricians and general practitioners: the need for role clarification. *Midwifery*, **1**(2), 102–113.
Robinson, S. (1985c) Maternity care: a duplication of resources. *Journal of the Royal College of General Practitioners*, **35**, 346–7.
Robinson, S. (1986a) Career intentions of newly qualified midwives. *Midwifery*, **2**(1), 25–36.
Robinson, S. (1986b) Midwifery training: the views of newly qualified midwives. *Nurse Education Today*, **6**(2), 49–59.
Robinson, S. (1986c) The 18 month training: what difference has it made? *Midwives Chronicle*, **99**(1177), 22–9.
Robinson, S. (1989a) Caring for childbearing women: the interrelationship between midwifery and medical responsibilities. In S. Robinson and A. Thomson (eds) *Midwives, Research and Childbirth Vol. 1*. Chapman & Hall, London.
Robinson, S. (1989b) The role of the midwife: opportunities and constraints. In M. Enkin, M. Keirse and I. Chalmers (eds) *Effective care in pregnancy and childbirth*. Oxford University Press, Oxford.
Robinson, S. (1990) Maintaining the independence of the midwifery profession: A continuing struggle. In J. Garcia, R. Kilpatrick and M. Richards (eds) *The politics of maternity care: services for childbearing women in twentieth-century Britain*. Clarendon Press, Oxford.
Robinson, S. (1991) Preparation for practice: the educational experiences and

career intentions of newly qualified midwives In S. Robinson and A. Thomson (eds) *Midwives Research and Childbirth Vol. 2.* Chapman & Hall, London.

Robinson, S. (1993) Combining work with caring for children: Findings from a longitudinal study of midwives' careers. *Midwifery*, **9**, 4.

Robinson, S., Golden, J. and Bradley, S. (1983) *A study of the role and reponsibilities of the midwife.* NERU report No 1. Nursing Education Research Unit, Kings College, London University.

Robinson, S. and Owen, H. (1989) Career intentions and career patterns of midwives. In J. Wilson-Barnett and S. Robinson (eds) *Directions in nursing research: ten years of progress at London University.* Scutari Press, London.

Robinson, S., Owen, H. and Jacka, K. (1992) *The midwives' career patterns project: Phases 1, 2 and 3.* Report to the Department of Health. Nursing Research Unit, King's College, London University.

Royal College of Midwives (1964) *Statement of Policy on the Maternity Services.* RCM, London.

Royal College of Midwives (1977) *Evidence to the Royal Commission on the National Health Service.* RCM, London.

Royal College of Nursing (1942) *Report of the Nursing Reconstruction Committee* (Chairman: Lord Horder). RCN, London.

Royal College of Nursing (1964) *A Reform of Nursing Education* (Chairman: Sir Harry Platt). RCN, London.

Royal College of Obstetricians and Gynaecologists (1944) *Report on a National Maternity Service.* RCOG, London.

Royal Commission on the Health Service (Chairman: Sir Alec Merrison) (1978) HMSO, London.

South Bank University (1992) *Midwifery Update Modules 1–9.* Distance Learning Centre South Bank University, London.

Standring, J. (1989) Return to practice courses. *Nursing Standard*, **3**(42), 42–5.

Stewart, A. (1981) The present state of midwifery training. *Midwife, Health Visitor and Community Nurse*, **17**(7), 270–72.

Sugarman, E. (1988) The case of the disappearing midwives. *Nursing Times*, **84**(8), 35–6.

Uncles, M.D. (1988) *Longitudinal data analysis: methods and applications.* Pion/Methuen, London.

United Kingdom Central Council for Nursing Midwifery and Health Visiting (1986) *Project 2000: a new preparation for practice.* UKCC, London.

United Kingdom Central Council for Nursing, Midwifery and Health Visiting (1990) *The report of the post-registration education and practice project.* UKCC, London.

Waite, R., Buchan, J. and Thomas, J. (1989) *Nurses in and out of work.* IMS Report 170. Institute of Manpower Studies, University of Sussex, Brighton.

Waterton, J. and Lievesley, D. (1986) *Attrition in a panel study of attitudes.* Paper available from: Social and Community Planning Research, London.

Winson, G. (1993) Career paths of nurse graduates. *Senior Nurse*, **10**(1), 50–55.

CHAPTER NINE

Midwifery training and employment decisions of midwives

Rosemary Mander

There are any number of ways in which the idea for a research project may be initiated. The study reported in this chapter, on the employment decisions of newly qualified midwives, originated in personal experience, when a midwife responsible for a small midwifery school was perturbed at the numbers lost to midwifery as soon as they qualified. This midwife's concern and her wish to investigate and, perhaps, offer a remedy were translated into a series of questions. These are described in this chapter, together with some of the methodological issues encountered in the study and the findings that emerged.

The study took place in Scotland during the period when post-registration midwifery education was extended from 12 to 18 months. Concern about retention after qualification was in fact one of the main reasons for introducing the longer course as it was hoped that a greater proportion of those who completed the longer course would remain in midwifery (Stewart, 1981). Consequently the study took the form of a comparison of a cohort of midwives who followed a 12 month course with a cohort who followed an 18 month course. A range of other changes that affected the profession were also taking place when the study was undertaken; these included reaction to a continuing decline in the midwife's level of responsibility, changes in women's expectations of the experience of childbirth, and the start of experimental schemes to enable men to qualify as midwives. At the time that the research was undertaken, the term 'midwifery training' was used rather than 'midwifery education'. This was reflected in the wording of the research instruments used and is retained here in the presentation of the project's methods and findings.

The aims of the research encompassed three main areas and were developed from the initial concern about retention of midwives and from a preliminary literature review.

1. To draw up a profile of student midwives in Scotland in order to describe who starts midwifery training in Scotland and why; to examine

the reasons for entering the course, the relationship of those reasons to employment intentions and whether change in intentions occurred during the course.

2. To study the potentially complex relationship between employment plans and actual employment (Vroom, 1964) in the context of retention in midwifery and in view of hopes and expectations concerning the longer course, to study its effect, if any, on planned and actual employment.

3. To examine factors influencing midwives' employment, particularly those associated with the course, in the hope that this might lead to recommendations for managers as to strategies that might increase retention in midwifery.

The design of the study, the content of the questionnaires and the interpretation of the findings were informed by a wide body of literature drawn from a variety of disciplines. Reviews of this literature have been included in a number of publications arising from the study and so are not included in this chapter. The areas include retention in midwifery (Mander, 1987b); related work on retention in nursing (Mander, 1987b); occupational socialization (Mander, 1989c); relationship between employment intentions and practice (Mander, 1989b), the relevance of occupational theory to women's careers (Mander, 1989a), and combining family responsibilities with work in the health service (Mander, 1989a). The structure of the chapter is as follows: first the need for evaluation of the extended midwifery course is discussed, followed by the methods employed in the study together with some of the problems that they raised. Selected findings are then presented together with a consideration of their implications for midwifery.

EVALUATING THE EXTENSION OF POST-REGISTRATION MIDWIFERY EDUCATION

A useful definition of evaluation is provided by Goldberg and Connelly (1982); 'assessing the worth or value of an object or activity'. Although evaluation is regarded by some planners as an integral component of the planning process (Bennett and Lumsdaine, 1975), the Central Midwives Board for Scotland's 'Guidelines for the extension of training' (CMBS, 1977) omitted any form of evaluation to follow this momentous change. Such an omission tends to support the view stated in the Perrin Report (DHSS, 1978) on the management of resources in the NHS: 'Evaluation is more frequently recommended than practised'.

This disparity between practice and recommendation in relation to evaluation raises the question of why is it considered to be so necessary? The reasons given for its importance include assisting resource allocation, assessment of effectiveness, cost-effectiveness analysis, monitoring of the process/system and, lastly, preventing changes with long-term implications being introduced on a whim of fashion (Goldberg and Connelly, 1982). The subjéct of the evaluation may be a person, programme, product or an institution. In the study described in this chapter, the subject of evaluation was the extended midwifery course. Goldberg and Connelly state that the problems inherent in the evaluation of a programme, especially one involving a person acquiring new skills, are that it may verge on evaluation of the person. This invidious form of evaluation also risks the potential inconsistencies inherent in any programme, such as when a: 'generally effective and viable programme may turn out an unfortunate product . . . the black sheep of a good family or college' (Bennett and Lumsdaine, 1975). It must be accepted that the reverse may also occur.

Programme evaluation thus raises a range of problems, which may serve to explain the tendency for its avoidance. Another factor which may contribute to this tendency is the view that clearly formulated objectives for the programme are needed against which its effectiveness can be assessed. Although this need for objectives is neglected in much of the work on evaluation, Abramson (1974, p. 23) considers these to be vital for the assessment of the effectiveness of any programme: 'for adequate evaluation the goals must be stated very specifically'. He goes on to state that the development of such goals is an essential part of the planning process. Evaluation of a programme in the absence of clearly stated objectives also needs to be considered however; other authors mention the need for evaluative criteria against which the success of a programme may be measured, but do not specify the need to develop these criteria prior to the implementation of the new programme (Bennett and Lumsdaine, 1975; Goldberg and Connelly, 1982). Despite the fact that evaluation of the extension to the post-registration midwifery course did not feature in the original CMBS guidelines, the programme may still be evaluated with validity.

In assessing the success of a programme, a range of outcome measures may be employed. A variety of aims were held in relation to extending the midwifery course although the only aim stated by the official guidelines was that of reciprocity with other European Community states. Despite this dearth of officially stated aims it is important to assess the extent to which widely held expectations have been achieved and so assess the overall success of the extension of the course. Expectations widely held among midwives were that the longer course would lead to greater confidence in clinical skills and an increase in the proportion who wished to practise (Stewart, 1981) and that retention of new midwives in midwifery would improve (Williams, 1979); it was this that was used as the evaluative criterion in this study.

METHODS

The research design comprised a longitudinal study of two cohorts of midwives; the first followed a 12 month course, the second an 18 month course. There were three phases of data collection.

1. A questionnaire sent to each member of the two cohorts at the start of the course (referred to as the 'Beginners' Questionnaire').
2. A questionnaire sent at the end of the course to those students who had completed it (referred to as the 'Completers' Questionnaire').
3. Examination of notification of intention to practise records held by the statutory body, in order to ascertain which members of the cohort had notified their intention to practise immediately after qualifying and on subsequent occasions. The significance of notification of intention to practice in this context, which makes it a suitable outcome measure and a proxy for midwifery employment, is that it is an absolute measure of the number of qualified midwives in the UK requiring the midwifery qualification for their work. This is because a midwife working as such is statutorily required to notify (United Kingdom Central Council, 1983, p. 17) and only midwives in practice are permitted to notify.

The rationale for this design

A survey was chosen in order to provide much needed information on the characteristics of the then current population of student midwives in Scotland, on their experience of training and their employment decisions. The survey was analytical as well as descriptive, however, in that it included items designed to determine the outcome of a process (i.e. the extension of the course) and factors relating to that outcome.

In attempting to relate changing employment intentions to other factors, particularly personal characteristics, it was decided that a longitudinal design was more appropriate than a cross-sectional design. Although the latter design had been used during a pilot study to test the instruments, the need to link findings from study members over time precluded its use in the main study. Essentially, a longitudinal study involves collecting data from the same people at different times and has the advantage of not having to make assumptions about comparability of data collected from different groups (Fox, 1982). A disadvantage of a longitudinal design is the prolonged period of data collection, in this case 12 and 18 month intervals between sending the questionnaire to the cohort at the beginning and at the end of the course. This problem could have been overcome by a cross-sectional design and using a 'single shot' questionnaire on completion of training, like Robinson (1986). However, it was decided that the subjects' views **at the time** were crucial and that the recall of views held 12, let alone

18, months earlier would have been too inaccurate to permit valid conclusions (Moser and Kalton, 1979). The longitudinal approach included not only the questionnaires at the beginning and end of the course, but was extended, with the co-operation of the statutory body, to include scrutiny of the Notification of Intention to Practise.

The study design entailed two kinds of longitudinal surveys; a panel study which assessed changes associated with taking the midwifery course and a trend study which evaluated the extension of the course. The distinction between panel and trend studies depends on the subjects involved. A panel study involves questioning the same people over a period of time, regardless of how they and their occupations change; in this case student midwives at the beginning and at the end of their course. In a trend study, however, the members of the population will inevitably change, as they are recruited solely by virtue of their being in that particular situation: 'a trend study among students at a state university will reflect a different population of students each time a survey is conducted' (Babbie, 1973, p. 63). In this study one population was the cohort taking the 12 month course and the second population the cohort taking the 18 month course.

Composition of the study groups

The cohort for the 12 month course (referred to as the Stage I respondents) comprised all student midwives beginning training in Scotland on the earliest convenient date, December 1980, (n = 303). There was some urgency to start the study by this date as later groups might have included more students avoiding the longer course and whose views differ from those who had taken the 12 month course in earlier years. The cohort for the 18 month course (referred to as the Stage II respondents) was chosen to replicate Stage I and, initially, comprised only students beginning in December 1982. Administrative changes, however, resulted in a small intake and necessitated including the March 1983 intake also, making a total of 397 students. In order to reduce the possibility of group characteristics differing between intakes, the December intake had been chosen for both Stages of the study. There was a possibility that differences might be present between the Stage II December and March intakes, as the former did not include smaller peripheral schools, and so data from these respondents were subject to an assessment as to whether the two intakes differed. The two cohorts may be described as purposive samples, as specialist knowledge was employed to decide which groups should be approached (Nachmias and Nachmias, 1981). Obviously they were non-random samples and so suffer the major disadvantage of not being representative; any deficiencies in this respect, however, may be compensated for by the size of the samples. 'The larger the sample the less the sampling variation, i.e. the less the likelihood that the sample will be a misleading one' (Abramson, 1974, p. 31).

The questionnaires

A postal questionnaire was chosen for data collection because of the limited time available, together with the wide geographical spread of midwifery training institutions. The questionnaires were developed specifically for this study and had been pretested with appropriate groups of student midwives in the course of a pilot study (Mander, 1980). The format of the Beginners' and the Completers' questionnaires were similar; they comprised five parts, each probing a different area. The Completers' questionnaire included a Likert-type scale to probe the students' veiws of midwifery, in an attempt to reveal positive or negative attitudes towards the profession. A number of items included were based on those used in earlier studies of student midwives (Ramsden and Radwanski, 1963; Golden, 1979; Robinson, 1986).

A disadvantage of the self-administered questionnaire is its inability to probe a topic in depth. Although the questionnaire was admirably suited to collecting data on employment intentions, it was less well suited to probing any changes in attitude associated with changing intentions. To counter this problem open-ended questions were included that provided an opportunity to express opinions and reduce the respondents' perceptions of an emphasis on forced choice. The volume of material obtained from these open-ended questions suggests that they were successful in achieving these aims.

Before going on to describe methods of data collection and the response rates, some consideration is given to the way in which the criteria of replicability, reliability and validity were addressed in the study, and the extent to which the design represented an experiment.

Replicability, reliability and validity

Replicability is defined (Fox, 1982, p. 82) as 'repeating it with all the essential elements of the original study retained'. The possibility of achieving Fox's ideal would depend on the interpretation of 'essential', but replication is invariably more difficult for researchers in the social sciences than for their colleagues in the physical sciences, due to the nature of the research environment and the measuring tools. This raises the question of whether replication is ever possible in social science research, as in research involving human beings no two groups can ever be identical, thus challenging the basic criterion for replicability (Fox, 1982). This means that a redefinition of replicability is required that includes samples which are not necessarily identical, but which have been drawn from the same population using the same sampling technique.

The reasons for the significance of replicability in this research are twofold. First, to facilitate further work in the same area that would serve as a check on findings from this study, and second in order to replicate the design of earlier studies on the subject so that the extent to which findings remain consistent over time can be assessed. Ramsden and Radwanski (1963) and Robinson and colleagues (Golden, 1979; Robinson, 1986, 1991) probed the views of midwives and students respectively and focused on career intentions and views about midwifery and midwifery training. As noted earlier, selected items from the questionnaires used in these studies were incorporated into the research instrument for this study and, although this limited form of replication may not meet the standard set by Fox, it enabled useful comparisons to be drawn.

Reliability is 'the accuracy of the data in the sense of their stability of repeatability' (Fox, 1982, p. 255). This stability is determined by the measuring instrument; possible errors are either in the instrument itself or in the way it is used by the researcher. The latter was unlikely in this study due to the number of closed items in the questionnaire and to the involvement of only one researcher. The instrument itself should have been assessed for reliability using many testers to exclude human error and employing techniques such as test-retest reliability and Kuder-Richardson reliability (Fox, 1982).

Validity, or the ability of the instrument to measure what it actually sets out to measure, was assessed during the pretest in the form of content validity (Mander, 1980). The limited value of assessing content validity is increased if a jury is used, but ideally predictive validity would be tested if any predictive validity is to be claimed. This was not feasible in view of the time it would have required. An assessment of concurrent validity, in which two groups with established, differing characteristics test the instrument to assess its discrimination, was both valuable and feasible. In summary, assumptions of knowledge, reliability and validity were areas which would have benefited from closer attention, had more time been available for pretesting the instrument.

Experimental design

Each stage of this research project compared the employment intentions of a group of students at certain times, i.e. prior to and on completion of training, and employment practice when employment had begun. Some similarities between this design and that of the classical experiment were apparent. These similarities deserve some scrutiny in order to assess the extent to which the study may be regarded as experimental and may therefore claim the power associated with such experiments.

> The controlled experiment is a powerful design for testing hypotheses of causal relationships among variables. Ideally the experimenter throws into sharp relief the explanatory variables in which he is interested, controlling or manipulating the independent variable and observing its effect on the dependent variable and minimising the effects of the extraneous variables which may confound his result. (Riley, 1963, p. 612)

In the research setting, power is increased by identifying and controlling extraneous variables to avoid any inconsistency in the data due to the variable's inconstant effects. Manipulation is essential to the experiment, but the concept of control is less clear, some even regard the two as synonymous. Manipulation is the more active process, whereas control comprises the measures taken to prevent any spontaneous alteration in the variables other than the dependent variable.

A midwifery training study, running twice, may be regarded as the first of the experiments in this study; the independent variable was midwifery training and the dependent variable was the employment decision. The other experiment was the evaluation of the extension of training. The extension constituted the independent variable, with the employment decision again as the dependent variable. In this experiment (Figure 9.1) Stage I, the 12 month course, was the control group and Stage II, the 18 month course, was the experimental group.

An important limitation in regarding the present study as experimental, is the absence of either control or manipulation by the researcher, making it more comparable with a natural experiment. This is defined in terms of the researcher's lack of control: 'Some force clearly unrelated to the dependent variable causes the variation in the independent variable' (Simon, 1969, p. 121). This deficit may be regarded as a disadvantage of 'real life' experiments: 'One samples situations instead of producing them' (Anderson, 1969, p. 24).

Anderson recognized the possibility of the manipulation in a natural experiment being by a third party. This endorses its application here, as in

Figure 9.1 Extension of training experiment.

	Before		After
Control	Stage I Beginners		Stage I Completers
Experiment	State II Beginners	Extended Training	Stage II Completers

Source: complied by the author.

this study, manipulation, such as it was, was by the statutory body. Thus, although the present study failed to meet rigorous criteria of the classical experiment, it corresponded with a natural experiment. Claims of strength must be moderated accordingly.

Data collection

The 'before and after' design of the survey sought the 'uncontaminated' views of the new student prior to any exposure to midwifery, apart from obstetric and maternity care courses. This was facilitated by the staff of the Central Midwives Board for Scotland (CMBS) distributing the Beginners' questionnaire with documents routinely sent to each new student prior to the start of the course. A disadvantage of this arrangement may have been the possibility of the questionnaire being perceived as issuing from the statutory body, constituting some pressure on the student to complete it.

A covering letter was enclosed with the questionnaire, which also gave information about the purpose of the study, assured anonymity and confidentiality, indicated the non-involvement of the statutory body, discounted any repercussions of responding, gave instructions about replying and mentioned the right not to participate. This letter aimed to create a positive impression with the student, allowing her to make a free, fully informed decision about participating, while avoiding a personal response (Treece and Treece, 1986).

The Completers' questionnaire was distributed at the end of the course and was accompanied by a similar letter. As the student midwife was being approached as a private individual, not as an employee, the employing health boards were not involved in recruitment and, as the survey had no immediate implications for client or patient care, it was unnecessary to contact medical ethics committees. Senior managers and senior tutors were informed that students were being recruited into the study. The statutory bodies, initially the CMBS and latterly the Scottish National Board for Nursing, Midwifery and Health Visiting (NBS), provided access to the student, and their student registration number was used for identification. The student midwives were asked to provide this number on both questionnaires in order that these could be linked and comparisons made of information provided at the start of the course with that provided at the end.

Response rates

Response rates for both cohorts separately and together are shown in Table 9.1 (page 242), along with the number of respondents who provided their student registration number on each occasion.

According to Treece and Treece (1986) a response rate of 72%, as

Table 9.1 Study response rates

	Stage I (12 month course)	Stage II (18 month course)	Total
Beginners' questionnaires			
Number sent out	303	397	700
Number returned	241	260	501
Response rate	80%	66%	72%
Number of respondents giving (MB[S]) number (Beginning identifiers)	215	207	422
Completers' questionnaires			
Number sent out	266	380	646
Number returned	179	197	376
Response rate	67%	52%	58%
Number of respondents giving (MB[S]) number (Completing identifiers)	124	102	226
Number of respondents who gave their (MB[S]) number in both questionnaires (Double identifiers)	102	65	167

Source: compiled by the author.

achieved for the Beginners' questionnaire, is high for a postal survey. The lower response for the Completers' questionnaire highlights a major problem of longitudinal studies; namely that of attrition at subsequent sweeps (see Robinson and Owen in Chapter 8 of this volume). Non-response, if major, may result in unrepresentative data and reduce the possibility of generalizing the findings (Atkinson, 1988). Consequently every effort must be made to keep it to a minimum. The presentation of the covering letter is crucial in creating a positive attitude in potential respondents and the wording, neatness and quality of the paper are all thought to influence whether the potential respondent does reply (Treece and Treece, 1986). Other methods of encouraging response are more questionable. They include 'persuading' potential respondents by applying pressure in the form of using 'someone important . . . to ask for co-operation, on the stationery of a prestigious institution' or offering 'gifts or payment to the respondents' (Simon, 1969, p. 119). These methods are hardly consistent with the concept of 'freely given and informed consent'

(Royal College of Nursing, 1977, p. 2). Moreover this type of pressure may have an effect on the answers which the reluctant respondents eventually give; as Babbie states 'you must be careful not to change the subjects' answers' (1973, p. 119).

If it is not possible to achieve a 100% response at the outset, the researcher may attempt to remedy the situation by using follow-up techniques; this involves sending reminders to tardy respondents to stimulate responses. This was not possible in this study as the researcher did not have respondents' personal details, such as home addresses, and so there was difficulty in obtaining access to the members of the two cohorts.

It cannot be assumed that non-respondents are randomly distributed among the study population and it is therefore important to ascertain whether non-respondents differ from respondents, in order to assess the representativeness of the latter. However, it was not possible to undertake such an investigation within the constraints of this project. Other studies of midwives' careers have shown that non-respondents have been much less likely to practise midwifery than respondents (see Robinson and Owen in Chapter 8 of this volume).

Considerable importance was attached to maintaining both respondents' anonymity and confidentiality in the hope that this would encourage them to respond and to be more forthcoming in their response. Maintaining anonymity may have exacerbated problems caused by non-response and it also hindered comparison of some Beginners'/Completers' responses. Non-identification manifested itself in three ways. First, a large proportion of respondents gave no identification number and they apologized for the omission. A second group gave a number other than the student midwife registration number; probably due to concurrent changes in the organization of nursing and midwifery in the UK the new Personal Identification Number (PIN) (United Kingdom Central Council, 1984) was frequently provided by Stage II Completers. A third, small group of respondents was unable to accept the researcher's assurance of confidentiality and anonymity and realized, correctly, that by stating the student registration number they would be traceable; for this reason they were not prepared to identify themselves. Data from respondents who did not identify themselves in both the Beginners' and the Completers' questionnaire could not be included in the analyses of changes in employment intentions, but did contribute to the overall group profile.

FINDINGS

The study generated a substantial volume of findings; some of which are included in this chapter, others have been reported elsewhere (Mander, 1987a, 1987b, 1989b, 1989c).

The findings in this chapter relate to:

- profile of the respondents;
- reasons for undertaking midwifery;
- student midwives' employment intentions at the start of training;
- changes in employment intentions made during course;
- factors influencing employment decisions at end of course;
- personal characteristics associated with practising midwifery;
- confidence in midwifery skills and its relationship to employment.

As shown in Table 9.1 (page 242) the cohorts comprised several sub-groups of respondents and the findings relate to several of these. In order to facilitate understanding, these subgroups are listed, together with the total number in each (Figure 9.2).

Figure 9.2 Study sub-groups.

Title	Definition	Number
Beginners	Those who returned the questionnaire sent to them at beginning of course	501
Beginning identifier	Those who returned the questionnaire sent to them at beginning of course and also provided their student registration number	422
Completers	Those who returned the questionnaire sent to them at end of course	376
Completing identifiers	Those who returned the questionnaire sent to them at end of course and who provided their student registration number	226
Double identifiers	Those who returned both questionnaires and provided their student registration number on both occasions	167
Notifying beginner	A respondent who had identified herself, by stating her student midwife registration number, when beginning the midwifery course and subsequently notified her intention to practise to her local supervising authority, indicating that she was practising as a midwife	261

Source: complied by the author.

Profile of the respondents

Information on aspects of the respondents' age, sex, marital status and educational and nursing background was obtained at the beginning of the course for two reasons. First to enable comparisons to be made with other studies of newly qualified midwives and, second, in order to determine

Table 9.2 Sex of respondents

	Stage I		Stage II		Total	
	%	No.	%	No.	%	No.
Female	96	231	96	249	96	480
Male	2	6	–	1	1	7
No answer	2	4	4	10	3	14
Total	100	241	100	260	100	501

Source: compiled by the author.

whether any particular characteristics appeared to be associated with subsequent retention.

Sex. Only seven of the 501 respondents were men (Table 9.2). They undertook their training at the one college in Scotland that participated in the experimental training scheme for male midwives (Speak and Aitken-Swan, 1982), and so were not evenly distributed throughout the two cohorts. The numbers were too small to allow for comparisons between the training experiences of male and female midwives or between their subsequent careers. The training experiences and careers of male midwives, however, have been the subject of a large-scale study, which included all those men who had qualified or who were students as at September 1987 (Lewis, 1988, 1989, 1991). In due course it will be interesting to see whether the progress of men in nursing is being replicated in midwifery. Male nurses' employment decisions have been shown to be different in terms of their nature, probably relating to their domestic responsibilities (Nuttall, 1983), and also their effects on females' decisions (Pollock and West, 1984).

Age. Respondents' age on completion of training is shown in Table 9.3. The small decrease in the proportion of Stage II respondents who were under 23 at this time is probably due to the extension of the midwifery course by six months rather than older students being recruited. In both cohorts the proportion of respondents who were 24 or over is smaller than that found in the study of midwives qualifying from 12 and from 18 month courses in England and Wales (Robinson, 1986, 1991). Table 9.3 (page 246) shows that in this study 32% and 33% of the two groups were over 24 at the time of completing their midwifery course, whereas the corresponding figures in Robinson's study were 42% and 49%.

Table 9.3 Age-group of respondents

	Stage I		Stage II		Total	
	%	No.	%	No.	%	No.
Under 23	24	58	16	43	20	101
23–24	41	99	48	124	44	223
Over 24	32	78	31	80	32	158
No answer	3	6	5	13	4	19
Total	100	241	100	260	100	501

Source: compiled by the author.

Marital status. Just under a quarter of the respondents were married (23%) at the time of starting their midwifery course. The Stage I respondents were slightly more likely to be married than their Stage II counterparts: 28% (67) compared with 19% (48).

Education. Table 9.4 shows respondents' educational background in terms of the highest level attained prior to starting their midwifery course. The data shows a significant increase in the proportion of Stage II respondents who had Highers or 'A' levels ($\chi^2 = 6.635$, $p < 0.05$, df = 2) suggesting that the educational background of student midwives may be rising.

Table 9.4 Educational background of respondents

Qualification	Stage I		Stage II		Total	
	%	No.	%	No.	%	No.
Higher/'A' levels	42	101	61	158	52	259
'O' levels only (or grade O in 1 above)	34	83	15	40	24	123
Other/no answer	24	57	24	62	24	119
Total	100	241	100	260	100	501

Source: compiled by the author.

Nursing background. All but a very few respondents were registered general nurses; 14 held the RSCN certificate, ten were qualified registered mental nurses and seven held other nursing qualifications. Information obtained on nursing experience prior to starting the course included length of time employed as a nurse and highest grade reached (Table 9.5). The figures show that the majority of respondents had practised as a nurse, about half of whom had done so for more than a year. These findings are similar to those found in the English and Welsh Study (Robinson, 1986, 1991).

Table 9.5 Nursing employment prior to midwifery training

	Stage I		*Stage II*		*Total*	
	%	No.	%	No.	%	No.
None	13	31	10	27	12	58
Under 1 year						
Staff nurse	37	89	46	120	42	209
Over 1 year						
Staff nurse	37	89	36	94	36	183
Over 1 year						
Sister/CN	5	13	5	14	5	27
Australian Sister	3	8	–	–	2	8
Other	5	11	2	5	3	16
Total	100	241	100	260	100	501

Source: compiled by the author.

Reasons for taking midwifery training

The students' primary and secondary reasons for beginning training were probed in a closed item that incorporated some of the reasons suggested in an earlier study by Ramsden and Radwanski (1963). The list of reasons offered to students is shown in Table 9.6 (page 248), as is the proportion of respondents who cited each as their main reason for beginning training. The findings show that the two cohorts differed little in the proportion to cite each reason. Overall these data support findings from earlier studies, in that only a minority seek the midwifery qualification because they wish to practise as midwives (Ministry of Health *et al.*, 1949; Ramsden and Radwanski, 1963; Robinson, 1986, 1991).

A total of 30% cited career goals outside of midwifery: 11% to achieve promotion, 9% as a precursor to health visitor training and 11% to work abroad. The two largest proportions related to more personal reasons; either a desire to complete or round off their general nursing training or to satisfy their own interest. A small number of respondents were unable to state a single reason, and these responses have been combined, in Table 9.6, with those who gave reasons such as 'liking babies', 'preparing for own childbearing' and 'for a change of job'.

Each of the reasons was cited more frequently than shown in Table 9.6 when the respondents were asked to indicate their secondary reason (or reasons) for taking midwifery training; thus midwifery practice was cited by 21%, promotion by 21%, health visitor training by 21%, work abroad by 19%, complete training by 44%, satisfy interest by 43% and other by 48%.

Table 9.6 Main reason for taking midwifery training

	Stage I		Stage II		Total	
	%	No.	%	No.	%	No.
Midwifery practice	12	28	15	38	13	66
Promotion	11	27	11	29	11	56
HV training	8	20	10	27	9	47
Work abroad	10	25	11	29	11	54
Complete training	25	60	20	53	23	113
Satisfy interest	22	54	19	49	21	103
Another reason/no single reason/DK	11	27	14	35	12	62
Total	100	241	100	260	100	501

Source: compiled by the author.

Student midwives' employment intentions

A closed item question, based on that used in an earlier study (Golden, 1979; Robinson, 1986, 1991), sought information about short- and long-term employment intentions, with a view to showing any differences, between Beginners', and Completers' intentions. Figure 9.3 shows the short- and long-term intentions expressed by both cohorts at the beginning of the course.

Taking the two cohorts together, then a small majority (56%) plan to work as midwives on completion of their course, either in hospital or in the community. This may not be realistic, as in practice it is usual for those who intend to find work as community midwives to be required to obtain

Figure 9.3 New student midwives' employment intentions.

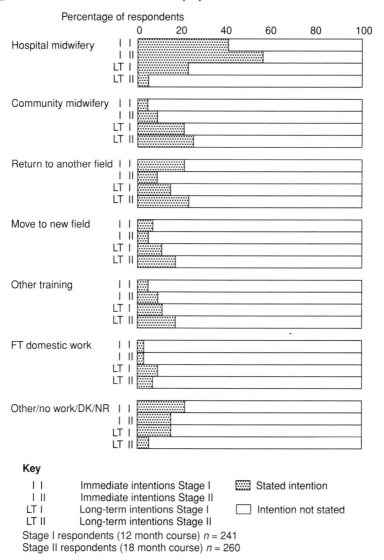

Key

| | | Immediate intentions Stage I
| || | Immediate intentions Stage II
LT I | Long-term intentions Stage I
LT II | Long-term intentions Stage II

Stated intention

Intention not stated

Stage I respondents (12 month course) *n* = 241
Stage II respondents (18 month course) *n* = 260

Source: compiled by the author.

hospital midwifery experience first. The data suggest that the Stage II respondents (those who took an 18 month course) are more likely than Stage I respondents (those who took a 12 month course) to plan to practise as midwives immediately after qualifying. However, only a small proportion of student midwives intend to practise as midwives on a long-term basis and this is especially marked for the Stage II respondents in relation to hospital midwifery.

The attraction of community work is clearly apparent from these data; 20% of respondents intend to undertake a health visiting course and this implies almost inevitably an intention to work as a health visitor. Small numbers gave this as their immediate employment intention, but a larger proportion (16%) stated that health visiting is their long-term plan. Including those hoping to take a health visiting course, a total of 150 respondents (30%) indicated their intention to undertake further training. This may be interpreted to mean that midwives perceive the need for further or continuing nurse education, but in view of the use in the questionnaire of the term 'training', as opposed to course or education, one may conclude that these respondents plan to obtain further nursing certificates, providing an illustration of the lateral movement syndrome (Hardy, 1983).

Factors influencing employment decision at end of training

The Completers' questionnaire, returned by 443 of those who completed the course, contained an open-ended question which asked 'what are the main factors which influenced you in making the decision about what you are going to do next?'

The categories shown in Table 9.7 were developed from the information obtained and then each respondent's answer was allocated to one of them. The figures indicate the percentage who mentioned the factor, but not whether it was viewed positively or negatively. An example of this is 'Satisfaction' which was mentioned or implied by 6% of the respondents, but who between them held a variety of feelings about midwifery and differing intentions about practising.

Table 9.7 shows that a large proportion (24%) of new midwives consider it necessary to gain experience in the area in which they have just qualified, although this was the case for fewer of those who had taken the longer course: 22% compared with 26%. The figures show that job availability had become more important as the research progressed, rising from 4% to 25%. References to job availability usually implied the difficulty the respondent had, or expected to have, in finding work. The number claiming that money was an influencing factor declined from 5% to 1%. Of the ten 12 month course respondents who mentioned finance, only one had no intention of ever working as a midwife. Among the 18

Table 9.7 Factors influencing the employment decision

	Stage I		Stage II		Total	
	%	No.	%	No.	%	No.
Experience/consolidate	26	55	22	51	24	106
Enjoyment	23	50	15	35	19	85
Domestic	13	29	13	29	13	58
Job available	4	9	25	56	15	65
Promotion/previous commitment	6	12	7	16	6	28
Satisfaction	8	17	5	12	6	29
Money	5	10	1	2	3	12
No/other response	15	33	12	27	14	60
Total	100	215	100	228	100	443

Source: compiled by the author.

month course respondents there were fewer and briefer references to finance. The factors cited as influencing employment decisions are not easily amenable to action by midwifery managers. This applies particularly to a perception of a deteriorating economic situation which appeared to exert an increasing influence on new midwives' employment decisions.

Changes in employment intentions made during training

Information provided by those respondents who identified themselves and also returned a questionnaire at the beginning and at the end of the course (referred to as the Double Identifiers) provided an opportunity to examine whether employment intentions changed during the course. Table 9.8 (page 252) shows employment intentions expressed at the beginning and at the end of the course.

The McNemar test, used to show the significance of changes in individual's views, suggests that they are largely favourable to midwifery (Siegel, 1956). These data show that of the 98 Beginners intending to practise midwifery, 22 had changed their minds, and by the end of the course intended not to practice. Only 17 of the 49 Beginners intending not to practice continued with that intention. Fourteen of the 20 uncertain Beginners were intending to practise by the time they had completed the course. It is apparent that a small majority of students do not alter their employment plans during midwifery training and, of those who do alter

Table 9.8 Double Identifiers' immediate employment plans

Completers	Intend to practise		Don't know		Intend not to practise		Total	
	%	No.	%	No.	%	No.	%	No.
Beginners								
Intend to practise	43	71	3	5	13	22	59	98
Don't know	8	14	0.6	1	3	5	12	20
Intend not to practise	18	30	1	2	10	17	29	49
Total	69	115	5	8	26	44	100	167

NB: Percentages shown are for the total group of respondents ($n = 167$)
Source: compiled by the author.

their plans, more change in favour of midwifery than decide against it. The same finding was demonstrated in Robinson's study (Robinson, 1991).

Factors associated with practising midwifery

Midwives who intend to practise have to notify their intention to do so with the statutory body (United Kingdom Central Council, 1983, p. 17); in this study therefore, as in others, notification was used as a measure of midwifery employment (Willcocks, 1968; Moores, 1980).

Data from this study was used to ascertain whether those who did notify an intention to practise differed from those who did not do so. This information was obtained from those who identified themselves in the questionnaire sent to the two cohorts at the beginning of training (the Notifying Beginners), as their number could then be linked to notification to practice records ($n = 261$). Findings for educational background showed that those who had attained Scottish Certificate of Education Highers or 'A' levels were significantly more likely than those who had not done so to notify an intention to practise ($\chi^2 = 4.70$, df $= 1$, $p < 0.05$). Findings on marital status, age and nursing experience did not reach the 0.05 level of significance, although there was some indication that respondents who were married were more likely to practise than those who were single, those in the younger age groups were more likely to practise than their older counterparts and those with less nursing experience were more likely to practise than those who had nursed for longer.

Confidence

Increased confidence in practice and, thus, improved practice and retention were generally considered to be reasons for the extension of post-registration midwifery training from 12 to 18 months (Stewart, 1981; Robinson, 1986). Consequently information about the confidence of the 12 month course respondents (Stage I) and the 18 month course respondents (Stage II) in relation to 12 essential midwifery tasks was obtained and its relationship to midwifery employment was examined. The list of tasks was based on that developed for the study by Robinson and colleagues (Golden, 1979; Robinson 1986, 1991).

Confidence in midwifery practice. Findings on respondents' confidence in some of the 12 tasks deemed essential to midwifery are shown in Figure 9.4. The group are the 376 midwives who completed the questionnaire at the end of the course (179 from Stage I and 197 from Stage II). Comparison of the 12 month cohort (Stage I) with the 18 month cohort (Stage II) show decreasing confidence in domiciliary midwifery; these data are combined under the heading of 'Home care'. The possibility of this being a chance result in a list of 12 items cannot be excluded. The decrease in confidence is most obvious in 'Home confinements' (not shown separately), but confidence is also lacking in basic domiciliary care. Whether this reduction in confidence is associated with the decreased proportion of community experience in the extended course merits further attention. This decline in confidence should be a source of concern to midwife managers as the duration of hospitalization of postnatal women decreases and the importance of community midwifery care increases (see Murphy-Black in Chapter 6 of this volume). These findings compare interestingly with those obtained by Robinson and colleagues (Golden, 1979; Robinson, 1986, 1991). They found that the cohort who had taken the 18 month course were as likely as the cohort who had taken the 12 month course to lack confidence in home confinements but more likely to feel confident in providing antenatal and postnatal care at home. Findings from both studies showed an increase in the proportion of respondents who felt confident about teaching; this may have reflected the increased emphasis placed on the principles and practice of teaching in the 18 month syllabus.

Confidence and employment practice. Of prime concern is the possible association of confidence in midwifery practice with employment as a midwife and indeed this may serve as one form of evaluation of the extension of training. Findings on the relationship between confidence and employment practice from this study suggest, however, that there is no difference in confidence levels between those who take up midwifery

Figure 9.4 Confidence of completers in certain midwifery tasks.

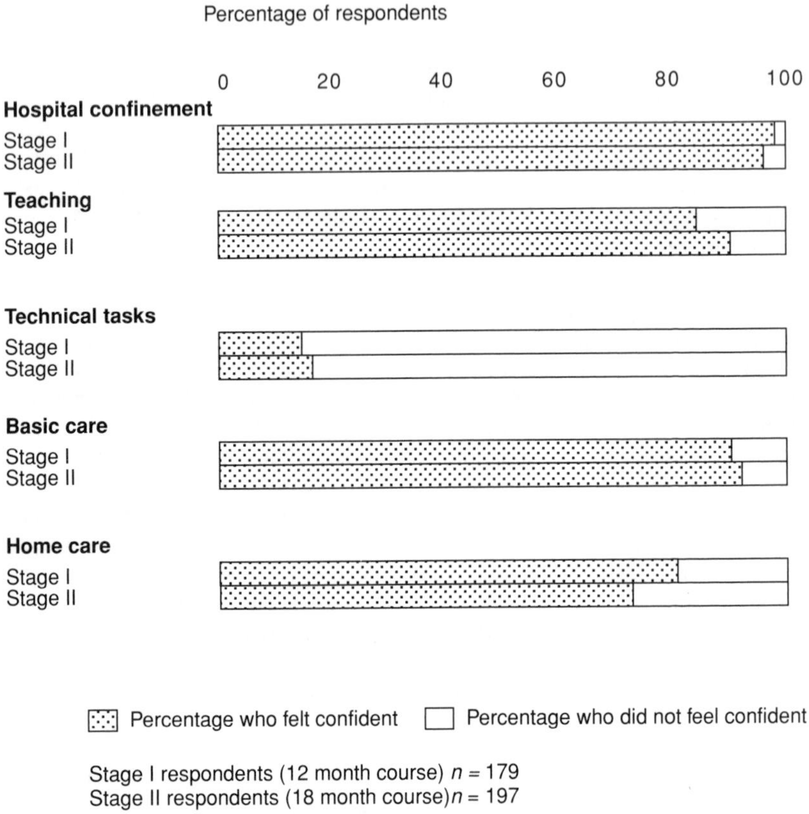

Percentage of respondents

Hospital confinement
Stage I
Stage II

Teaching
Stage I
Stage II

Technical tasks
Stage I
Stage II

Basic care
Stage I
Stage II

Home care
Stage I
Stage II

Percentage who felt confident   Percentage who did not feel confident

Stage I respondents (12 month course) *n* = 179
Stage II respondents (18 month course)*n* = 197

Source: compiled by the author.

employment and those who do not. These findings are discussed in detail in Mander (1989c). The relationship between confidence in practising as a midwife and midwifery employment is more complex than is sometimes assumed and a variety of other variables may affect, and perhaps play a more significant role than, confidence in the new midwife's employment decision.

The findings reported in this chapter relate only to immediate employment intentions and practice. Had the study ended at this stage it would have failed to identify the return of investment that might be produced by those students undertaking midwifery training with no intention of practising midwifery immediately, but intending to return to it at a later date (possibly after their own childbearing) making midwifery their secondary career. However, a follow-up study involving scrutiny of notification to practice records at subsequent intervals has provided such information. These findings are reported in Mander (1989b).

DISCUSSION

In this final section some of the implications of the findings for midwifery are discussed. The study provided a profile of the personal, domestic and occupational characteristics of student midwives in Scotland. Points of particular interest included considerable nursing experience prior to starting the course and the increased proportion of 18 month students who held Scottish Certificate of Education Highers or 'A' levels. Reasons given for undertaking the course showed that only a minority did so because they wanted to practise midwifery. This indicates that nurses were still using midwifery training as a 'stepping stone' to achieve goals which did not relate to midwifery. These included enhancing nursing career prospects and training to be a health visitor. The study therefore supported findings from other studies of reasons for training as a midwife (Ministry of Health *et al.*, 1949; Ramsden and Radwanski, 1963; Golden, 1979; Robinson, 1986, 1991). The combined weight of evidence from these studies has been a contributory factor in the decision to introduce pre-registration midwifery education (see Radford and Thompson, Chapter 10 in this volume).

Findings on career plans showed that these tended to be vague and in some cases subject to change during the midwifery course. Moreover those who had completed the course were sometimes exposed to sudden changes in domestic and, particularly, occupational arrangements which required abrupt revision of employment plans. The possibility that this domestic vulnerability may be a characteristic of female employment cannot be ignored and needs to be taken into account in workforce planning. Revisions of plans may result in a shortfall between the number of new midwives who intend to practise and the number who actually notify their intention to do so.

Other findings, reported elsewhere, showed that satisfaction with the midwifery course is high, regardless of its duration (Mander, 1989c). However, the increase in confidence and, consequently, retention which was expected to accompany it (Stewart, 1981) failed to materialize.

New midwives' employment decisions are influenced by a range of variables. The more intrinsic variables include personal characteristics such as higher education qualifications; such midwives were more likely to wish to practise midwifery. Findings from the study therefore indicated that criteria for selection of candidates may contribute to remedying the problem of retention. However, there are many aspects of maternity care that are also amenable to action to improve retention.

Other factors unique to midwifery were also taken into account by new midwives in their employment decisions; these included changes in the midwife's role, and also certain aspects of the organization of midwifery, which were widely perceived as making midwifery less attractive to new entrants. Certain extrinsic phenomena, affecting the decision were also identified in the study; these included the employment climate, UK membership of the EC and, to a lesser and decreasing extent, financial remuneration. Two factors of particular importance were the deteriorating role of the midwife and the undifferentiated salary structure; these two factors are not unconnected, as remuneration reflects the value ascribed to midwives' work, by both midwives and other personnel.

It may be suggested that the close, perhaps interdependent, relationship between midwives' salaries and their role is likely to continue until the work of midwives can be shown to be qualitatively different from that of the nurse grade to which it is initially linked. By the same token, it is unlikely that midwives will reassert themselves to regain their role until they are confident that the increased responsibility inherent in their proper role will be recognized in both salary and status. The close relationship between these motivators suggests that a piecemeal remedy is not a long-term answer, but that a comprehensive solution, addressing role, remuneration and retention, is required (Mander, 1987a).

Such a solution would adopt a theoretical framework such as that developed by Vogt and her multidisciplinary team to retain professional nurses (Vogt *et al.*, 1983). These workers sought to alleviate non-retention in nursing by revision of the occupational role, appropriate remuneration and a holistic approach to care. A comprehensive approach to midwifery would, while satisfying midwives' aspirations and the need for efficiency, also take account of the increasing desire among consumers for some degree of control over their care. Such an approach would have three main components: retention, role and remuneration.

Retention. Retention is a problem which could be addressed by more focused selection of student midwives, together with strategies to increase subsequent retention. For example, unrealistic expectations held by new student midwives indicate the need not only for amendments to the maternity care module in nurse training, but also for the provision of better career advice for nurses. The provision of effective careers guidance might also assist sound, durable employment decisions, preventing the kind of reversals demonstrated in this study and perhaps the associated personal trauma.

Lack of recognition of the student's previous nursing experience was also revealed as a source of considerable dissatisfaction. The great variation in this experience must make its recognition difficult, but in view of the discontent aroused an attempt to do so may be worthwhile. The association between non-recognition of nursing experience and the disinclination of more experienced nurses to remain in midwifery is an area which warrants further research. More efficient selection and better retention would reduce the need for a large student contribution to the service workforce.

Role. The midwife's role could develop along the lines sought by many and introduced by a few (Flint and Poulengeris, 1986; Flint, 1991). This would involve midwives working in small groups and taking responsibility for all aspects of care, with the exception of women exhibiting or developing high-risk conditions. Flint and Poulengeris (1986) and Flint (1991) demonstrated that not only is continuity of care by midwives feasible (as long as midwives are sufficiently flexible), but also that it is greatly welcomed by consumers. Since this research has been completed many moves in this direction have been made in the UK. It is sometimes suggested that much of the work undertaken by midwives could be undertaken by less qualified personnel, but this may not be consistent with the general desire for better continuity and more holistic care. Finally the midwife's role as a teacher and communicator could be further expanded, and this would have implications for the curriculum of the midwifery course.

Remuneration. Remuneration should increase to be commensurate with the midwife's increasing responsibility and this could be financed by both a reduction in wasted midwifery education costs if selection was more focused and a decrease in duplication of the midwife's work by other qualified staff.

In conclusion this study has provided a substantial volume of findings on many aspects of post-registration midwifery education and midwives' employment decisions, and indicated directions for future research on this important topic. Moreover, the study provides a useful examination of the methodological problems encountered in undertaking research of this kind.

REFERENCES

Abramson, J.H. (1974) *Survey methods in community medicine.* Churchill Livingstone, Edinburgh.

Anderson, B.F. (1969) *The psychology experiment.* Wadsworth, Belmont.

Atkinson, F.I. (1988) Non-response rates in nursing research. *Senior Nurse*, **8**(5), 23.

Babbie, E.R. (1973) *Survey research methods*. Wadsworth, California.

Bennett, C.A. and Lumsdaine, A.A. (1975) Social program evaluation: definitions and issues. In C.A. Bennett and A.A. Lumsdaine (eds) *Evaluation and experiment*. Academic Press, New York.

Central Midwives Board for Scotland (1977) *Guidelines for extension of training*. CMBS, Edinburgh.

Department of Health and Social Security (1978) Royal Commission on the National Health Service: *The Management of Financial Resources in the NHS*. Research Paper No 2. (The Perin Report) HMSO, London.

Flint, C. (1991) Continuity of care provided by a team of midwives – the Know Your Midwife Scheme. In S. Robinson and A.M. Thomson (eds) *Midwives, research and childbirth*, Vol 2. Chapman & Hall, London.

Flint, C. and Poulengeris, P. (1986) *The 'Know Your Midwife' report*. 49 Peckarmans Wood, Sydenham Hill, London.

Fox, D. (1982) *Fundamentals of research in nursing*. Appleton Century Crofts, Connecticut.

Golden, J. (1979) *The views of newly qualified midwives*. Occasional Paper No 1, Chelsea College, London.

Goldberg, E.M. and Connelly, N. (1982) *Evaluative research in social care*. Policy Studies Institute, Heinemann, London.

Hardy, L.K. (1983) An exploration of the career histories of leading female nurses in England and Scotland. Unpublished Ph.D. Thesis, University of Edinburgh.

Lewis, P. (1988) Men in midwifery. *Research and the Midwife Conference Proceedings for 1987*. Nursing Research Unit, Kings College, London.

Lewis, P. (1989) Male midwives: reasons for training and subsequent career paths. In J. Wilson-Barnett and S. Robinson (eds) *Directions in midwifery research*. Scutari Press, London.

Lewis, P. (1991) Men in midwifery: their experiences as students and as practitioners. In S. Robinson and A.M. Thomson (eds) *Midwives, research and childbirth*, Vol 2. Chapman & Hall, London.

Mander, R. (1980) The development and pretest of questionnaires to be used for a study of the employment decisions of newly qualified midwives. Unpublished M.Sc. Dissertation, University of Edinburgh.

Mander, R. (1987a) A study of the employment decisions of newly qualified midwives. Unpublished Ph.D. thesis, University of Edinburgh.

Mander, R. (1987b) Change in employment plans. *Midwifery*, **3**(2), 62–71.

Mander, R. (1989a) Carers' careers – contingencies and crises. *Midwives Chronicle*, **102**(1212), 3–8.

Mander, R. (1989b) Who continues? A preliminary examination of data on continuation of employment in midwifery. *Midwifery*, **5**(1), 26–35.

Mander, R. (1989c) 'The best laid schemes . . .': An evaluation of the extension of midwifery training in Scotland. *International Journal of Nursing Studies*, **26**(1), 27–41.

Ministry of Health, Department of Health for Scotland, Ministry of Labour and National Service (1949) *Report of the working party on midwives*. (Chairman: Mrs M. Stocks) HMSO, London.

Moores, B. (1980) Towards rational midwifery service planning. *Journal of Advanced Nursing*, **5**, 301–9.

Moser, C.A. and Kalton, G. (1979) *Survey methods in social investigation*, 2nd edn. Heinemann, London.

Nachmias, C. and Nachmias, D. (1981) *Research methods in the social sciences*. Edward Arnold, London.

Nuttall, P. (1983) Male takeover or female giveaway? *Nursing Times*, **79**(2), 10–11.

Pollock, L. and West, E. (1984) On being a woman and a psychiatric nurse. *Senior Nurse*, **1**(17), 10–13.

Ramsden, D. and Radwanski, P. (1963) *Some aspects of the work of the midwife*. Dan Mason Research Committee of the National Florence Nightingale Memorial Committee, London.

Riley, M.W. (1963) *Sociological research I: A case approach*. Harcourt, Brace & World, New York.

Robinson, S. (1980) Are there enough midwives? *Nursing Times*, **76**(17), 726–30.

Robinson, S. (1986) The 18 month training: what difference has it made? *Midwives Chronicle*, **99**(1177), 22–9.

Robinson, S. (1991) Preparation for practice: the educational experiences and career intentions of newly qualified midwives. In S. Robinson and A.M. Thomson (eds) *Midwives, research and childbirth*, Vol 2. Chapman & Hall, London.

Royal College of Nursing (1977) *Ethics related to research in nursing*. RCN, London.

Siegel, S. (1956) *Non-parametric statistics*. McGraw-Hill, New York.

Simon, J.L. (1969) *Basic research methods in social science*. Random House, New York.

Stewart, A. (1981) The present state of midwifery training. *Midwife, Health Visitor and Community Nurse*, **17**(7), 270–72.

Speak, M. and Aitken-Swan, J. (1982) *Male midwives: a report of two studies*. DHSS, London.

Treece, E.W. and Treece, J.W. (1986) *Elements of research in nursing*, 4th edn. CV, Mosby, St Louis.

UKCC (1983) *Handbook of midwives rules*. UKCC, London.

UKCC (1984) *Personal identification number*. UKCC, London.

Vogt, J.F., Cox, J.L., Velthouse, B.A. and Thames, B.H. (1983) *Retaining professional nurses*. CV Mosby, St Louis.

Vroom, V.H. (1964) *Work and motivation*. John Wiley, New York.

Willcocks, A.J. (1968) The staffing of the maternity services. In G. McLachlan, (ed.) *Problems and progress in medical care*. Nuffield PHT/Oxford University Press, Oxford.

Williams, S.M.K. (1979) Student nurses attitudes towards midwifery. *Nursing Times*, **75**(10), 41.

CHAPTER TEN

A study of issues concerning the implementation of direct entry midwifery education

Nancy Radford and Anne Thompson

INTRODUCTION

Legally it has always been possible to become a midwife in England without first qualifying as a nurse. Practically, by the mid 1980s it had become impossible for all but the tiniest handful of determined candidates as there was only one remaining school in the country for direct entrants to midwifery. This situation gave rise to a growing disquiet, both inside and outside the midwifery profession. Despite the fact that the English National Board (ENB), the then Department of Health and Social Security (DHSS), the Royal College of Midwives (RCM) and a variety of other organizations (such as the Association of Radical Midwives) had all expressed commitment to an increased provision of direct entry courses, very little progress had been made in this respect. In Spring 1987 therefore the English National Board commissioned the study described in this chapter with a remit to investigate what was inhibiting the implementation of direct entry courses and to recommend how development in this area could be fostered. The DHSS funded the study, which was carried out by the Department of Educational Studies of the University of Surrey.

The chapter looks first at the historical background of non-nurse midwifery education in England before describing the project's aims and methods. The findings are then presented in the form of series of important practical and philosophical issues which emerged in the course of the research and which those contemplating the provision of direct entry midwifery courses will need to address.

It could be argued that the study is now of historical interest only, insofar as a growing number of direct entry courses have subsequently been implemented (22 at the time of writing). These courses are themselves the subject of an evaluation study however (Kent and Maggs, 1992), and it will be of considerable interest and importance in due course to see how the issues identified in the feasibility study reported here, have been addressed in practice.

One of the difficulties which faced the researchers from the outset was to find a universally acceptable and convenient term for the longer midwifery training. 'Direct entry midwifery training' was the term most commonly used, both in the press and by respondents and interviewees. It was immediately understood and covered options such as part-time or degree courses which may last longer than three years. However, representatives of the ENB felt this term carried undesirable connotations and meant the new course would be associated with previous direct entry courses which were felt not to have kept pace with educational and technical developments. They therefore favoured the use of the term 'three year midwifery training'. This was found to be a somewhat awkward phrase, especially when referring to part-time or longer (e.g. degree) courses. It was not as well understood by the respondents and the general public as 'direct entry'. Another term suggested was 'non-nurse midwifery training' – this had the advantage of being easily understood by the general public. On the other hand, it was not a phrase in common usage, and again was felt to have negative connotations. All three terms were in fact used in the course of the study. Since the research was completed the term most commonly used is 'pre-registration midwifery education'.

In most research projects the identification of firm objectives and design of the project are agreed between the funding or commissioning body and the contractor before the project commences. This means that the ideological assumptions of both can be examined and recognized, some background work can be undertaken, contacts developed, a timetable drafted, budgets agreed and a consultation mechanism created. The preparation and discussion of proposals can take many months or even years before a project commences. In the case of this study, funding was made available only a very short time before the project was to start and a timetable of one year was set; from the beginning of April 1987 to the end of March 1988. Therefore, the project had to be designed within strict financial and time constraints. The design had to be formulated within the timetable of the project rather than before, and of necessity much of it developed as the study progressed. The various constraints and the way they affected the project are discussed in the aims and methods section.

Although this meant the research team could be more flexible in responding to developments in the areas covered, it also meant that less time could be spent on background work and piloting. To overcome this limitation various consultation mechanisms, formal and informal, were devised. These routes of communication ensured that the researchers were aware of policy decisions and changes, as well as relevant events, and were given informed advice on appropriate fields of research. The research team, however, was independent and the final report consisted of their own findings, conclusions and recommendations (Radford and Thompson, 1988).

The subject of the next section has a twofold purpose: first it brings together, from a variety of disparate sources, the history of non-nurse midwifery education; second it provides a context for the commissioning of the study and its aims, and for the findings that emerged.

Midwifery education for non-nurses: some historical perspectives

The following account is based on a literature review that was ongoing throughout the study; it drew on a wide range of sources that included the Annual Reports and Rules of the Central Midwives Board (CMB), various statutes and official reports on the maternity services, as well as written and verbal accounts of witnesses to the development of midwifery. The history of midwifery has been well documented by a number of authors (Donnison, 1977; Bent, 1982; Robinson, 1990); in particular the opposition to state certification in midwifery mounted by both the nursing and the medical professions. What is not so clear is the later development within midwifery itself of hostility towards the access of non-nurses to the profession. Although Fenney (1954) states that 'at no time in its history has the Central Midwives Board considered the exclusion of such women (i.e. non-nurses) from training', opinion within the profession seems frequently to have been divided on this.

Until 1916 there was a single path into midwifery for nurses and non-nurses alike. The 1902 Act required the Central Midwives Board to regulate training, examination and admission to the roll of women wishing to practise as midwives, and the first Rule Book of 1903 established the length of training at three months for non-nurses and nurses alike. From the beginning this was recognized as far too short a time, but since pupils had to pay for training the Board could not be too demanding in the early days.

The first Annual Report of the CMB (1908) highlighted a fact which was to give rise to concern until the present day, namely that fewer than 60% of successful candidates intended to practise as midwives. In its Report for 1913 the Board comments 'the majority . . . seek the Board's certificate for collateral purposes'. Although State Registration for nurses was not to happen until 1919, nurse training was well organized in schools throughout the country and, more importantly, the conditions of service and pay of the nurse, as well as her social standing, were much better than those of the midwives. It was not asking much of a woman who may already have completed three years of training in hospital nursing to spend three months learning the elements of midwifery and gaining a place on the roll of midwives, if those months were likely to enhance her career prospects. This, in fact, had already become the 'inherited wisdom' of the nursing profession. Dual certification was seen as a pre-requisite for promotion or obtaining a post overseas.

In 1916 the Board acknowledged the pressures put on the training system by this enthusiasm for dual qualification, by doubling the length of midwifery training to six months for non-nurses while, for the first time, offering a remission for those who had an appropriate background (a minimum of three years training) in general nursing. Such nurses were only required to do four months midwifery training, while those who had, in the course of their nurse training, completed a three month course in gynaecology or children's nursing were only required to do three months' midwifery training (Central Midwives Board, 1916, *Rules*, p. 5). From now onwards a structural distinction (in terms of educational preparation) was made in entrants to the midwifery profession, between those with a nursing qualification and 'others', as the Board's tables call them. The term 'direct entry' seems not to have been current in 1916.

Ten years later the training requirements were again doubled. In 1926 the CMB promulgated new rules which specified that training was to be not less than 12 months for the non-nurse, while the qualified nurse was required to complete six months training. This was in response to recommendations made in a series of reports on maternal and child health and midwifery education and practice published by the Ministry of Health under the chairmanship of Dr Janet Campbell (1917, 1923, 1924).

A year after the new rules of training, in 1927, Janet Campbell was urging a further extension of the training which she claimed could not yet be considered adequate. It should, she claimed, be:

> . . . further extended and improved until it is at least equal to the training given in the best midwifery schools in, say, France or Holland or Denmark. (Campbell, 1927, p. 43).

With even more prescience she adds:

> . . . it is idle to contemplate extending the training unless and until we can offer the midwife training conditions sufficiently attractive to encourage an educated woman to choose this profession, and, sooner or later, we shall probably be compelled to reconsider the whole question of the training, supply and subsequent employment of midwives. (p. 43)

Campbell goes on to suggest that there should be two types of certification for midwives, one for the practising midwife, 'whose training cannot be too good or too thorough', the other, a certificate for obstetric nurses 'should be restricted to nurses who had already taken hospital training'. These latter certificates could not be obtained by otherwise untrained women (p. 46). She does, however, show a certain ambivalence in going on to say, 'Municipal midwives should, wherever possible, be trained nurses'. Throughout these and other reports of the period one of the main arguments for recruiting more and better-trained midwives was the need to provide a service for the poorest women, among whom maternal mortality levels were unacceptably high and who could scarcely afford the services of a doctor.

In 1929 a report on the Training and Employment of Midwives was published, based on the deliberations of a committee chaired by Sir Robert Bolam. It made recommendations about the standardization of selection procedures in order to recruit students who were fit for the 'arduous and responsible duties which midwifery practice entails'. Nurse-trained candidates for the six month course were to be exempt from the proposed entry test. The report continues:

> It has been stated by many witnesses that as an ideal to be arrived at in the future all midwives should be required to possess the general nursing qualification . . . There is no doubt but that if such an end could be brought about it would be for the good of the profession as a whole and to the community at large . . . but we have grave doubts as to its practicability . . . and we feel that it would be injudicious to disturb the existing arrangements. (Ministry of Health, 1929, p. 21)

By the time this Report was published fewer than 10% of all midwifery candidates were non-nurses.

The years of the depression saw few changes in education and training. In a memorandum to the Minister of Health the CMB (1934), in discussing the proposed new Section B of the Midwives Rules, explicitly addresses the question of non-nurse candidates for midwifery in the following terms:

> After giving careful consideration to the suggestion, which has frequently been made, that every pupil midwife should possess a general nursing qualification, the Board has come to the conclusion that *it is not practicable* to introduce such a requirement at the present time.

In the next paragraph, however, the Board notes, that:

> . . . over the past 10 years the number of candidates at its [i.e. the Board's] examinations who did not hold a nursing qualification has steadily decreased. It is of the opinion there is likely to be a further marked decline when the service of salaried midwives has been established.

Significantly, at no point does the Board express an opinion about the **desirability** of retaining a non-nursing portal of entry into midwifery. Its views are limited strictly to the **feasibility** of such a move.

The 1936 Midwives Act, which greatly improved the conditions under which midwives worked by establishing a proper salaried service nation-wide under Local Authority supervision, also laid the ground for a major revision of midwifery education. The proposals incorporated many of the ideas explored by the reports of previous decades. In 1938, the length of midwifery education was doubled for the third time; the non-nurse was to complete two years training and the qualified nurse one year. The training was, however, to be divided into two distinct parts. Both parts were to be separately examined and certified by the CMB and training institutions were normally to be approved to conduct one or other parts of training. Part I, 18 months for non-nurses, six months for qualified nurses, was to provide a solid training in a hospital setting, in the theory and practice of midwifery. Part II six months for all candidates, was designed to confirm the student in her practice as a midwife with a minimum three months experience 'on the districts'.

The restructuring of the arrangements for certification was designed to reduce wastage from those seeking dual qualification for career advancement purposes. In fact, the extension of training for non-nurses acted as a disincentive to older women with family commitments and the numbers of 'direct entrants' in training dropped still further. In 1939, the last examination under the old Rules, only 8.1% (270) of the 3273 successful candidates were not nurses. By 1940, the first examination under the new Rules, all but one of the 1366 successful candidates were state registered nurses. The situation was made more acute by the war, despite midwifery being given the status of a form of National Service. In 1942 the CMB Annual Report, noting that only 58% of those enrolled in 1940 were still practising a year later, concluded that a permanent solution would only be achieved by a generous improvement in salaries, conditions of service and public regard for midwives.

Towards the end of the war the provision of an adequate maternity service was causing sufficient concern for the Royal College of Obstetricians and Gynaecologists to publish a report (Royal College of Obstetricians and Gynaecologists, 1944) urging greater concentration of resources in maternity centres which also integrated the services of general medical practitioners. In its comments on midwifery education, the report criticised the multiplicity of 'petty training schools' throughout the country and recommended, as part of the establishment of a National Maternity Service, a rationalization of training in 'a few select training schools in large maternity centres distributed evenly throughout the country'. The obstetricians go on to state 'we are of the opinion that every midwife should be a state registered nurse', although they note the existence of the alternative: a European system of midwifery training, where 'the pupils have no connection with the nursing profession'.

By the end of the war just over 52% of practising midwives on the Roll were general trained nurses. This is in contrast with the student midwives, of whom 91% taking Part I and 89% taking Part II training were state registered nurses (Central Midwives Board, 1945, *Annual Report*). The pace of change accelerated even more rapidly as more and more of the non-nurse midwives came to the end of their professional careers and were replaced by dually certificated women.

The problem of the supply of an adequate number of suitably-trained midwives was addressed in 1947 by a Government Working Party chaired by Mrs Mary Stocks. This detailed and sensitive report (Ministry of Health *et al.*, 1949) explored issues related to the midwife's place in the health care team (then under threat from the workings of the new NHS Act of 1948 – see Wood, 1963; Bent, 1982; Robinson, 1990), her training, pay and promotion, her working and living conditions, recruitment and wastage. The report still makes relevant reading today. Among the many significant statements made by the Working Party the following stands out as witness to its perspective on the profession:

> . . . it is clear that, if the midwifery profession is to attract and hold the type of woman that it requires, then the midwife must be given such training and conditions of service as will enable her to become and remain a professional woman as are the doctor, the teacher and the civil servant. (p. 103)

On the subject of the non-nurse candidate for midwifery the Committee adds:

> Our own investigations and the evidence we have heard have convinced us that there are fundamental differences between midwifery and nursing.

They go on to elaborate these differences in terms of accountability and independent decision making, as well as a field of practice related more to normal childbearing than to illness:

> The midwife and nurse have different objects in view, and what is exceptional in the midwife's world is normal in the nurse's. It is important to maintain this vital difference in outlook between the two professions and, we think that, except in comparatively few cases *it is neither necessary nor desirable for a midwife to become a SRN before she starts the specialised training.* (p. 112)

They also note the number of women who have positively no wish to become nurses who would never have become midwives at all if they had first to survive a general nurse training. Nonetheless, after further reflection the Report, considering whether two portals of entry to midwifery should be retained, states 'no part of our proposals have cost us more anxious thought and detailed discussion'. The committee lists three main considerations before proceeding to its conclusions.

1. the increased complexity of midwifery seriously disadvantages the singly qualified midwife;

2. the non-SRN midwife is getting very scarce and there are difficulties in training with regard to comparative academic skills and the degree of ward responsibility which can be delegated;

and worst of all

3. 'the non-SRN midwife has today no prospects of promotion whatever'. Despite holding the same certificate, having passed the same professional examination as her dually qualified counterpart the non-nurse midwife is denied access to posts including ward sister, tutor or supervisor of midwives.

Because they have been frequently misinterpreted we report the Committee's conclusions in full.

Paragraph 117. After much careful and sympathetic discussion we have come to the conclusion that there is at present little chance of improving these conditions permanently and that it is almost dishonest to train women, give them a statutory qualification and then use them in a permanent position of inferiority. As stated above, this does not imply that we regard a full nursing qualification as necessarily an essential prelude to midwifery – if our training proposals are accepted the midwife will again become 'S.C.M. only'. But with a different and longer training.

Paragraph 118. For all these reasons we think that the time has come to bring to an end this long and honourable chapter in midwifery. We recommended that the training of midwives without the SRN or SRCN (or, in Scotland, SRFN) qualification be discontinued but, and this we urge most emphatically, to those who already hold the qualification of SCM only, and have the necessary experience, all midwifery appointments should be open on their merits and no distinction in advertisements, pay, or anything else, should be made. (Stocks, 1949, p. 29)

Stocks foreshadowed the Briggs report (Department of Health and Social Security, 1972) and Project 2000 (United Kingdom Central Council, 1986) by suggesting a path out of the 'multiple qualification' dilemma by proposing a common basic training for nurses and midwives alike, carrying no qualification, which could be followed by specialization within the candidates' chosen field (p. 138). In this, the Working Party was adopting the proposals of the contemporaneous Nurses' Working Party which also included separation of schools of nurse education from the general hospital system, student status and grants for nurses in training. The proposals met much the same response from the profession as was later to greet Briggs and Project 2000 – midwifery on the whole saw its identity as an independent profession put at risk by the sharing of a common preparation for practice with its sister profession.

Stocks speaks of closing a 'long and honourable chapter' in midwifery by discontinuing non-nursing candidates. By a fairly narrow squeak this did not happen. By 1949, 31% of practising midwives were not nurses and by 1982 only 7.2% of midwives on the register were singly qualified. As for students, in 1949 only 4% were not nurses. This figure dropped to 0.6% by 1983, according to the ENB's index of students. Regrettably no further figures for non-nurse midwives in practice are available, due to the present system of data analysis used by the UKCC for its professional register. The figures must, however, have dwindled still further as since 1985 the potential output of non-nurse midwives had dropped to the eight candidates a year being trained by the one remaining training school for non-nurses.

The two immediate post-war decades may be considered the nadir of the non-nurse midwife. With a few admirable exceptions, she had the worst of all possible worlds in terms of professional preparation. On the whole she seems to have suffered a poorly constructed, discriminatory curriculum which did nothing at all to improve the status of those with no nursing qualification behind them. All too often the two years were spent in variants of the recipe: Preliminary Training School (General Nursing), general wards, Part I midwifery training twice, then Part II. This may be a parody of what the best schools offered but sufficient midwives still practising today gave evidence of this system, the only advantage of which must surely have been that it was a relatively cheap way of producing midwives.

In the 1960s, the gateway to midwifery was widened further to admit enrolled nurses to yet another form of shortened course lasting 18 months. These, confusingly, were also to be known as 'direct entrants', although they held a nursing certificate. These were, on the whole, women whose academic background did not equip them to undertake full RGN studies, thus reinforcing the increasingly poor status of the 'direct entrant' midwife.

Ten years after the Stocks report, the Report of the Maternity Services Committee (Ministry of Health, 1959) appeared, and spoke briefly of the non-nurse midwife. In its evidence to the Committee the CMB pointed out that although only 5% of student midwives were not nurses some 23% of midwives in practice had no nursing qualification. It was stated that they tended to stay in midwifery for about 12 years and were drawn from an older group of women either with family or from other professions. Despite the continuation of very poor promotion prospects they were stated to be among 'the best recruits to the profession'. The committee made no recommendations about their training.

The mid-sixties to mid-eighties witnessed a much wider debate about the structure and function of the NHS and of the reform of nurse educa-

CArm CyansK

tion in general. A stream of documents, culminating in Project 2000 from the UKCC (1986), usually included midwifery within the ambit of nurse education. Nonetheless control of the midwifery profession remained solely in the hands of the CMB until the National Boards and UKCC took over in 1983 under the terms of the unifying Nurses, Midwives and Health Visitors Act of 1979. The midwifery profession retained its distinct identity within the statutory framework. Direct entry received little or no overt consideration throughout the early part of this period. In 1970 a committee was set up under the chairmanship of Professor Asa Briggs, to review the role, education and training of nurses and midwives (Department of Health and Social Security, 1972). Although the Colleges of Nursing and Midwifery recommended by Briggs had not materialized in England and Wales at the time of this study, many of the other recommendations had or were being implemented. The 1979 Nurses, Midwives and Health Visitors Act brought under a single statutory control the multiplicity of nursing, midwifery and health visiting certifying authorities.

Although the Briggs Committee says categorically 'we note that most midwives are already nurses and we recommend that in future all midwives should be nurses' (DHSS, 1972, para. 626) it does acknowledge that, in giving evidence, both the CMB and RCM said that they wished to continue to see entry to the profession either through midwifery or through nursing (para. 246). The Briggs recommendations for nurse/midwife education consisted basically of an 18 month common core curriculum for all students leading to a Certificate in Nursing Practice, which could be followed by a further 18 month course leading to specialist registration. Midwives would be among such specialists, although the Committee stated that the initial education of midwives should not be separate from that of nurses (para. 253g). To meet European Community requirements Briggs proposed that there should be a year's post-registration supervised practice prior to eligibility for practice as a midwife in Europe. Briggs, in fact, saw most midwives preparing for practice by an alternative course. They would, normally, take the full three year path to registration as a general nurse, and then complete their training as a midwife with 12 months specialist integrated course. Those who used the first path, i.e. certification followed by 18 month Midwifery Registration and Higher Certificate, would not be eligible to work as nurses, should they wish to, without a further conversion course.

Some 13 years later, after a series of NHS reorganizations, a Royal Commission on the NHS and the erection of a totally new statutory framework for the regulation of nursing and midwifery practice, a clutch of major documents appeared on the future of nurse education. The first (in April 1985), the Royal College of Nursing's report on the education of nurses chaired by Harry Judge (Royal College of Nursing, 1985) had little to say about direct entry midwifery training, but did not exclude the possibility in its proposals for a two year common foundation course. In May 1985 the ENB published a consultation paper on professional education/training courses which, while also promoting a health-based common core course, positively favoured a direct entry approach to midwifery education and training. It noted with enthusiasm that midwifery students are prepared to deliver care in the community as well as in hospital and that midwife teachers combine the roles of teacher and practitioner. An analysis of the 796 responses to the consultation (Dodd, 1985) showed that 61% of respondents agreed with the view that the direct entrant element in midwifery should be increased. A small minority commented that an RGN qualification was essential for midwifery. Events, public opinion and professional opinion had evidently countered Brigg's position that all midwives should hold a nursing qualification.

Another relevant development in the late 1970s saw a swing away from the medicalized model of childbirth. Writings by authors such as Oakley (1984), Kitzinger (1988), Cartwright (1979) and Inch (1982), as well as an increasingly high media profile for childbirth related topics and the feminist lobby all contributed to a swing towards the previously unfashionable non-nurse midwife. The Association of Radical Midwives, started in the mid seventies, actively took up the challenge of promoting the cause of direct entrants and set up a working party for this purpose.

In 1981, in response to the EEC Midwifery Directives, the CMB lengthened training to 18 months for RGNs and three years for non-nurses (Central Midwives Board, 1980, *Rules*, Rule 24). By 1983 just two schools of midwifery had taken up the challenge of providing the new style three year education. One of these two schools only trained a single set of students, who qualified as midwives in 1985.

In May 1986, Project 2000 (United Kingdom Central Council, 1986) was published. Sweeping reforms of nurse education were proposed. Midwifery, with due recognition of its 'specialness', was nonetheless subsumed as a 'branch', one of five of the 'tree of nursing'. In common with other educational documents, supernumerary status was claimed for the students and a health-based Common Foundation Programme of two years proposed. Although there was mention of a possible experimental three year course, most midwives were still envisaged as post-registration, with their course remaining at 18 months duration.

The midwifery profession reacted with surprising vigour to these proposals. Following consultation with the professions, Project 2000 took cognisance of the midwifery profession's strong feelings about its distinct professional identity and abandoned plans for incorporating midwifery as a branch of nursing in the final Project 2000 strategy sent to the Minister of Health. Midwifery, seemingly challenged and stimulated by the Project 2000 debate, moved on rapidly to develop alternative projects, centering mainly around amalgamation of schools in one form or other and the development of direct entry training. The Association of Radical Midwives (ARM) produced its suggestions for the future of midwifery education and practice in a document entitled, *The Vision* (December 1986) and, in January 1987, the Royal College of Midwives published a report on the Role and Education of the Future Midwife in the United Kingdom (Royal College of Midwives, 1987). The RCM document did not mention the direct entrant explicitly but, in its educational ideology, spoke of preparing the midwife for her specific role and, even more significantly, outlined a curriculum content for a three year education of the midwife, with no reference to alternative courses. Both the ARM and RCM documents described the practice of the midwife as they envisaged it for the future, before discussing a possible educational programme. With its emphasis on fully-exercised practitioner-status, direct referral systems, team and group practices, that picture makes a marked contrast to the reality of midwifery practice as documented by Robinson *et al.* (1983). The ARM *Vision* opens its brief paragraphs on education bluntly with the statement that 'midwifery training will be primarily by a three year direct entry course'.

Several major lines of argument were evident in the views expressed by the proponents of direct entry. They asserted that direct entry would result in a more independent practitioner who was less 'doctor orientated', and more confident. They felt that such a midwife would bring a more critical approach to practice, be more effective as an agent for change and be more sensitive to women's health care needs and open to client participation in that care. Other arguments focused on economic, demographic and manpower considerations; it was maintained that direct entry courses would appeal to an older candidate, the retention would be improved and that the whole enterprise in terms of providing practising midwives would be cheaper than the current system.

Direct entry supporters frequently used a combination of these arguments. The problem lay in the fact that such a wide-ranging variety of assumptions was largely unexamined and virtually unproven.

As a result of this renewed interest in a distinct identity for the midwifery profession, a refocusing of midwifery practice on the needs of the well woman and her family and, inevitably, growing concern about adequate recruitment via the traditional post-RGN route, the ENB held a meeting in the Autumn of 1986 to promote the concept of the direct route into midwifery. This study is, to some extent, a sequel to that discussion and attempted to provide a more solid basis for the important choices which lay before the midwifery profession in the late 1980s.

AIMS AND METHODS

The initial phase of the project consisted of reviewing literature and formulating the aims and design of the project. During the course of the study, a great deal of unpublished material from professional and personal archives was made available to the researchers. There was, however, little concrete information, published or unpublished, on direct entry midwifery. This lack of firm data indicated that information gathering was a priority in order that the promotion of direct entry could be based on knowledge of the existing situation. The project commenced in April and the objectives agreed at the Advisory Group meeting on May 1 1987 were as follows:

1. To collate available information on direct entry (and relevant other subjects), to identify gaps in existing information, and to try and fill those gaps.
2. To promote the development of direct entry courses, create greater awareness of direct entry, discover the inhibiting factors and to provide useful tips on the establishment of such courses. (Radford and Thompson, 1988)

In the course of the initial phase of the project, these aims were refined as follows:

- to describe the national situation concerning provision of and planning for direct entry courses;
- to discover the factors inhibiting or encouraging the development of such courses;
- to advise on the issues which those thinking about planning such courses should consider;
- to recommend ways in which direct entry midwifery education could be developed and established more rapidly.

A problem appeared at an early stage of the project when the researchers realized that many people expected the study to return some form of verdict about direct entry. That was never our remit. As described in the previous section, policy decisions in favour of promoting the development and availability of such courses had already been taken at a national level well before the study was set up (ENB, 1986; Department of Health and Social Security, 1986).

Data colletion comprised the following:

1. surveys by questionnaire of regional and district health authorities and schools of midwifery;
2. survey by questionnaire of potential applicants for non-nurse midwifery courses;
3. interviews with a range of individuals by means of personal visits and telephone.

The research team met regularly with an Advisory Group whose members were drawn from relevant professional and statutory bodies, educational researchers and midwifery service and education departments. The researchers also had frequent contact with professional officers (midwifery) at the ENB and UKCC, the nursing officer (midwifery) at the then DHSS, the education officer at the ENB, and with representatives of the RCM and midwives involved in service and education. Consultation was extensive and continued throughout the project.

Survey by questionnaire of regional and district health authorities and schools of midwifery

The aim of the first survey was to provide information about the current situation regarding direct entry midwifery training and to identify those factors inhibiting or encouraging its development. It was hoped that alternative methods of dealing with potential obstacles and innovative schemes would be discovered. Three similar questionnaires were designed for regional health authorities, district health authorities and midwifery schools; they included questions on the following aspects of course provision:

- current policy;
- investigation of feasibility including cost;
- factors that had encouraged courses to be considered, planned and run (including staffing needs, demand for courses and staff attitudes);
- the importance of potential obstacles to running, planning, or considering courses (including supply of candidates, staff attitudes and adequate resources in terms of funds, educational expertise and availability of clinical experience). (Those respondents who identified obstacles were asked if they would be prepared to discuss them with the research team in interview at a later date);
- whether advice had been sought concerning obstacles to course provision;
- factors that had contributed to a decision not to consider course provision or to reject it after consideration (these included demand, poor career prospects, staff attitudes, resources) and how important each of these were in relation to a reconsideration;
- what would help course provision (e.g. advice on costing, advice on curriculum development, financial assistance).

Questionnaires for regional health authorities asked whether a strategy for midwifery and for midwifery education had been developed. Questionnaires for district health authorities and midwifery schools also included questions on collaboration with other institutions/districts over direct entry course provision and the latter also included a question on the effect that providing direct entry courses might have on the size of 18 month post-registration courses.

Direct entry midwifery education

Table 10.1 Response rates for institutional questionnaires

	Regions	Districts	Schools
Total number of questionnaires sent	14	194	144
Completed questionnaires	13	162	139
Letter explaining current situation	1	15	3
Total responses	14	177	142
	(100%)	(91%)	(99%)
No answer	—	17	2
Total	14	194	144

Source: compiled by the authors.

As time constraints ruled out piloting, the draft questionnaires were sent instead to relevant individuals and representatives of statutory and professional bodies, then discussed in detail with them and with the Advisory Group. The questionnaires were redrafted and recirculated, then finally revised and approved by the Advisory Group. The regional health authority questionnaire was sent to the Regional Nursing Officer and the school of midwifery questionnaire to an Approved Teacher of Midwifery. The district health authority questionnaire was sent initially to the District Nurse Advisor (DNA) as an overall district perspective was required, and she or he was asked to forward it for someone else to complete if this was thought to be appropriate. In 20 of the 162 cases, the questionnaire was in fact completed by the Director of Midwifery Services (DMS). The rest were completed by the DNA, either alone or in consultation with the DMS.

Following two reminders, excellent response rates of 100%, 91% and 99% were achieved for the three surveys respectively (Table 10.1). There were no major problems reported by respondents in the completion of the questionnaires; nearly all were completed correctly.

Survey by questionnaire of potential applicants

The aim of the second questionnaire survey was to try and find out more about potential applicants for direct entry courses. This survey had not been considered in the initial design of the project; but the literature review highlighted the dearth of information on quantity and quality of possible candidates. The design and administration of this postal survey were done in a rapid and *ad hoc* fashion in order to fit in to the time scale of the project. There was not time to circulate drafts by post, so an initial list of possible questions was discussed with as many appropriate people as possible.

Questions included the following:

- demographic profile (age, sex, family responsibilities);
- academic and employment profile;
- reasons why want to train as a midwife;
- whether discussed plans with a midwife, other health worker and/or careers adviser;
- in which region want to train;
- full- or part-time course preferred;
- how long prepared to travel to course centre;
- how long prepared to wait for a place;
- immediate plans (i.e. apply for place at Derby School of Midwifery (the only school running a direct entry course at the time of the study), wait for another course, do something else).

Again the final draft was seen, discussed and approved by the Advisory Group. The English National Board Careers Advisory Centre (ENBCAC) had offered to send out a questionnaire, explanation and freepost envelope to anyone writing to them requiring information on direct entry midwifery courses. This offer was gratefully accepted and 365 questionnaires were sent out by the ENBCAC.

Schools of midwifery were also asked, via the Education Advisory Group of the Royal College of Midwives, if they would like to participate – due to other pressures on tutors, few did so. However, several schools who did not participate directly referred enquiries to the researchers, or sent the names of those interested to them. The Association of Radical Midwives (ARM) also provided a list of names and addresses. These methods accounted for 48 questionnaires. To avoid duplication (e.g. an individual may have received a form from the ENBCAC and a school), a slip was attached to the questionnaires asking the respondent to tick a box and return the questionnaire uncompleted if she or he had previously completed one. No reminders were sent, due to the shortage of time, and the variety of ways the questionnaire was administered.

The response rates varied with the method of administration. Those administered by the ENBCAC showed a response rate of 30%, those sent out by the schools or as a result of referrals from the schools showed a response rate of 58%. This did not include ten late responses and four duplicates. This poor response was disappointing but not altogether surprising. First of all, the questionnaire was sent to those enquiring about direct entry midwifery training, not merely those expressing a firm commitment to doing such a training. Many of those writing (particularly to the ENBCAC) may also have been enquiring about alternative careers. If the idea of a midwifery career had been rejected, there was little incentive to complete the questionnaire.

Interviews and visits

The questionnaire surveys gave a broad outline, but to gain in-depth information and to add flesh to the bare bones of the statistics, interviews and visits were made. These fell into two groups. The first group were semi-structured interviews with various people at schools of midwifery (including service colleagues), usually in person, but occasionally over the telephone. The second category consisted of unstructured personal or telephone interviews with a wide range of people to clarify or supplement information received via questionnaires, the semi-structured interviews or the grapevine. These conversations were also used to formulate a costings guide, models of recruitment and selection and fill out the historical and current picture of direct entry midwifery education.

Schools of midwifery. The criteria for the selection of places to visit and the topics to cover in the semi-structured interviews were formulated by the researchers, discussed with relevant people and after consideration, approved by the Advisory Group. The schools visited were:

- the one running a three year course;
- some with projects planned;
- some where projects had been abandoned or shelved;
- some beginning to consider the option of direct entry;
- some who had rejected the option.

The researchers tried to ensure a reasonable geographical spread and to include schools in a variety of surroundings (inner city, rural, etc.). Due to the financial and time constraints mentioned earlier the visits had to be cost effective, therefore in some cases information was gathered by telephone rather than by a visit. Although schools in each of the above groups were visited, there were proportionally more in certain groups in which there was more information to be gathered or more people to be seen. Table 10.2 illustrates the groups and shows the number visited or contacted.

The following topics were covered in the interviews with school personnel:

1. organizational background: this included – amalgamations, (actual/ envisaged), sites and distances between them, number of deliveries per year;
2. philosophy – e.g. why direct entry? Why now? Type of midwife needed;

Table 10.2 Schools' intentions by interviews

Schools	Questionnaires returned	Interviewed	
		By visit	By telephone
Not considering three year training	22	2	3
Considering (undecided)	29	2	4
Want to but no action	30	4	4
Planning	9	6	3
Want to but could not	16	4	3
Decided against	11	3	1
Other	22	4	3
Total	139	25	21

Source: compiled by the authors.

3. demand for direct entry: evidence? Comments?
4. problems and solutions – finance and costings/funding, education, in terms of curriculum, staffing levels, experience and preparation of staff, availability of learning areas, attitudes to direct entry, career development;
5. advice and help about course provision: has any been received? If so what and from whom? Is advice wanted, and if so what and from whom?

Information about Derby Midwifery School. As the only school running a direct entry course, at the time of the study, Derby School of Midwifery was naturally of particular interest. However, it was felt that to concentrate too much time and effort on Derby would blinker people to the range of alternative options for direct entry. Therefore, rather than trying to evaluate the present course, the researchers endeavoured to obtain a picture of the situation in Derby and draw out useful pointers as to problems which may arise and possible solutions. This was done by studying existing literature, gathering perceptions of Derby from interviewees and respondents nationally and by extensive interviews and telephone conversations with a wide range of staff and students at Derby. Correspondents and ENB officials provided supplementary data and gave added insights.

Other interviews. Close contact was maintained throughout the project with key people in the statutory bodies, as was mentioned earlier. Personal and telephone interviews were used to investigate modes of recruitment and selection (e.g. police, army, Manpower Services Commission), to devise a costings guide, and study other experimental courses which could provide useful tips (e.g. Portsmouth and their mature entrants course). Other contacts included relevant bodies such as the Royal College of Midwives, Association of Radical Midwives, National Childbirth Trust, Midwives Information and Resource Service and the Institute of Manpower Studies. Individuals who play or had played a key role in midwifery and/or the campaign for direct entry were interviewed.

Data analysis

The quantitative data were analysed using SPSSX (the revised version of the Statistical Package for Social Sciences) and the Lopez-Velastin-Radford Interface (Lopez *et al.*, 1985). Analysis was done for each survey group as a whole and then for various subsets. For the 'institutional' questionnaires the data from districts and schools were split by policy decision and then by region. For the 'enquiries' questionnaires, the results were grouped by age, place of enquiry, qualifications and dependants and each subset was then compared.

The majority of respondents to both questionnaire surveys had written copious comments, which were too valuable a resource to waste. All the comments were read and similar ones grouped together, which enabled some form of quantitative value to be assigned. In some cases, the responses were able to be coded and analysed using SPSSX. This method was also used for analysing data from the interviews. Whenever feasible, quantitative analysis was done, but the most valuable contribution of the interviews was the added insight they gave into the complexity of the situation. The material gathered in the interviews confirmed the data obtained from the questionnaires.

Dissemination

A final draft of the full report was prepared for the Advisory Group in mid-February, and it was then presented to the ENB for circulation to the March meeting of the midwifery committee. The researchers hoped that it would then go to the ENB, when publication would be approved. This timetable would have allowed printing and a launch to take place within the lifespan of the project. In the event, the midwifery committee wished to discuss the report further and it went to the ENB in June. The ENB endorsed the report and arranged its publication and distribution.

FINDINGS AND RECOMMENDATIONS

The format employed for the presentation and discussion of findings in this chapter differs from that usually followed in this series of books. Instead of presenting the findings from each phase of the data collection (the institutional surveys, the potential applicant survey and the interviews), followed by a final discussion section, the findings and recommendations are presented in terms of the five main issues that emerged from the data when considered as a whole. This approach is consistent with the research team's brief, which was to identify factors hindering or encouraging the implementation of direct entry courses, to advise on issues that should be considered by those intending to implement courses and to make recommendations relating to each. A number of topics were considered in the study which are not included in the findings reported here. A costings formula for example was prepared during the study; information about this and the detailed findings for all the issues considered are available in the full report of the project (Radford and Thompson, 1988).

Before looking at the five main issues to emerge from the data, the national picture as indicated by the study is briefly outlined. The findings showed that there was a great deal of interest in the idea of direct entry midwifery, but that at the time of writing the report, only 13 areas had taken positive steps towards implementing such programmes. Many of these were at a very early stage, and only two courses had gained ENB approval in principle. It seemed that people in most areas were waiting for someone else to set up a course first and see how they got on, before committing themselves to such a venture. Findings from questionnaires and from interviews showed that the factors inhibiting the development, like those encouraging it, were pragmatic, historical and/or ideological. The major pragmatic reason encouraging direct entry courses was a present and/or predicted shortage of midwives. Practical factors identified as inhibiting course developments were organization of funding, shortage of tutors, and lack of information on matters such as the supply of candidates, and the structure and organization of the course. The historical and ideological factors that have promoted or inhibited the development of direct entry programmes have already been highlighted in the second section of this chapter. They revolve around the status of the direct entrant, the relationship of midwifery to nursing and differing perceptions about the ideal role of the midwife; ranging from that of an independent practitioner who is the 'guardian' of normal childbirth, to someone who assists medical staff in the management of an event that is 'only normal in retrospect'.

Turning now to the five issues identified as essential for consideration in the implementation of direct entry courses; these were:

1. what sort of midwife will be needed?
2. recruitment and selection to the course;
3. what sort of educational programme should the course comprise?
4. resources needed to initiate and run courses;
5. staff attitudes to direct entry midwifery.

Each is discussed in turn.

What sort of midwife will be needed?

The most important issue, and one which had not been adequately addressed at the time of the study, is agreement on what kind of midwife is needed and consequently on what kind of preparation she required. Although the project had no specific remit to examine the midwife's role, no discussion of a new direction in midwifery education could entirely ignore the issue and it was therefore explored in the course of the literature review and the interview study.

A number of studies (e.g. Robinson *et al.*, 1983; Robinson, 1985; Garcia and Garforth, 1991), had documented the extent to which the midwife's role had been eroded, primarily by the increasing involvement of medical staff in normal maternity care. The mid 1970s onwards had seen a gradual heightening of the midwife's profile in terms of debate in the profession and in the media. Much of the growing enthusiasm for direct entry had been underpinned by arguments centring on the proper role and responsibilities of the midwife and the assumption that the proposed new form of education would foster the qualities needed by the 'better' midwife that some supposed would emerge (Flint, 1986; Downe, 1988).

The literature review and the study interviews undertaken indicated a degree of polarization about the role of the midwife. This is not surprising, given the historical background of the profession, nor is it unique to the United Kingdom (Ris, 1986; Kitzinger, 1988; Simonot, 1989). In England, as in many of the 'developed' nations, midwifery debate centres round the degree to which the profession should be the guardian of childbirth as a normal, non-medical, family-centred event (Van Daalen, 1988). This gives rise fairly frequently to the medical profession, specifically obstetricians, being cast in an adversarial role.

To some extent, the sharper picture of the midwife's identity that was emerging seemed closely linked to beliefs held about the relevance and value of nurse education as an appropriate precursor of midwifery education. Those respondents who emphasized the feature of a community-based, family-centred model of care, offering maximum choice to the client, a full range of independent practice to the midwife, personalized systems of care delivery and accountability by the midwife to her clients as well as to her employing authority, were concerned that the ethos of nurse education, with its then still identifiable bias towards a medical mode of care, cannot prepare the candidates they need for such practice. Certainly most of the direct entrant midwives who were interviewed stated that they would not ever have wanted to be nurses; their sense of midwifery as a distinct profession was striking. Recent trends towards a health-based model for nurse education (English National Board, 1985; United Kingdom Central Council, 1986) did not seem to have allayed anxieties among midwives looking for a more assertive, independently-minded practitioner. At least one senior tutor welcomed the prospect of non-nurse learners because it would save her having to help her students to 'unlearn' some of the lessons of their initial training.

Although such views were frequently encountered, there were alternatives. A number of midwives in both service and education voiced their disquiet about the expansion of the direct entry initiative. They argued strongly for general nurse training as an essential prerequisite for midwifery education, if standards of practice were to be maintained. Replies to the questionnaires recognized the commonality of many concepts necessary to preparation for either midwifery or nursing, and while some preferred that such preparation should be done in some form of joint shared-learning venture, others felt equally keenly that direct entry is and would remain 'only second best', as one tutor put it.

Faced with such a lack of consensus it was evident that in order to design any coherent educational strategy for the future, the profession needed to clarify its intent in terms of which type of midwife was desired. If midwifery practice was to continue in the mode identified by studies such as that by Robinson *et al.* (1983) then there was an economic argument to support a shorter, cheaper direct preparation. If, however, midwives now wished to assume a more independent professional stance, then the necessary educational investment would have to be greater in terms both of quality and of quantity as otherwise the singly qualified midwife would be permanently disadvantaged by comparison with her nurse-trained counterpart, regardless of just how much of the initial training was directly relevant to good midwifery practice. Developments within midwifery, for example the response to the Project 2000 proposals described earlier in this chapter, indicated that it was this more independent practitioner that the profession wished to foster. Moreover, in the period since this project was completed, the move towards greater professional independence has gathered momentum, as recently exemplified in the recommendations of the Winterton Report (House of Commons Select Committee, 1992).

Decisions about the kind of midwife needed underpin the next two issues discussed in this section – recruitment and selection of candidates, and the kind of course that should be provided.

Recruitment and selection

The literature review on direct entry midwifery training gave the impression that there was a great 'demand' for it and that increasing the number of courses would result in an enlarged recruitment pool and improved retention. Data obtained in the course of this study indicated that assertions in the literature did not seem to be based on factual evidence. It was difficult to obtain information about the numbers of people who would be available for and interested in direct entry midwifery training. Firstly, the direct entry option is not widely known, which is not surprising as there was only one course available at the time of the study. Secondly, it was found that few centres kept detailed records about those enquiring about such courses; that the staff tended to overestimate the number of enquiries that they had received, and in some instances to draw conclusions about the kind of person interested in direct entry on the basis of a handful of letters. The study highlighted the need for detailed records of enquiries. It is important that information is collected locally, as areas vary in their demographic composition. A draft format for this purpose was designed by the team, that could be adapted to local circumstances. There was little consensus amongst those interviewed as to the type of person who would be considered suitable for such a course. This is the most crucial question, for unless one can define the target recruitment group, its size cannot be estimated nor can effective recruitment methods be devised.

For the reasons outlined in Section 3, the postal survey of those enquiring about direct entry midwifery training only gave a partial picture of any potential recruitment pool. It did however, provide some useful findings; these are reported in full in Radford and Thompson (1988). Three of the main issues are highlighted here. Firstly, the characteristics of the respondents varied greatly and certain of these, such as age and dependants, influenced the type of course desired. For example, those with dependants were more likely than those without to prefer a part-time course and to be prepared to wait longer for a place to become available, but were less likely to be willing to move in order to obtain a place. Secondly, many of the respondents seemed unaware that midwives looked after women throughout pregnancy, labour and the postnatal period. Before the potential supply of candidates can be assessed, there must be greater public understanding of the role of the midwife. Moreover, it is important that candidates' expectations are realistic or there is a danger of a high wastage rate during the course. Finally the study highlighted the importance of selection as not all those who expressed an interest in midwifery would be suitable as candidates for the course.

What steps then should be taken when assessing the recruitment pool, considering the type of course to run, and devising recruitment and selection procedures? First the aims of the course must be clarified, and certain issues addressed. The process will only be successful if a clear idea of the desired result of direct entry education (i.e. the role of the qualified midwife) has been drawn up in advance. This may seem unnecessary, but in interviews and from comments it was obvious that the profession itself has widely varying ideas of what midwives could and should do. The other issue to address is what are the ideal characteristics of a direct entry student? Guidelines are needed as to age range, educational ability and qualifications, recruitment area, physical requirements and domestic commitments, as well as the more hazy character traits and skills such as communication etc. Such a profile must take care not to fall foul of the Equal Opportunities legislation. Once the decision on the type of person required has been made, the second step is to set up a recruitment strategy.

To set up a strategy, the local supply of candidates must first be assessed. Each school will have different needs. Some will already take most or all of their students from the local area. Others, such as some in inner city areas, are accustomed to looking further afield. Each school which wants to run a direct entry midwifery course should research the potential local recruitment pool by advertising in the local press, visits to secondary schools and visits to groups such as the National Childbirth Trust, community centres, etc. The size and composition of this potential source of applicants should then be matched to the local requirements for replacement midwives and the desired ratio of direct entry midwives to post-registration students. Should the supply of possible direct entry midwifery candidates appear inadequate, then either the ratio of post-registration places offered could be increased or the course opened to non-local candidates. Once the needs of each school have been established, the advertising mix can be worked out. Advertising takes two main forms, general awareness/corporate and specific needs. General or corporate advertising raises peoples' awareness of a topic or issue; in this case the role of the midwife and the availability of direct entry midwifery education. Specific need advertising is done when the issues are clear and all that is needed is to sell a product/service, e.g. places on a specific direct entry midwifery course. It may be worth considering the creation of a specific midwifery or direct entry recruitment team either on a formal, national level or on an informal local level. These teams could carry out visits to clubs and societies, and even schools. The source of funding for recruitment activities must be clarified – will it be the Department of Health, the regional or district health authority or the midwifery school?

Once an effective recruitment strategy has been devised, the next step is to design relevant selection procedures. The selectors will have to determine whether candidates:

- are temperamentally suited to the job and training;
- are physically capable;
- are likely to remain in post long enough to recover the cost of training;
- are educationally able for the course.

One of the concerns of respondents to the institutional questionnaire was that selection of appropriate direct entry candidates would be crucial and more complex than for post-registration ones. This is because many, if not all, post-registration candidates would have some obstetric experience and their time in nursing would have already weeded out most of those

mentally, physically or emotionally unfit to undertake midwifery education. Few post-basic midwifery courses include formal training in recruitment and selection of candidates and staff. Prior to instituting a direct
entry course, all those involved in selection should be properly trained.

When investigating the alternative models of recruitment, the researchers
discovered that those with the lowest wastage rates had properly trained
selection staff using a combination of interviews, psychometric and physical testing.

The evidence from the postal surveys and interviews indicated that
unless effective recruitment and selection methods are devised and fully
implemented, there is little point in investing money and effort in establishing a direct entry midwifery course. Unless appropriate candidates are
chosen, high wastage rates and/or lower standards may well result, neither
of which will benefit midwifery or childbearing women and their babies.

What sort of educational programme?

Education for any profession takes place within a more or less clear framework of strategy and structure. Because of the far-reaching implications of
extending availability of direct entry courses, the study investigated the
existing and proposed structures for midwifery education and sought information about strategies for the future at national, regional and local levels.

The National Health Service provides the physical environment in which
the clinical and theoretical components of education are carried out, according to ENB approved norms. Until recently this has effectively meant each
one of about 144 distinct midwifery schools developing its own curriculum
and seeking its own resources, financial and other, usually from the district
health authority's maternity unit budget. The picture is changing rapidly,
the institutional questionnaires showed that some 42% of schools were
already collaborating with others in some form and a further 37% said that
they were willing to do so. Overall a significant proportion of the country's
schools were willing to undertake major organizational change in order
to provide an improved educational service. Such pooling of resources,
coupled with an increasing willingness to develop links with higher and
further education, should improve the educational opportunities available
to staff and students alike. The postal survey also showed that while only
16% of schools were collaborating with institutions of higher and further
education some 71% were willing to do so in the future.

Clear, consistent evidence of the development of an educational strategy was less easy to come by. At the time of the study it was known that
the DHSS had indicated that there should be at least one direct entry
project developed in each region. Simultaneously the regions were working out a massive scheme of rationalization for the provision of nurse

education. This re-organization, in terms of consortia linking schools of nursing, the creation of colleges of nursing and other alternatives affected midwifery education, if only because of its responsibility for providing the maternity care component in the RGN syllabus and the common dependence of nursing and midwifery students alike on access to specific clinical learning areas. All this, together with the then imminent introduction of the demonstration schemes for the Project 2000 preparation for nursing created a climate in which coherent strategic planning was an enormously difficult task. This might explain why, at the time of the study, only 21% of the regions had completed a strategy for midwifery education.

Whatever the reasons, uncertainty about both the structures and the strategies of the future played an important part in the anxieties felt by those exploring the possibility of developing direct entry courses. The study looked in some detail at the problems of planning and communication identified in this area (Radford and Thompson, 1988). This chapter, however, looks at some of the other issues which, in the eyes of the schools, either encouraged or discouraged them in their plans for direct entry. Data from the institutional questionnaires showed that the assurance of financial support would be a major incentive, together with firm evidence of the extent of demand for such a course. Encouragement from the ENB and the health authorities was felt to be a further important factor. On the other hand, lack of tutorial time, the demands of student supervision and support and the shortage of funding acted as major disincentives to 74% of the schools answering this question. Inadequate educational resources and perceived lack of demand were other reasons for schools not developing courses. It is worth noting that nearly 20% of the respondents felt that career prospects for direct entrants were so poor as to warrant their not providing a course.

The data provided by the questionnaires were confirmed and amplified during the visits to the schools, in which lengthy discussions with service, school and planning personnel provided a rich source of insight into their concerns with regard to direct entry education. Since only one school of midwifery had any current experience of direct entry, it was not surprising that a fair amount of apprehension was detectable. What was more unexpected was the relatively widespread positive response to the challenge of providing such education. Recruitment, retention and staffing problems seemed to act as a spur to direct entry project development. The anxiety expressed by tutorial staff seemed to have less to do with teaching 'new' areas of curriculum than with their awareness of the huge additional demands on very limited resources made by curriculum planning for such a project. This was especially true as the study took place at a time when many schools were deeply involved in developing curriculum proposals for ENB course re-approval for 18 month courses and in complex discussions across health districts and within regions about potential amalgamations. Understandably, many were cautious of pressing forward with direct entry plans until the educational infrastructure which would be needed to support them was assured.

For all the above reasons, only a handful of schools were identified in which curriculum planning had developed to a recognizable stage. In practical terms this presented problems with long-term planning, since without at least a broad curriculum outline it is not possible to present a realistic analysis of the resources needed in terms of staff, premises, accommodation, equipment, as well as student numbers. Costing the course is an impossibility in such circumstances and no remotely accurate bid for funding could have been made to the health authority or other source.

In those schools in which planning was more advanced, directly educational issues were receiving due attention. Opportunities for shared learning were being explored, both within the NHS and in the wider educational system of local polytechnics or universities. Some of the assumptions about direct entrants were having an impact on the style of curriculum being planned. It seemed widely accepted that, in some centres at least, such a course would correspond to the needs of an older candidate who would bring her (or his) own fuller life experience to the course and, ultimately, to the profession. A philosophy of student-centred, self-directed learning, clearly focused on a study of the health care needs of childbearing women and their babies in their local environment was central to planning. A few schools were beginning to recognize just how much a well-tried and familiar system must become flexible if it is to accommodate and hold a new generation of people who have not been socialized into its ways through years of earlier training, and whose values and priorities may not automatically sit comfortably with established NHS patterns. There was talk of part-time programmes, credit accumulation, the provision of crèches, supernumerary status. A few were already looking to the development of a degree course, partly because of the feeling that the time was right (if not overdue) and partly in an attempt to exorcise the ghost of the old-style, Cinderella image of direct entry.

The widespread recognition of the need to assure educational excellence led often to the discussion of two other related issues, the clinical learning environment and the adequate preparation of both tutors and trained staff for the new style course. There is insufficient space to expand on these here, but the importance of a detailed local feasibility study as a preliminary planning step becomes very obvious when faced with widespread variations in the provision of specialist experience such as paediatrics, psychiatry and theatres. As an increasing number of courses in the NHS turn their focus on the community that, in its turn, risks becoming an educational bottleneck. While only 3% of respondents felt that arranging appropriate medical experience for direct entry students would be 'nearly impossible' the figure rose to 19% for paediatrics. Such difficulties, however, led to some imaginative alternatives from the traditional placements.

Awareness of the extra support such students would need led to requests for greater access to courses such as the ENB Teaching and Assessing in Clinical Practice, 997/998, as well as the Advanced Diploma in Midwifery. Enthusiasm for an initiative which was often seen as a new chance for midwifery education was tempered by a realistic grasp of the extra demands it would make on both educational and service staff.

Resources

One of the aims of the study was to gather information about the resources needed and available for direct entry midwifery training. This information was sought by means of the institutional questionnaires and by interviews during site visits or by telephone. The first problem was that there was little consensus on the composition of the ideal direct entry course. The second was that few of those responsible had any idea of the cost of present training or of how to calculate the likely cost of any other training. Staff establishments were often based on historical precedent. Only some schools had considered which clinical experience circuits would be available. In addition, tutors were uncertain whether the ENB would approve the proposed circuits.

The lack of consensus as to the composition of the course made any attempt to estimate resources difficult, if not impossible. For example, some centres envisaged a university or polytechnic based course, others that all teaching would take place within the midwifery services, and still others envisaged a combined course with nurses. The service contribution expected from the direct entrant ranged from 0% to 90% of a staff midwife over the three years of the course. The proposed amount of ward/community based teaching and who was to do it also varied.

Faced with almost infinite variation on a theme, the research team felt it would be nonsensical to state that one would need X number of tutors and extra staff and that a direct entry midwifery course would cost X amount of money. Rather more useful would be guidance for those considering setting up courses to enable them to estimate their own resource needs. The recommendations made by the team, with input from the Advisory Group, are discussed in the next two paragraphs.

The first step is to decide on the aims and objectives of the course. A core planning team should then be set up with representatives from finance/administration (probably at district level), service and education, each member of whom should be senior enough to have the full information required and to make decisions. A rough curriculum would then be drawn up, involving the ENB education officer at an early stage; and once this was done investigation into resources could begin. An inventory of available accommodation (classroom and residential), staff (clinical, tutorial and secretarial), and support facilities such as audio-visual aids, library, office equipment and experience circuits should be made, if this is not already available. The needs of the next course can be roughly estimated by considering the draft curriculum. There must be adequate provision made for pre-course activities such as designing the full curriculum, investigating resources, devising and implementing recruitment and selection procedures, and staff preparation.

The existing and required resources could then be compared. If there was an enormous shortfall which could not be corrected by rationalization of training, either the existing scenario must be altered (e.g. increase the service contribution or decrease the number of students, etc.) or additional funds sought. If the first option is ideologically unacceptable or impractical and there is no source of extra funds, the plan to implement direct entry midwifery training in such a situation would not be feasible. If initial investigations proved the idea possible, the team would then move on to more detailed investigations and costings. This could either be done as a project with its own specific funds and staff or as extra duties for existing staff. The first option is more costly, and there is the possibility that if 'an outsider' is bought in, that communication may not be so effective. However, the second option would put great strain on already overstretched resources and a possible new course would have less priority than existing commitments. The preferred option would be to nominate an existing tutor to investigate the course and hire a replacement. Extra secretarial staff should also be provided. A costings guide is included in the full report (Radford and Thompson, 1988).

In summary adequate investigations and preparation must be undertaken prior to the implementation of a direct entry midwifery course, otherwise there are bound to be problems.

Staff attitudes

Some information about the attitudes prevailing towards direct entry students and their education has already been mentioned. The subject is of such critical importance to the ultimate success or failure of direct entry that it was with regret that the researchers had to admit that their investigation of this element of the project would have to be limited. There was compensation, however, in the knowledge that an extensive study of attitudes was underway at the time (Downe, 1988) because its experience of direct entrants, students and midwives, was contemporary, Derby City Hospital was the focus of a significant proportion of our discussions on this subject. We interviewed the full range of people involved in the training, including the RGN students undertaking their 18 month midwifery course concurrently with the direct entrants and the non-midwifery specialists from areas such as accident and emergency and gynaecology. On the whole their response was strongly favourable to the direct entry students. They were seen as 'bringing a breath of fresh air'. Some felt they were important agents for change in the profession. Their commitment and tenacity was recognized, since most had had to wait a considerable amount of time for a place in the school. But even in Derby there was some ambivalence, with reflections such as 'they are a nuisance on a busy ward' (ward sister), or demands for a distinctive insignia from the RGN students who felt that their already-qualified status went unnoticed.

In other places with only a dim memory, if any at all, of direct entry training, the ambivalence and occasional opposition was more overt. Comments such as 'How would she cope with a PPH (postpartum haemorrhage) . . . diabetic coma . . . epileptic fit . . . etc., etc.?' came from auxiliaries and consultants alike. The 'Cinderella effect' of an often poor educational foundation was obvious. Some very senior members of the profession still felt that it would be vital to retain post-RGN training, despite the present huge wastage to other parts of the NHS and elsewhere, because, in just such an emergency, only the dually certified midwife could be relied on to cope. There was the unspoken and totally unsupported assumption that no form of non-nurse preparation for midwifery practice could reliably equip its students to deal with the really difficult situations in the way that an RGN certificate could. The need for a concerted effort of staff development in relation to the planning of a direct entry curriculum was obvious. As Marion Young, Senior Tutor of Derby School of Midwifery, pointed out (personal communication), no amount of support, protection and encouragement from the tutors is going to make up for negative attitudes on the wards, and it is the clinical areas where learning for practice takes place. Positive role-models are even more vital to novice learners in the NHS than to the post RGN students who may well have developed a wealth of survival skills in a still fiercely hierarchical world. Without really positive staff attitudes the mythology of 'improved retention' for direct entry students could swiftly be converted into the worst wastage rates in the NHS.

CONCLUSION

Most research projects raise more questions than they answer; this was certainly true of this study. One question which it did answer was 'Why is the development of direct entry midwifery so slow?' One reason is the lack of information about all aspects of the proposed courses. Another is the lack of consensus within the profession as to what exactly a direct entry course should consist of and the status of the direct entrant. Thus the research raised the question of what the profession wishes to achieve through direct entry. The answer to this question will affect who should be recruited, whether there is an adequate supply of candidates, what the course will cost and what funds will be required.

The researchers made various recommendations which would encourage the development of direct entry courses, such as improved co-ordination, increased support, research providing more detailed information, clearer lines of communication and responsibility, rationalization of funding and decision making mechanisms and wider publicity. However, unless the profession can come to a consensus on the future of midwifery and the role the direct entrant will play, progress will continue to be slow. If there is a real wish to separate midwifery from nursing, there needs to be major changes in service delivery as well as education. An effective way to increase the proportion of direct entry midwives will be gradually to reduce the remission given to nurses until all entrants, regardless of background, do the same course. At the moment a direct entrant gets no remission if she chooses to do nurse training and this anomaly lowers the status of the direct entrant.

Direct entry is not a panacea for all midwifery's ills, as many would argue. It must be taken as an integral part of the programme to move midwifery away from an illness-centred philosophy ('no birth is ever normal except in retrospect') and to make the independent practitioner status a reality. Changes in training alone will not achieve this unless they are accompanied by changes in service delivery, staff attitudes, public expectation, management and financing.

Since the research reported in this chapter was completed, a growing number of what are now known as pre-registration midwifery education courses have been introduced and more are planned. In time this development may have far reaching effects on the composition of the workforce, the practice of midwifery and on career pathways of individual midwives. The importance of continuing research into all aspects of this major development in midwifery education in England cannot be over-emphasized.

REFERENCES

Association of Radical Midwives (1986) *The Vision: proposals for the future of the maternity services*. ARM, London.

Bent, A. (1982) The growth and development of midwifery. In P. Allan and M. Jolley (eds) *Nursing, midwifery and health visiting since 1900*. Faber & Faber, London.

Campbell, J. (1917) *Reports on the physical welfare of mothers and children*. Carnegie Trust, Tinling & Co., London.

Campbell, J. (1923) *Reports on public health and medical subjects No 21. The training of midwives*. Ministry of Health, HMSO, London.

Campbell, J. (1924) *Reports on public health and medical subjects No 25. Maternal mortality.* Ministry of Health, HMSO, London.

Campbell, J. (1927) *Reports on public health and medical subjects No 48. The protection of motherhood.* Ministry of Health, HMSO, London.

Cartwright, A. (1979) *The dignity of labour.* Tavistock Publications, London.

Central Midwives Board (1903, 1916, 1926, 1937, 1980) *Midwives Rules.* CMB, London.

Central Midwives Board (1908, 1913, 1916, 1934, 1939, 1940, 1942, 1945) *Annual Reports.* CMB, London.

Department of Heath and Social Security (1972) *Report of the Committee on Nursing* (Chairman: A. Briggs). HMSO, London.

Department of Health and Social Security (1986) *Midwifery leaflet NLO29.* HMSO, London.

Dodd, A. (1985) *Key to the professions response to the ENB.* Consultation document. ENB, London.

Donnison, J. (1977) *Midwives and medical men.* Heinemann, London.

Downe, S. (1988) Direct entry midwifery training – the future for English midwifery. *MIDIRS,* **7** April.

English National Board For Nursing, Midwifery and Health Visiting (1986) *Reasons for development in direct entry midwife training,* (mimeo, ENB, AS/LB). ENB, London.

English National Board for Nursing Midwifery and Health Visiting (1985) *Professional Education/Training Courses.* ENB, London.

Fenney, R. (1954) *Historical notes in midwifery.* (Unpublished paper.)

Flint, C. (1986) Should midwives train as florists? *Nursing Times,* **82**(12), 21.

Garcia, J. and Garforth, S. (1991) Midwifery policies and policy-making. In S. Robinson and A.M. Thomson (eds) *Midwives, research and childbirth Vol II.* Chapman & Hall, London.

Grant, J. (1988) Clearing the way for direct entry. *MIDIRS,* **9**, November.

House of Commons Select Committee (1992) Sessions 1991–1992. *Second Report. Maternity Services* (Chairman: Nicholas Winterton). Vol. 1. HMSO, London.

Inch, S. (1982) *Birthrights: a parents guide to modern childbirth.* Hutchinson, London.

Kent, J. and Maggs, C. (1992) *An evaluation of pre-registration midwifery education in England: a research project for the Department of Health. Working Paper 1 – Research design.* Maggs Research Associates, Bath.

Kitzinger, S. (1988) *The midwife challenge.* Pandora, London.

Lopez, M., Radford, N. and Velastin, S. (1985) *Information on training: a data collection and handling package.* HCRA, University of Surrey, Guildford.

Ministry of Health (1929) *Report on the Departmental Committee on the training and employment of midwives* (Chairman: Sir Robert Bolam). HMSO, London.

Ministry of Health (1959) *Report of the Maternity Services Committee* (Chairman: The Earl of Cranbrooke). HMSO, London.

Ministry of Health, Department of Health for Scotland, Ministry of Labour and National Service (1949) *Report of the Working Party on Midwives* (Chairman: Mrs M. Stocks). HMSO, London.

Oakley, A. (1984) *The captured womb.* Blackwell, Oxford.

Radford, N. and Thompson, A. (1988) *Direct Entry: A preparation for midwifery practice.* University of Surrey, Guildford/ENB, London.

Ris, M. (1986) Obstetrical care in the Netherlands. The place of midwives and specific aspects of their role. In M. Kaminski and G. Brearty *et al.* (eds) *Perinatal care delivery systems. Description and evaluation in European Community Countries.* Oxford University Press, Oxford.

Robinson, S. (1985) Midwives, obstetricians and GPs: the need for role clarification. *Midwifery,* **1**, 102–13.

Robinson, S. (1990) Maintaining the independence of the midwifery profession: a continuing struggle In J. Garcia, R. Kilpatrick and M. Richards (eds) *The politics of maternity care.* Oxford University Press, Oxford.

Robinson, S., Golden, J. and Bradley, S. (1983) *A study of the role and responsibilities of the midwife.* NERU Report, Chelsea College, London.

Royal College of Midwives (1987) *The role and education of the future midwife.* RCM, London.

Royal College of Midwives (1988) *Towards a healthy nation.* RCM, London.

Royal College of Nursing (1985) RCN Commission on Nurse Education. *The education of nurses: a new dispensation* (Chairman: Harry Judge). RCN, London.

Royal College of Obstetricians and Gynaecologists (1944) *Report on National maternity service.* RCOG, London.

Simonot, D. (1989) Personal communication.

UKCC (1986) *Project 2000: a new preparation for practice.* UKCC, London.

Van Daalen, R. (1988) Dutch obstetric care. *Health Promotion,* **2**(3), 247–55.

Wood, A. (1963) The development of the midwifery service in Great Britain. *International Journal of Nursing Studies,* **1**, 51–8.

CHAPTER ELEVEN

Research into some aspects of care in labour

Ann M. Thomson

A number of small-scale studies investigating various aspects of midwifery care for women in labour are the subject of this chapter. Although not extensive enough to warrant a separate chapter each, they are nonetheless of sufficient importance to merit inclusion in the series. Papers describing the studies were first presented at Research and the Midwife conferences but the conference proceedings are not necessarily readily available. The studies are of artificial rupture of the membranes in labour (Henderson, 1985), the use of a chair in the second stage of labour (Hillan, 1984; Romney, 1984; 1987), postpartum haemorrhage (Moore and Levy, 1982; 1983) and women's reaction to delivery by caesarean section (Kirchmeier, 1985). Each study is described, the findings presented and discussed in the light of some studies which have been reported since the original studies were concluded. However, no attempt has been made to review all the literature in each area. Lessons which can be learnt and implications for practice and further research are discussed in a final section.

ARTIFICIAL RUPTURE OF THE MEMBRANES: WHOSE DECISION?

Whilst undertaking a course leading to a higher degree Henderson (1984, 1985) read of the continuing dissatisfaction of the consumers of the maternity services (Oakley, 1980; Macintyre, 1982; Kirkham, 1983) and of the absence of job satisfaction experienced by midwives (*NM News*, 1981; Robinson *et al.*, 1983). In exploring these issues further Henderson found that one of the reasons given for both these problems was the introduction of technology into the maternity services (Meredith, 1983; Maternity Services Advisory Committee, 1984). At the same time Kirkham (1983) reported that women were not consulted on the type of care they would like – they were just told what would be done. In an attempt to examine midwives' job dissatisfaction and women's dissatisfaction with maternity care Henderson (1984, 1985) decided to investigate one aspect of the midwife's role – the influences and interactions surrounding the midwife's decision to rupture the membranes during labour. The hypothesis she tested was that 'the decision to rupture the membranes of a woman in normal labour is made by the midwife without consulting the woman'.

Artificial rupture of membranes (ARM) is a technique which has been in existence for a considerable number of years and certainly since the 1920s (Kreis, 1928). Proponents of the technique suggest that there are two advantages. Firstly, ARM allows the fetal head to descend so that there is increased pressure on the cervical os which in turn increases the strength of the uterine contraction leading to more rapid cervical dilatation. Secondly the fact that the membranes have been ruptured means that the liquor can be observed for colour and quantity (O'Driscoll and Meagher, 1980). The advantages of leaving the membranes intact are that there is a reduced risk of infection, even hydrostatic pressure to the whole fetal surface is applied and fetal distress is less likely because the intact amniotic sac discourages major degrees of retraction of the placental sight (Donald, 1969; Caldeyro-Barcia *et al.*, 1974). Discussion on the value of ARM at a Royal College of Obstetricians and Gynaecologists' conference suggested that the rates of ARM have been controlled by changes in fashion (Beard *et al.*, 1975). However, the almost routine use of ARM in labour coincided with the rise of active management of labour. As doctors are not present during all labours, midwives have become involved in the routine practice of ARM in labour.

The questions that Henderson (1985) asked were, 'In performing an artificial rupture of membranes in labour:

1. does the midwife consult the woman?
2. what guides the midwife in her decision?
3. what is the woman's understanding of what happens?'

Methods

Henderson undertook the study at the hospital in which she was working as a midwife teacher. She described the area as an inner city area and said that it served a multiracial, socially deprived population where the majority of the women were in social classes four and five.

In order to answer the research questions two methods of data collection were employed. Firstly, observation of vaginal examinations on labouring women where it was known that the membranes were intact. Secondly, in order to capture the thoughts of the women and the midwives a semi-structured interview schedule was devised to be administered to each immediately after the procedure had been undertaken.

The inclusion criteria for the women were that they should be English speaking, belong to social classess four and five, and 18 to 40 years, in spontaneous labour where it was known that the membranes were intact, and that they should be willing to participate. The midwives were also asked if they were willing to participate.

When it was known that a vaginal examination was to be undertaken on a labouring woman with intact membranes, Henderson approached the midwife to ascertain that the woman fulfilled the inclusion criteria and that the midwife was willing to take part. Henderson then approached the woman and asked her if she also would be willing to take part.

Findings

Twenty-eight women were approached and a vaginal examination on each one was observed and an artificial rupture of membranes was performed during each examination. The women were all caucasian and mainly multiparae. Twenty-two midwives participated.

Of the 28 vaginal examinations observed explanation and consent was only observed on two occasions (Table 11.1). Explanation was given, but no consent obtained, on 17 occasions. Of those women whose consent was not obtained, none refused consent to the examination, but the midwife appeared to take the woman's silence as agreement to the procedure. Henderson was not able to discern any differences between the midwives or between the women to indicate why some women were given an explanation and asked for their consent and others were not. It appeared that as long as the woman did not object the midwife assumed that consent was given.

A similar situation existed with artificial rupture of the membranes (ARM). On only two occasions was consent to ARM obtained before the procedure. However when Henderson questioned the women after the

Table 11.1 Observed explanation and consent to vaginal examination

Explanation and consent to vaginal examination	No.
Explanation given/consent given	2
Explanation given/no consent obtained	17
No explanation/no consent given	3
Not present to see	6
Total	28

Source: compiled from Henderson (1985).

procedure many of them said that this had been done in a previous labour, did not express any anxiety or objection, and accepted the decision without question. The majority of the women said that they were happy for the midwife to take the decision and did not think there should be any discussion. On two occasions the women had asked the midwives not to tell them what they, the midwives, were going to do. When the midwives were questioned about the absence of observed consent to the procedure three said that they had discussed this with the women earlier in the labour and had told the women that they would be carrying out an ARM at the next vaginal examination. Whilst this is possible because Henderson was not present for the whole labour, but only for the vaginal examination, it is also possible that the midwife thought she had explained and obtained consent when in fact there was no previous discussion or the midwife may have thought she had discussed when in fact all she had done was 'tell', for example,

> Midwife: Just going to examine you as before, you're getting on
>   well. Just going to break waters and put clip on, OK?
>   [Did not wait for a reply]
>   Water's gone now. This is the clip I was talking about.

Henderson gained the impression that there was a general acceptance by the women that what the midwife was going to do was in the best interests of the mother and baby. However, the midwives' replies to the question 'Why did you not discuss your decision to rupture membranes?' give cause for concern and would lead one to question whether the midwives' actions were in the best interests of the woman and her baby. Eight of the midwives did not discuss the procedure because the women did not ask any questions and six midwives said that they never discuss ARM with the women (Table 11.2). On being asked whether they would ever discuss whether or not to rupture the membranes with the woman, 19 said they would only do so if the woman asked about it. This suggests that the midwives thought either that the women did not want to know, or already knew about the procedure and did not need any further information. However, the midwives failed to recognize that for some labouring women it is not possible to ask questions. They feel vulnerable, particularly if lying on their back, are in pain and are tired. Some women feel that if they ask questions they may be seen as being ignorant. What happened in the majority of the vaginal examinations that Henderson observed is illustrated by the following quote from a midwife:

> You come to the mother and say 'I'm just going to examine you and
> break your waters', and she usually accepts.

This latter quote suggests that ARM is routine policy but that the woman might have a chance to object. Henderson recognized that there might be

Table 11.2 Midwives replies to 'Why didn't you discuss your decision to rupture membranes?'

Midwive's replies	No.
Woman did not ask	8
Never discuss	6
She knew about it, 'usually had it done before'	4
Did discuss	2
Didn't think of it	2
Doctor told me to do it	2
No time, going to be busy	1
Lack of understanding	1
Mother said 'water' already gone	1
Discussed previously	1
Total	**28**

Source: Henderson (1985).

Table 11.3 Midwives' stated reasons for rupturing the membranes

Reason	No.
Progressing in labour, therefore rupture to accelerate	14
Doctor said to do it	4
Bulging membranes	4
To apply fetal scalp electrode	3
Poor external trace	2
Policy	1
Total	**28**

Source: Henderson (1985).

other factors affecting the midwife's decision whether or not to rupture membranes. The presence of a doctor who might override the midwife's expertise or a unit policy requiring that the membranes be ruptured would take the decision away from the midwives. The reasons given by the midwives for ARM are shown in Table 11.3. Henderson suggested that the midwives appeared to be making the decision and possibly, she suggests, with good reason. However when the situations and question responses of the 14 midwives who said they ruptured the membranes to accelerate a progressing labour are examined (Table 11.4) a different picture emerges. It would appear that there was some underlying policy which was affecting the midwives' decisions. Why when the cervical os was three cms dilated and labour was progressing satisfactorily would the midwife rupture the membranes? Four midwives had been told by a doctor to rupture the membranes but there was no apparent reason for doing so. Another quote from a midwife illustrates the prevailing attitude:

Question: 'You ruptured the membranes. What made you make that decision?'

Midwife: 'Nearly second stage, so might as well'.

Question: 'Is there a policy?'

Midwife: 'No policy, but usually rupture them if in established labour'.

Because of the control exerted by the medical profession Henderson asked five obstetricians (four consultants and one senior registrar) for their views on vaginal examination, ARM and consultation. All stated that they would rupture the membranes once cervical dilatation had begun and none would

Table 11.4 Midwives replies to question 'is there a policy about ARM?' and the cervical dilatation at which they were seen to carry out ARM

No.	Reason for ARM	Dilatation of os
4	No policy	3, 3, 5, 8 cm
4	No policy, up to midwife	4, 5, 6–7, 8 cm
2	No policy *but* if os 3 cm rupture membranes	3, 4 cm
1	No policy. I use my own judgement *but* if os is 3 cm dilated, doctors ask 'why not ruptured?'	4 cm
1	No definite policy. Between midwife and woman. If os 3 cm dilated rupture membranes	3 cm
1	No policy, left to midwife's discretion. If ruptured *too* early it is not good. Get on better if left a while. Some doctors do not agree and argue with you.	4 cm
1	If os 3 cm – rupture membranes	2 cm
14		

Source: compiled from Henderson (1984).

discuss this with the women. They expressed the opinion that the fact that the woman had come to the hospital for delivery implied consent. The obstetricians had obviously forgotten that in the early 1980s it was extremely difficult for women to have their baby anywhere except a hospital.

Discussion

Henderson's study had a small sample and only included caucasian women. The data collection was only undertaken in one hospital, therefore it is not possible to generalize the findings. However, her findings did support her hypothesis that midwives ruptured the membranes in labour without reference to women and there are some lessons that we can all learn from this study. The greater proportion of the midwives were undertaking an intimate, invasive procedure without apparently consulting the women. The midwives were deceiving themselves as to the reasons for their actions. They were under the impression that they exercised autonomy and clinical judgement when in fact they were carrying out a routine procedure. Their actions were either directly or indirectly affected by medical staff. In view of the consultants' responses this is not really surprising.

Since Henderson undertook her study three studies investigating rupture of the membranes in labour have been reported (NCT, 1989; Fraser *et al.*, 1991; Barrett *et al.*, 1992) and another is in progress (Tasker *et al.*, 1991). The first is a survey of women's experience of amniotomy in labour. In no way can the sample used be considered to be representative of women throughout the UK because the women were recruited through National Childbirth Trust classes. However, 3000 women filled in the questionnaire and of these 3000 708 also wrote letters describing their experiences; 53% (1588) had an ARM and 46% (1366) had spontaneous rupture of the membranes. Of those who had ARM 56% (886) said that the only reason for this was acceleration of labour. In the letters that were sent with the questionnaires many women wrote that when ARM was suggested they frequently asked for it to be delayed. In some cases women reported having to resist quite considerable pressure in order not to have an ARM. The letters also stated that rupture of the membranes sometimes occurred during vaginal examination and suggested that the number of vaginal examinations/or the manner in which they were undertaken influences the time in labour at which the membranes are ruptured. Six per cent (168) of the sample had had a home confinement and as the proportion of home births was greater than could be expected in the general population comparison between home and hospital deliveries could be made. Whereas 54% of those who delivered in hospital had an ARM only 28% of those who deliverd at home did so.

The second study is a randomized controlled trial of amniotomy in labour versus the intention to keep the membranes intact in nulliparae at low obstetric risk (Fraser *et al.*, 1991). During the study period 278 women were elligible to participate, but only 97 actually took part in the study. Forty-seven women were randomized into the early amniotomy group and 50 into the group where membranes were to be conserved. There was no difference between the groups in the lengths of the first and second stages, fetal heart rate trace abnormalities, the proportion of babies with low Apgar scores or abnormal cord pH.

The third study is also a randomized controlled trial (Barrett *et al.*, 1992). A total of 362 women in spontaneous labour were studied. Two hundred and six were multiparous and 156 were primiparous. One hundred and eighty-three women were allocated to have ARM and 178 (97%) of them had an ARM. Of the 179 women allocated to the non-intervention group 83 (46%) had an ARM. There was a significant ($p = 0.05$) decrease in the length of labour in primiparae in the ARM group (mean 8.3 hours, SD 4.1 hours) when compared with the non-intervention group (mean 9.7 hours, SD 4.8 hours). There was no difference in the length of the second stage between the two groups. There was a statistically significant ($p = 0.01$) increase in the proportion of women who used epidural analgesia in the ARM group ($n = 63$, 34%) when compared with the non-intervention group ($n = 39$, 22%). Not all women had continuous fetal monitoring in labour. Three hundred and forty-four traces were available, 172 in each group. There was a statistically significant ($p = 0.04$) increase in the proportion of women in the ARM group who had fetal heart rate abnormalities recorded the last hour of labour (10%, $n = 18$) when compared with the non-intervention group (4%, $n = 7$). There were no differences in the conditions of the babies at delivery. The advantage of a labour of one hour less has to be balanced against the need for extra analgesia with the potential long-term effects of backache (MacArthur *et al.*, 1991). The concerns engendered by an abnormality of the fetal heart rate do not seem to be necessary when the baby is not disadvantaged at birth by having the membranes left intact until the beginning of the second stage.

Fraser *et al.* (1991) acknowledge that one of the reasons they were unable to demonstrate a significant difference in length of labour was because their sample size was too small. However, Barrett *et al.* (1992) achieved their projected sample size, found a statistically significant decrease in the length of labour in the group which had early amniotomy but also found side effects, namely abnormal fetal heart rate patterns and an increase in the use of epidural analgesia.

THE USE OF THE DELIVERY CHAIR IN THE SECOND STAGE OF LABOUR

Two studies describing research on the use of the birthing chair in the second stage of labour were presented at the 1983 Research and the

Midwife conference (Hillan, 1984; Romney, 1984). Romney (1987) subsequently presented a follow-up study at the 1986 conference.

The end of the 1970s and in the early 1980s witnessed a recognition that requiring a woman to lie on her back in labour was not necessarily the best position for her. At that time it appeared that the health professionals caring for labouring women found it difficult to allow a labouring woman to 'roam free'. There appeared to be a feeling that the woman had to be 'contained', preferably on a bed. As it was recognized that an upright position was better, in particular for delivery, than a recumbent position the birthing chair was designed. It was based on the design of the birthing chairs and stools used in Europe in the seventeenth and eighteenth centuries but was made of modern steel and plastics. Whilst assisting the woman to maintain an upright position it also allowed the accoucheuse/ accoucheur the greater access which was considered necessary to achieve a controlled delivery. The methods and findings of each trial are presented separately, the discussion relates to findings for all three trials and those from another two subsequent trials.

Methods and findings of Hillan's (1984) trial

Hillan's study was a randomized controlled trial comparing delivery in bed, where the woman could be propped up to an angle of 20° from the horizontal, with delivery in a delivery chair where the back was maintained 15–20° from the horizontal. The inclusion criteria were that the women had to have a singleton pregnancy with a cephalic presentation at 37–42 weeks gestation. Women whose labour was to be induced were included. Women were recruited in the antenatal clinic, parentcraft classes, antenatal wards or on admission to the labour ward. The women were encouraged to remain mobile in the first stage. Randomization occured towards the end of the first stage of labour. At the onset of the second stage all women had a vaginal examination to assess the station and position of the fetal head. All spontaneous deliveries were undertaken by a group of midwifery sisters who had expressed an interest in the study and who had previously gained experience in delivering women in the chair.

A sample size of 500 was used with equal numbers of primiparae and multiparae. Although Hillan states that the women were randomly allocated to deliver in one of the two groups it is surprising that there were equal numbers of women in each of the chair and bed groups and equal numbers of multiparae and primiparae within each group.

There were no differences between the four groups in age or gestational age and there was no difference in use of analgesia in the first stage between the chair and bed groups (Table 11.5, page 302). However, fewer primiparous women who delivered in the bed had an induced or augmented labour (Table 11.5). There was no difference between the groups in the

Table 11.5 Comparison of women participating in study (Hillan, 1984)

	Primiparae		Multiparae	
	Chair (n = 125)	Bed (n = 125)	Chair (n = 125)	Bed (n = 125)
Age (yrs)				
Mean	25.2	24.0	28.5	27.4
Range	16–36	16–33	18–41	18–38
Parity				
Mean	0 + 0	0 + 0	1.6	1.5
Range			1–5	1–5
Gestation (weeks)				
Range	37–42	37–42	37–42	37–42
Labour				
Induced labour	51 (40%)	36 (29%)	53 (11%)	65 (13%)
Augmentation of labour	20	15	11	13
Length of 1st stage				
Mean (hrs)	8	8.15	4.75	4.75
SD	3.5	3.4	3.0	2.7
Analgesia				
None	16 (13%)	11 (9%)	63 (50%)	60 (48%)
Pethidine	41 (33%)	44 (35%)	52 (42%)	47 (38%)
Pethidine – mean dose				
(mgs.)	107	108	80	84
Epidural	68 (54%)	70 (56%)	10 (1%)	18 (4%)
Posture in 1st stage				
Bed	50 (40%)	52 (42%)	18 (14%)	14 (11%)
Ambulant	75 (60%)	73 (58%)	107 (86%)	111 (89%)
Ambulant till 2nd stage	17 (22%)	14 (19%)	50 (47%)	20 (18%)

Source: compiled from Hillan (1984).

length of the second stage between the chair and bed groups (Table 11.6, page 303). However, when the duration of active pushing was considered a different picture emerged. The mean duration for pushing of primiparae delivering in the chair was 43 minutes compared with 51 for those who delivered in the bed ($t = 2.387$, $p < 0.05$). For multiparae delivering in the chair the mean length of pushing was 15 minutes compared with 19 minutes for those delivering in the bed ($t = 2.108$, $p < 0.05$). There was no difference between the groups in the mode of delivery for multiparae, but there was a statistically significant difference in the proportion of

Table 11.6 Comparison of outcomes in Hillan's (1984) trial

	Chair		Bed	
	Primip. (n = 125)	*Multip.* (n = 125)	*Primip.* (n = 125)	*Multip.* (n = 125)
Length 2nd stage				
Mean (mins)	86	19	81	23
SD	67	30	56	22
Length of active pushing				
Mean (mins)	43	15	51	19
SD	27	14	26	16
Mode of delivery				
Normal	99 (79%)	122 (98%)	82 (66%)	119 (95%)
Forceps	23 (18%)	2 (2%)	42 (34%)	6 (5%)
Caesarean	3 (2%)	1 (<1%)	1 (<1%)	0 —
Blood loss				
Mean (mls)	346	263	300	182
SD	360	244	194	145
Loss > 500 mls	12	12	11	4
Perineal damage				
None	24 (19%)	39 (31%)	11 (9%)	33 (26%)
1° tear	23 (18%)	48 (38%)	4 (3%)	37 (30%)
2° tear	16 (13%)	20 (16%)	12 (10%)	17 (14%)
Episiotomy	61 (48%)	18 (14%)	98 (78%)	38 (30%)

Source: compiled from Hillan (1984).

primiparae delivering spontaneously in the chair (79%, 99) when compared with those who delivered in the bed (66%, 82) ($\chi^2 = 5.59$, $p < 0.05$). A total of five women were delivered by caesarean section. Forceps delivery had been attempted unsuccesfully for four of the women and in the fifth the head was so high that forceps delivery was not attempted. Postnatal X-ray pelvimetry confirmed cephalo-pelvic disproportion in all five women. Perineal damage was significantly increased for primiparae ($\chi^2 = 20.84$, $p < 0.001$) and multiparae ($\chi^2 = 4.36$, $p < 0.05$) who delivered in the bed (Table 11.6). For primiparae there was no difference between the groups in mean blood loss but multiparae delivering in the chair had a significantly higher mean blood loss ($t = 3.292$, $p < 0.01$) and an increased incidence of loss over 500 ml when compared with women who delivered in the bed

Table 11.7 Mode of delivery for primiparae who used an epidural for analgesia in labour

Mode of delivery	Chair		Bed	
	No.	%	No.	%
Spontaneous	45	66	34	48
Forceps for delay	15	22	32	46
Forceps for fetal distress	5	7	3	4
Caesarean section	3	5	1	1
Total	68	100	70	100

Source: compiled by Hillan (1984).

(Table 11.6). Sixty-eight primiparae allocated to deliver in the chair had used epidural for analgesia and 70 of those allocated to deliver in the bed. There was a statistically significant increase in the proportion of primiparae who used epidural and were delivered in the chair achieving a spontaneous delivery when compared with those who delivered in the bed ($\chi^2 = 7.32$, $p < 0.05$) (Table 11.7).

Methods and findings of Romney's (1984) study

The delivery chair was first introduced into the delivery unit at Northwick Park Hospital in April 1981. Romney (1984) states that its reception by the midwifery staff was 'mixed'. Women were shown the chair on visits to the delivery suite during pregnancy and they were told of its availability for use. Recognizing the need to evaluate this innovation in care a questionnaire was designed to be given to all women who delivered in the chair and to the midwives and doctors caring for the women. The staff considered conducting a randomized controlled trial but because the women would be denied the basic freedom of choice in such a trial the midwives decided it was 'ethically unacceptable to subject women to the recently introduced innovation'. A pilot study comparing the outcomes of 41 women who delivered in the chair with 41 who delivered in the obstetric bed was undertaken. Thirty-nine of the deliveries in the chair were spontaneous and although the majority of the midwives enjoyed delivering women in the chair a few stated that they did not feel in complete control because of the rapidity of the birth. Following the pilot study a further study comparing 100 women who agreed to deliver in the chair with 100 women delivering in the obstetric bed was undertaken. Information was collected on the use of analgesia in labour as well as outcome measures. The women, midwives and doctors were also asked for their opinions of the chair and bed.

The proportion of primiparae in the two groups and the proportion of women using the differing types of analgesia were comparable (Table 11.8). In this first study Romney did not report separate findings for primparae and multiparae (Romney, 1984). A greater proportion of women achieved a vaginal delivery in the chair than did in the obstetric bed (Table 11.9, page 306). Similar (small) proportions achieved an intact perineum but there were more episiotomies in the group that delivered in the bed (Table 11.9). Twice as many women had a postpartum haemorrhage when delivering in the chair ($n = 10$) when compared with women who delivered in the bed ($n = 5$). No information is given on the length of the second stage but Romney (1984) stated that clinical impression suggested 30 minutes of pushing in the chair equalled 60 minutes of pushing in the bed. The midwives and doctors were of the opinion that a greater proportion of women were able to exert 'very good' effort in the chair when compared with women in the bed (Table 11.10, page 306). When asked about their comfort the women stated they were equally comfortable in the chair or the bed (Table 11.11, page 307).

More women felt reassured on first sight of the chair than were reassured by the bed (Table 11.11). Only 22 of the women who delivered in the chair found it hard whereas 47 of those who delivered in the bed said it was hard. However, 91% of those who delivered in the chair and found it

Table 11.8 Proportion of primiparae and analgesia used in the first stage in the Chair and Bed groups in Romney's (1984) study

	Chair (n = 100)		Bed (n = 100)	
	No.	%	No.	%
Primiparae	53	53	52	52
Analgesia				
none	24	24	24	24
'Entonox'	20	20	7	7
pethidine	36	36	40	40
epidural	20	20	29	29

Source: compiled from Romney (1984).

Table 11.9 Outcome measures in Romney's (1984) study

	Chair (n = 100)		Bed (n = 100)	
	No.	%	No.	%
Spontaneous delivery	96	96	79	79
Intact perineum	10	10	10	10
Lacerations	15	15	15	15
1° tear	14	14	14	14
2° tear	8	8	6	6
3° tear	3	3		
Episiotomy	44	44	53	53

Source: compiled from Romney (1984).

Table 11.10 Midwives' and doctors' opinions as to the effort and comfort exhibited by the women

	Chair (n = 100)		Bed (n = 100)	
	No.	%	No.	%
Effort				
Very good	65	65	27	27
Good	34	34	45	45
Poor	1	1	28	28
Comfort				
Very comfortable	98	98	95	95
Uncomfortable	2	2	5	5

Source: compiled from Romney (1984).

hard and 83% of those who said the bed was hard found this to be an advantage (Table 11.11). Half of the women who delivered in the chair found they were restrained by it whereas only 31 of the women who delivered in the bed complained of this.

Table 11.11 Women's views of delivery in the chair (Romney, 1984)

	Chair (n = 100)		Bed (n = 100)	
	No.	%	No.	%
First impressions of chair				
Reassured	50	50	34	34
Indifferent	41	41	23	23
Frightened	8	8	33	33
Didn't know	1	1		
Chair/bed was hard				
Yes	22	22	47	47
Hardness was an advantage				
Yes	20	91	39	83
Felt restrained by chair/bed				
Yes	50	50	31	31
Backache in labour				
Yes	48	48	59	59
Backache relieved by chair/bed				
Yes	44	92	18	30

Source: compiled from Romney (1984).

Methods and findings of Romney's (1987) study

The findings of the first, non-randomized study of the use of the delivery chair appeared to show a benefit to the women who used it when compared with those using the bed. However, the midwives at Northwick Park Hospital recognized the dangers in not adequately evaluating a new practice and decided to subject the delivery chair to the rigour of a randomized controlled trial.

Inclusion criteria for the study were: women with a single fetus, cephalic presentation and gestational maturity greater than 36 weeks. Only women 'booked' under the care of one of the consultants at the hospital were recruited into the study. Women who expressed a preference for delivery in either the chair or the bed were not invited to take part. Women whose labour had been induced were included, induction of labour being achieved with the insertion of a prostaglandin pessary (3 mg) into the vagina. Amniotomy was performed as soon as the woman was in labour. During labour a policy of active management (O'Driscoll *et al.*, 1984) was followed for primiparae. Continuous electronic fetal monitoring was used when indicated. Progress in the first stage was assessed vaginally every two hours for primiparae and every four hours for multiparae. Delivery in the chair was conducted with the back tilted at an angle of 40° from the vertical. Delivery in the bed was in the dorsal position but the women could be propped by a pillow for comfort. A total of 638 women (288 primiparae) took part in the study. Random allocation to deliver in either the chair or the bed was by means of opening a sealed envelope before commencement of the second stage. The second stage of labour was diagnosed either at vaginal examination or if the vertex was visible. Statistical tests used were Student's *t* and Fisher's exact tests.

Two hundred and twenty-six women (111 primiparae) were allocated to deliver in the chair; 313 women (140 primiparae) were allocated to deliver in the bed. The women in the groups were comparable on maternal age, social class, gestational age, baby's birthweight and length of the first stage (Romney, 1987). Despite random allocation women did not always deliver according to allocation. Although informed consent to participate in the trial had been obtained five women insisted on being delivered in the chair. A further 92 women allocated to be delivered in the chair were delivered in the bed: 40 because they declined to be moved from the bed to the chair in the second stage of labour, 32 women delivered too quickly

Table 11.12 Outcome of treatment in Romney (1987) trial

| | Chair | | Bed | |
	Primip. (n = 111)	Multip. (n = 115)	Primip. (n = 140)	Multip. (n = 173)
Mean duration of 2nd stage (min)	58	20	20	19
Mean duration of pushing	45	43	20	19
Spontaneous delivery	87 (78%)	107 (93%)	107 (76%)	164 (95%)
Forceps	22 (20%)	6 (5%)	31 (22%)	7 (4%)
Caesarean section	2 (2%)	2 (2%)	2 (1%)	2 (1%)
Mean blood loss (ml)	317	275	280	257
Intact perineum	13 (12%)	26 (23%)	30 (21%)	61 (35%)
Perineal tear	39 (35%)	71 (63%)	26 (18%)	81 (47%)
Episiotomy	57 (51%)	16 (14%)	82 (58%)	29 (17%)

Source: compiled from Romney (1987).

to be moved to the chair and 20 were not moved to the chair, at the request of the obstetrician, because of complications such as fetal distress. Analysis of outcome was undertaken according to intention to treat.

There was no difference between the groups for both primiparae and multiparae in length of the second stage, the incidence of normal delivery, assisted vaginal delivery, caesarean section and episiotomy (Table 11.12). However, only 12% of primiparae and 23% of multiparae in the chair group had an intact perineum whereas 22% of primiparae and 36% of multiparae in the bed group achieved an intact perineum ($p < 0.05$) (Table 11.12). There was a significant increase among both primiparae ($p < 0.005$) and multiparae ($p < 0.025$) in the proportion of women in the chair group who sustained a perineal tear (Table 11.12). Although there was no difference between the groups in the mean blood loss at delivery (Table 11.12), 9% of women in the chair group and 4% of women in the bed group had a blood loss in excess of 500 mls ($p < 0.02$), primiparae experiencing a higher incidence of postpartum haemorrhage than multiparae. Only one baby whose mother was in the chair group and two babies whose mother was in the bed group had Apgar scores of less than 7 at five minutes post delivery.

Discussion

In discussing the need for evaluation of treatments and practices used in providing care for childbearing women Chalmers (1989) explains the need for systematic scientific evaluation of all care. The chair trials reported here support that statement. In the original non-randomized trial at Northwick Park Hospital (Romney, 1984) delivery in the chair appeared to be advantageous to the women in that a greater proportion achieved a vaginal delivery and there was a lower incidence of episiotomy in the chair. However, the subsequent randomized controlled trial did not show any difference in the incidence of spontaneous delivery and there was an increased incidence of vaginal tears in women in the chair group. It is interesting that before the first study was undertaken (Romney, 1984) it was felt it would be unethical to remove the element of choice from women. Because of this women were allowed to use an unevaluated treatment and were put at increased risk of postpartum haemorrhage and vaginal tears. Romney (1987) stated that subsequent to the RCT all women asking to use the chair for delivery were informed of its detrimental effect. Although women delivering in the chair in Hillan's (1984) study had a statistically significant shorter pushing time, it has to be questioned whether mean differences of eight and four minutes respectively for primiparae and multiparae are clinically significant.

In two subsequent studies (Stewart and Spiby, 1989; Currell et al.,

1991) the chair was found to have no advantage over delivery in the bed and delivery in the chair resulted in a higher mean blood loss (Stewart and Spiby, 1989) and a higher rate of postpartum haemorrhage (Stewart and Spiby, 1989; Currell *et al.*, 1991). The advantage of the Currell *et al.* (1991) study over the other studies described here is that the sample size was calculated to determine a specific reduction in the instrumental delivery rate. These authors can therefore be more confident in their findings and that the differences between the groups are even less likely to have occurred by chance.

POSTPARTUM HAEMORRHAGE

Although postpartum haemorrhage (PPH) is not as dangerous for women in the UK in the 1990s in terms of maternal mortality as it was at the beginning of the century, those caring for women in childbirth are concerned to ensure that women lose as little blood as possible at delivery. In this section of the chapter two issues in the management of the third stage of labour are considered; how the placenta should be delivered and the accurate measurement of blood loss.

Two midwife teachers noticed that there were increasing differences between what they were teaching in the classroom about delivery of the placenta and what was happening in clinical practice. Moore and Levy (1982, 1983) taught that when delivering the placenta, traction should be put on the cord as soon as the uterus had contracted without waiting for signs of placental separation. However, in clinical practice the midwives were waiting for signs of separation before applying traction to the cord. A survey of 33 midwives working in the delivery suite showed that 16 preferred to wait for signs of separation and descent of the placenta before applying traction to the cord, although some of the midwives did state that if they were supervising a student midwife they would teach the student to apply traction immediately as they, the midwives, knew this was the method taught in the school of midwifery. A review of the literature showed that Brandt (1933) had investigated separation of the placenta by injecting sodium iodide into the umbilical vein in 30 women after the delivery of the baby, and had taken an X-ray within three minutes of the baby's birth. In every case the placenta was separated and lying in the lower segment of the uterus. As a result of this Brandt (1933) recommended that after the baby was born the cord should be clamped and the cord held close to the vulva with one hand. The other hand should then push the uterus upwards to the umbilicus. If the placenta had separated there was only a slight tension on the cord and delivery of the placenta could be accomplished by supra-pubic pressure. Working independently Andrews (1940) came to the same conclusions and the Brandt-Andrews technique was widely used for many years. Spencer (1962) describes the practice of a modified Brandt-Andrews technique in the delivery of 1000 women experiencing normal delivery. Intravenous ergometrine (0.5 mg) was given with the delivery of the baby's anterior shoulder, the baby was delivered slowly, the cord was divided and the baby was passed to an assistant. Contraction of the uterus was ascertained and then steady upward and backward pressure was exerted on the uterus at the same time as 'controlled cord traction' (CCT) was applied to the cord. Nine hundred and seventy-three women experienced a normal third stage of labour, six had a PPH, 15 a manual removal of placenta and six both a PPH and manual removal of placenta. The mean blood loss was 91 ml (SD 81 ml) with 603 women having a loss of up to 100 ml and in only 51 women did the loss exceed 284 ml. However, despite the fact that Spencer (1962) describes this as a 'trial' she did not compare the modified Brandt-Andrews technique with any other method of care or management.

One problem in caring for women is accurately assessing the blood loss at delivery. Frequently blood is mixed with liqour and it also soaks into the sheets and pads. Making an accurate assessment of the amount of blood lost is thus very difficult and it is known that there is great variation between individuals. Brant (1967) calculated blood loss at delivery by direct measurement of loss and by measuring haemoglobin from soiled sheets. He compared his findings with the estimate of the accoucheuse/accoucher and found that in losses up to 300 ml estimates were fairly accurate but higher blood losses were more and more inaccurately assessed. In measuring loss and the haemoglobin from soiled sheets he found a PPH rate in women experiencing a normal delivery of 20%. In another attempt to be more accurate in measuring blood loss at delivery Haswell (1981) developed a drape and pouch which was placed under the woman's buttocks at delivery. He claimed that blood, but not liqour, was collected but did not explain how this was achieved.

In view of the differing views between what was being taught and what was being practised and the concerns over potentially inaccurate estimates of blood loss Moore and Levy (1982, 1983) felt there was a need for further investigation of these problems.

Methods

Two studies are reported here, a prospective study examining the effects of CCT before waiting for evidence of placental separation/descent compared with waiting for these signs before attempting CCT and a study to assess the accuracy of estimation of blood loss at delivery (Moore and Levy, 1982, 1983).

In the first study a prospective study of factors affecting the PPH rate in women whose placenta had been delivered by CCT was carried out between January and August 1981 (Moore and Levy, 1982). On a proforma midwives were asked to record whether the following factors were present prior to the application of CCT:

- contraction of the uterus;
- cord lengthening, had a third cord clamp been used to check this;
- trickle of blood *per vaginum*;
- uterus had risen in the abdomen;
- narrowing of the uterus;
- mobility of the uterus.

The estimated blood loss was recorded. The midwives were also asked to record whether they had waited for signs of placental separation and/or descent before they delivered the placenta, and the method they used to deliver the placenta.

The inclusion criteria were all women who had a normal delivery, whose placenta was delivered by CCT and who delivered between January and August 1981. A PPH was defined as a loss of 500 ml or more.

In the second study (Moore and Levy, 1983) assessing the accuracy of estimations of blood loss four units of date-expired blood were obtained from the haematology department. The blood was divided into four measured amounts – 100 ml, 300 ml, 500ml and 1200 ml. Two hundred ml of normal saline were added to each amount of blood to mimic a moderate amount of liquor. A quantity of blood and saline was poured on to one or two green towels and an incontinence pad (to imitate conditions at delivery), on four separate trolleys in the sluice. Some of the blood and saline was left in each jug, and the trolleys were labelled one to four.

A sample of convenience of those staff available in the delivery suite on the day the data were collected was used. One of the midwife teachers stood at the door of the sluice and recruited the participants while the other midwife teacher remained in the sluice. The participants were told that there were four measured amounts of blood, one on each of the trolleys, and that they were asked to estimate how much blood was on each trolley, including the amounts in the jugs, as they would do if they were estimating blood loss at a delivery. The participants were told that the blood was mixed with saline equal to a moderate amount of liquor and that the same amount of saline was mixed with each amount of blood. The participants were also told that the blood contained citrate and therefore would not clot. Participants were given disposable plastic gloves to wear so that they could handle the towels and incontinence pads if they so wished. After they had made their estimates the participants were told the actual amount of blood on each trolley.

Findings

Data collection sheets on 546 deliveries were received for the prospective study. However, only 489 could be analysed. The remaining 57 could not be used either because the data were incomplete or because the method of delivery of the placenta was other than CCT.

Thirty-four of the 489 (7%) women had had a PPH. Data were analysed comparing the findings for two groups:

Group 1 where signs of separation and descent were awaited, $n = 335$
Group 2 where signs of separation and descent were not awaited, $n = 154$.

Five per cent (16) of women in the group in which signs of separation were awaited experienced a postpartum haemorrhage (blood loss of 500 ml or more) compared with 12% (18) of those in the group where signs of separation were not waited for. This difference was significant ($\chi^2 = 7.791$, df = 1, $p < 0.01$). However in the latter group although the midwife did not await for signs of separation they did occur in 120 women. Of these 120 women 13% (16) experienced a PPH. Of the remaining 34 women where the midwives did not wait for signs of separation or descent, nor saw any, two women had a PPH.

Of the 335 deliveries where signs of separation and/or descent were awaited, lengthening of the cord was the sign noticed most frequently (Table 11.13) with a trickle of blood *per vaginum*, rising of the fundus in the abdomen, narrowing of the fundus and uterine mobility occuring in the frequency order. There was no difference in the mean lengths of the third stage (Table 11.14, page 314).

In the study of the accuracy of estimated blood loss, 12 midwives, two student midwives, one very experienced nursing auxiliary and one obstetric registrar took part, a total of 16 participants. The estimations are shown in Table 11.15 and support Brant's (1967) findings that the greater the blood loss the greater the under estimation. It should also be noted

Table 11.13 Signs of placental separation and descent observed during the third stage of labour

	(n = 335)*	
	No.	%
Lengthening of the cord	304	91
Trickle of blood *per vaginum*	294	88
Fundus rises	152	45
Uterus more mobile	76	23
Fundus narrows	48	14

* More than one sign exhibited by some women.
Source: compiled from Levy and Moore (1982).

Table 11.14 Mean lengths of third stage

Method of CCT	Mean length in min
Group 1 (waited)	5.0
Group 2 (did not wait)	4.3
Sub-group 2a (signs nevertheless seen)	4.4
Sub-group 2b (no signs seen)	4.0

Source: compiled by Levy and Moore (1983).

Table 11.15 Estimations of blood loss in ml

Amount of blood	Range of estimation	Mode	Mean	Error in mean estimation
100	20–400	100	111	+11
300	65–550	200	197	−103
500	125–750	250	307	−193
1200	450–2000	550	718	−482

Source: compiled by Levy and Moore (1983).

that most participants estimated the 1200 ml loss as 550 ml, less than half has its actual amount.

Discussion

Concern about dissonance between teaching and clinical practice led two midwife teachers to investigate two factors in the management of the third stage of labour, whether signs of separation and or descent should be awaited before applying CCT, and the accuracy of blood loss estimations. Their findings from the retrospective analysis of information from the third stage of labour would suggest that awaiting signs of separation and/or descent before applying CCT would reduce the amount of blood lost and the incidence of PPH. However, they did not undertake a randomized controlled trial. Although both Bonham (1963) and Kemp (1971) undertook studies into the management of the third stage of labour using CCT, neither assessed the value of waiting for signs of placental separation compared with applying immediate cord traction. It appears that this aspect of management of the third stage of labour still awaits scientific evaluation by a randomized controlled trial.

Concern for accurate estimation of blood loss is not confined to the midwifery profession. However, the findings from the small study on the estimation of blood loss at delivery suggest cause for concern. The over estimations could lead to women being at best subjected to unnecessary blood tests and at worst being subjected to unnecessary transfusion. The under estimation shown here, particularly in the two highest losses, is potentially, very debilitating for women.

INFLUENCES ON WOMEN'S REACTIONS TO CAESAREAN DELIVERY

In part fulfilment of her studies for a degree in sociology and psychology Kirchmeier (1985) undertook a study to investigate factors which affect women's perception of a delivery by caesarean section.

Despite the increase in the caesarean section rate at that time Kirchmeier found that there was very little research which had investigated the psychological effects of caesarean section on the mother (Marut and Mercer, 1979; Trowell, 1982; Cranley *et al.*, 1983). Using a sample of convenience Marut and Mercer (1979) compared the experiences of 30 primiparous women who had had a vaginal delivery (spontaneous and assisted) with 20 primiparous women who had had an emergency caesarean section under either regional or general anaesthesia. Trowell (1982) also used a sample of convenience of primiparous women and also compared women who had had a vaginal delivery (*n* = 18) with a group of women who had had an emergency caesarean section under general anaesthesia (*n* = 16). The study by Cranley *et al.* (1983) compared three groups of women, 40 who had had a vaginal delivery, 39 who had had an unexpected caesarean section and 43 who had had an elective caesarean section. This latter study again used a sample of convenience, included both primiparous and multiparous women and women who had had regional or general anaesthesia. These studies found that caesarean section was regarded as a serious deviation from the normal birth events and led to unmet expectations. Unmet expectations may result in feelings of guilt, failure, disappointment and anger; a sense of failure at not being able to fulfil the expected role as a natural mother; a sense of guilt at putting the baby in danger and depriving her partner of the shared experience of birth; and a sense of anger and disappointment at having been deprived of a natural birth herself (Marut and Mercer, 1979; Trowell, 1982; Cranley *et al.*, 1983).

There were two factors which may limit some of the negative feelings. Firstly, women who had a caesarean section under regional anaesthesia viewed their experience more positively than those who had a general anaesthetic and were therefore unconscious when their baby was born

(Marut and Mercer, 1979; Cranley *et al.*, 1983). Secondly, women who had an elective caesarean section viewed the experience more positively than those who had an emergency caesarean section in labour (Cranley, *et al.*, 1983). Kirchmeier (1985) suggests that because women who had an elective caesarean section know about this during pregnancy they are able to prepare themselves for the event. Using regional anaesthesia for the operative delivery means that the delivery approximates as closely as is possible to a vaginal delivery. A continuum from the normal (vaginal) method of delivery to the most abnormal is shown in Figure 11.1. This figure shows four groups representing the different types of caesarean section.

Apart from the work of Trowell (1982), which assessed maternal attitudes and behaviour at one month and one year post delivery, most of the research assessing women's reactions to caesarean section had concentrated on the first few days after delivery and there was no work assessing whether these reactions change over time. The first aim of Kir-

Figure 11.1 Continuum of four experimental groups arranged according to how nearly they approximate to a spontaneous vaginal delivery.

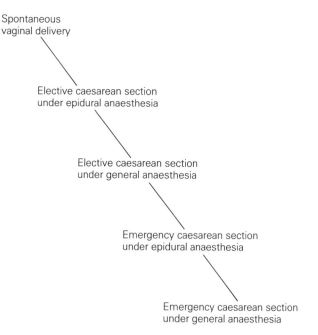

Source: compiled by Kirchmeier, 1985.

chmeier's study was to establish whether the reactions to caesarean section were the same for women in the four caesarean section groups and to compare their reactions to those of a control group of women who had had a vaginal delivery. The second aim of the study was to assess whether the reactions to caesarean section changed over a period of eight weeks.

Methods

A quasi-experimental design was used, utilizing the natural groupings of the four types of caesarean section and a control group of women who had delivered vaginally. Four methods of data collection were utilized and are summarized in Figure 11.2. At 3–4 days post delivery all women filled in a birth perception questionnaire and those who had had a caesarean section were also interviewed. Those women who had had a vaginal delivery and all those who had had an emergency caesarean section filled in a birth perception questionnaire adapted from that of Marut and Mercer (1979). This asked the women to answer questions such as 'Do you remember your labour as painful?', 'To what extent did your experience of having a baby go along with the expectations you had before labour began?' on a five point scale from 'not at all' to 'extremely'. All the women who had had an elective caesarean section were asked to fill in a perception of birth questionnaire adapted from that of Cranley *et al.* (1983). This again utilized a five point rating scale from 'not at all' to 'extremely' and asked questions such as 'How relaxed were you during the pre-operative procedures?', 'To what extent do you wish you could have experienced labour?' During the postnatal interview the women were asked questions to elicit demographic and pregnancy related data; how prepared the woman was for having a caesarean section and her initial reactions when told;

Figure 11.2 Summary of methods of data collection.

Time of administration	Data collection method	Groups responding
3–4 days post delivery	Perception of birth questionnaire – labour and delivery (from Marut and Mercer, 1979)	All types of caesarean section. Spontaneous vaginal delivery
3–4 days post delivery	Perception of birth questionnaire – pre-operative procedures and delivery (from Cranley *et al.*, 1983)	All types of caesarean section
3–4 days post delivery	Structured interview	All types of caesarean section
8 weeks post delivery	Postal questionnaire	All types of caesarean section

Source: compiled by Kirchmeier, 1985.

method of anaesthesia and whether chosen by the woman or prescribed by the anaesthetist; overall picture of the woman's reactions to having a caesarean section and how understanding her partner, relatives and friends were.

Because of time and money constraints it was not possible to interview the women who had had a caesarean section at eight weeks post delivery. Therefore, they were sent a questionnaire which attempted to assess whether their reactions had changed over time. This information was obtained in two ways. Firstly the women were asked to answer the following five questions:

1. What are your feelings now about having had a caesarean section?
2. Do you feel as though you are able to care for the baby adequately having had a caesarean section?
3. Does your partner understand the way you feel?
4. Do your relatives understand the way you feel?
5. How would you feel about needing a further caesarean section if it were necessary?

Secondly in an attempt to overcome busy mothers writing 'I feel fine' the women were asked to tick which statements of a provided list best described their feelings at that time.

Recruitment to the study was made by Kirchmeier and all women were very willing to take part.

Findings

Seventy-five women agreed to take part in the study, 15 in each of the caesarean groups and 15 in the spontaneous vaginal delivery group. All were between 38 and 42 weeks gestation at the time of delivery; 66 (75%) were married, six were not married but were living with their partner and three were single. The women came from a predominantly middle class socioeconomic group, thus reflecting the catchment area of the hospital where the data collection was undertaken. Both primiparous and multiparous women were included in the study.

Perception of birth. The findings from this study on perceptions of birth support those from the previous studies (Marut and Mercer, 1979; Trowell, 1982; Cranley *et al.*, 1983). The women in the two emergency caesarean section groups felt significantly less positive about their labour experience than did the women in the spontaneous vaginal delivery group ($t = 2.09, p < 0.05$). The women in both of the planned caesarean section groups felt significantly more positive about their labour/preoperative procedures and delivery experiences than did the women in the two emergency caesarean section groups ($F = 13.26, p < 0.01$). The women who knew they were going to have a caesarean section were significantly more positive about their delivery than those women who had an emergency caesarean section ($F = 8.93$, $p < 0.01$). As Kirchmeier (1985) stated 'forewarned was definitely forearmed'.

Again the findings on the effect of the different types of anaesthesia on birth perceptions support the findings of Marut and Mercer (1979) and Cranley *et al.* (1983). The women in the two groups whose caesarean section was performed under epidural anaesthesia had significantly more positive views about their delivery than did those women who were given a general anaesthetic ($F = 9.864$, $p < 0.01$). Also the women whose caesarean section was performed under epidural anaesthesia (both emergency and elective) were able to enjoy their initial contact with the baby significantly more than the women in the two groups who had general anaesthesia for their caesarean section ($F = 10.9$, $p < 0.01$).

Perception of caesarean section over time. There was a significant change in the women's perceptions over time to all five questions but these changes were not significantly related to the type of anaesthesia or whether the caesarean section was elective or an emergency (Kirchmeier, 1985).

Discussion

As in previous work on this topic the sample size was small and a sample of convenience was used. Therefore the findings cannot be generalized to a larger population. However, the findings of reactions to a caesarean section within the immediate postpartum period do support those of previous studies (Marut and Mercer, 1979; Trowell, 1982; Cranley *et al.*, 1983). Therefore it is suggested that there are some points which midwives should consider.

Women who had an elective caesarean section had more positive views than did those who had an emergency caesarean section. This is possibly because they were able to prepare themselves for this type of delivery. Books on childbirth do not always have the most up-to-date information about caesarean section. However organizations such as the National Childbirth Trust and the Caesarean Support Group have produced literature on the subject, as well as providing postnatal support for these women.

Women who had an epidural anaesthesia expressed fewer negative comments than did those women who had general anaesthesia. Kirchmeier (1985) suggests that epidural anaesthesia improves the quality of a caesarean delivery and allows a surgical operation to be as near as possible to a vaginal delivery. Being awake when the baby was born and being able to share the moment of birth with their partner were reasons given by women for choosing epidural anaesthesia. Another possible reason for the lower level of negative feelings in this group of women is that the women reported feeling involved in the decision on the type of anaesthesia. Whilst regional anaesthesia is still not available everywhere in the UK, for those women for whom it is an option, and where there is time to make this choice, Kirchmeier suggests that midwives and doctors should encourage women to choose regional anaesthesia for a caesarean section.

The women who expressed, at 3–4 days and at eight weeks post delivery, the most negative feelings about their delivery were the women who had an emergency caesarean section under general anaesthesia. Further research should be undertaken to assess whether there are any interventions, such as debriefing the women, which might reduce these negative feelings.

DISCUSSION

The studies reported in this chapter were small and some had methodological problems. In some of the studies the sample sizes were constrained because of the reason for undertaking the study, for example, in part fulfilment of a degree (Henderson, 1984, 1985; Kirchmeier, 1985). However, this does not mean that lessons cannot be learnt by those practising midwifery. Henderson (1984) questioned a routine practice which had extended from obstetric practice into midwifery. The sample size was small in that only 28 vaginal examinations were observed. Although the reader has been given information about the women experiencing the examinations there is no information about the demographic details of the midwives performing the examinations. It is not possible to generalize the findings but individual midwives should, as a result of this study, be stimulated to reflect on whether they are giving women enough information so that they, the women, can make an informed decision on whether a particular procedure is right for them. As a result of this study midwives should also have a heightened awareness of whether they are exercising autonomy over their practice or whether they are deluding themselves into thinking they are when in fact they are just carrying out an obstetric ritual. Since Henderson's study neither of the randomized controlled trials of routine amniotomy in a woman experiencing an uncomplicated labour have shown it to have any advantage over leaving the membranes to rupture spontaneously (Fraser *et al.*, 1991; Barrett *et al.*, 1992) and one has shown that there are disadvantages to this routine practice (Barrett *et al.*, 1992).

The studies of the use of a delivery chair in the second stage of labour (Hillan, 1984; Romney, 1984, 1987) demonstrate the importance of evaluating a new treatment before it is made generally available. Not only is it important to evaluate a treatment but it is important that the research methods used have validity. Romney's first study (Romney, 1984) was only an observational study, not a randomized controlled trial, and the findings appeared to suggest that there were advantages in using a chair for delivery when compared with the bed. However a subsequent randomized controlled trial did not support the earlier findings (Romney, 1987) and actually found disadvantages in using the chair when compared with the delivery bed. Although Hillan's (1984) study was reported to be a randomized controlled trial it is strange that the numbers of women in each group were equal, suggesting that allocation to each of the treatment groups was not random. In neither of these two latter studies (Hillan, 1984; Romney, 1987) were the sample sizes calculated to exclude type 1 and type 2 errors (Freiman *et al.*, 1978; Detsky and Sackett, 1985) therefore the validity of the findings must be questioned. However, one subsequent study has, using a sample size calculated to exclude type 1 and type 2 errors, shown that the chair has no advantage over the bed and that there is an increased incidence of postpartum haemorrhage in women delivered in the chair (Currell *et al.*, 1991).

Postpartum haemorrhage was the topic of the studies undertaken by Moore and Levy (1982; 1983). They examined two aspects, whether signs of placental separation should be waited for before CCT is applied and estimation of blood loss at delivery. In both studies samples of convenience were used and the sample sizes were small. Although randomized controlled trials of active versus physiological management of the third stage of labour have been carried out (Prendiville *et al.*, 1988; Begley, 1990) there have not been any studies that have examined a particular part of active management of the third stage, namely whether signs of placental separation should be awaited before CCT is applied. No further studies have assessed estimation of blood loss at delivery but midwives should be aware of the potential to underestimate blood loss, particularly where a large blood loss has occurred.

Caesarean section can be a life-saving operation and some may feel that women should be very grateful that they, the women, and their babies are alive and well after the procedure. However, Kirchmeier's (1985) study has shown that there are some actions that midwives can take which will enhance the woman's perception of the birth of her baby. Women who used an epidural anaesthetic had more positive views of the experience than did those who had a general anaesthetic. Encouraging women, when appropriate, to use this form of anaesthetic in preference to a general anesthetic will obviously improve postnatal perceptions. Where epidural anaesthesia is not available, because of funding and/or staffing inadequacies, midwives should be at the forefront of the fight to obtain these services for childbearing women. Women who had an elective caesarean section had more positive views than did those who had an emergency caesarean section, probably because they were able to prepare themselves. Whilst midwives would hope that all women would have a normal vaginal delivery a small proportion of women do have to be delivered by caesarean section and one way of reducing negative postpartum views of caesarean delivery may be to give all women antenatal education on the possibility of caesarean section. This aspect needs further research.

In his evidence to the House of Commons Health Committee on the Maternity Services in the UK (House of Commons, 1992) Iain Chalmers is reported as saying that midwives ask different questions from those asked by obstetricians. The research reported in this chapter supports that statement.

REFERENCES

Andrews, C.J. (1940) Third stage of labor with evaluation of Brandt method of expression of placenta. *Southern Medicine and Surgery*, **102**, 605–8.

Begley, C. (1990) A comparison of 'active' and 'physiological' management of the third stage of labour. *Midwifery*, **6**(1), 3–18.

Barrett, J.F.R., Savage, J., Phillips, K. and Lilford, R.J. (1992) Randomized trial of amniotomy in labour versus the intention to leave membranes intact until the second stage. *British Journal of Obstetrics and Gynaecology*, **99**, 5–9.

Beard, R., Brudenell, M., Dunn, P. and Fairweather, D. (1975) Discussion on augmentation of labour. In *Management of labour. Proceedings of the 3rd study group of the RCOG.* Royal College of Obstetricians and Gynaecologists, London.

Bonham, D.G. (1963) Intramuscular oxytocics and cord traction in the third stage of labour. *British Medical Journal*, **2**, 1620–23.

Brandt, M.L. (1933) The mechanisms and management of the 3rd stage of labour. *American Journal of Obstetrics and Gynecology*, **25**, 662–7.

Brandt, H.A. (1967) Precise estimation of post-partum haemorrhage difficulties and importance. *British Medical Journal*, **i**, 398–400.

Caldeyro-Barcia, R., Schwartz, R., Belizau, R. *et al.* (1974) Adverse perinatal effects of early amniotomy during labour. In L. Gluck (ed.) *Modern perinatal medicine.* Year Book Medical Publishers, Chicago.

Chalmers, I. (1989) Evaluating the effects of care during pregnancy and childbirth. In I. Chalmers, M. Enkin and M.J.N.C. Keirse (eds) *Effective care in pregnancy and childbirth.* Oxford University Press, Oxford.

Cranley, M.S., Hedahl, K.J. and Pegg, S.H. (1983) Women's perceptions of vaginal and caesarean births. *Nursing Research*, **32**(1), 10–15.

Currell, P., Elbourne, D., Ashurst, H., Garcia, J., Murphy, D. and Duigan, N. (1991) Delivery in an obstetric chair: a randomized controlled trial. *British Journal of Obstetrics and Gynaecology*, **98**, 667–74.

Detsky, A.S. and Sackett, D. (1985) When was a negative clinical trial big enough? How many patients you needed depends on what you found. *Archives of Internal Medicine*, **145**, 709–12.

Donald, I. (1969) *Practical obstetric problems*, 4th edn. Lloyd-Luke, London.

Fraser, W.D., Sauve, R., Parboosingh, I.J., Fung, T., Sokol, R. and Persaud, D. (1991) A randomized controlled trial of early amniotomy. *British Journal of Obstetrics and Gynaecology*, **98**, 84–91.

Freiman, E.A., Chalmers, T.C., Smith, H. and Kuebler, R.R. (1978) The importance of beta, the type 2 error and sample size in the design and interpretation of the randomised controlled trial. *New England Journal of Medicine*, **299**(193), 690–94.

Haswell, J.N. (1981) Measured blood loss at delivery. *Journal of Indiana State Medical Association*, **74**(1), 34–6.

Henderson, C. (1984) Some facets of social interactions surrounding the midwife's decision to rupture the membranes. Unpublished MA thesis, University of Warwick.

Henderson, C. (1985) Influences and interactions surrounding the midwife's decision to rupture the membranes. In S. Robinson and A.M. Thomson (eds) *Proceedings of the 1984 Research and the Midwife Conference*. Department of Nursing, University of Manchester.

Hillan, E. (1984) The birthing trial. In S. Robinson and A.M. Thomson (eds) *Proceedings of the 1983 Research and the Midwife Conference*. Department of Nursing, University of Manchester.

House of Commons Select Committee (1992) Sessions 1991–1992, Second Report. *Maternity services*. (Chairman: Nicholas Winterton) HMSO, London.

Kemp, J. (1971) A review of cord traction in the third stage of labour from 1963 to 1967. *Medical Journal of Australia*, **1**, 899–903.

Kirchmeier, R. (1985) Influences on mothers' reactions to caesarean birth. In S. Robinson and A.M. Thomson (eds) *Proceedings of the 1984 Research and the Midwife Conference*. Department of Nursing, University of Manchester.

Kirkham, M. (1983) Admission in labour: Teaching the patient to be patient? *Midwives Chronicle and Nursing Notes*, **96**(1141), 44–5.

Kreis, J. (1928) L'accouchement medical. *Review France Gynecology Obstetrics*, **19**, 604–16.

MacArthur, C., Lewis, M. and Knox, E.G. (1991) *Health after childbirth*. HMSO, London.

Macintyre, S. (1982) Communications between pregnant women and their medical and midwifery attendants. 1981 Sir William Power Memorial Lecture. *Midwives Chronicle and Nursing Notes*, **95**(1138), 387–93.

Marut, J.S. and Mercer, R.T. (1979) Comparison of primiparas' perceptions of vaginal and caesarean deliveries. *Nursing Research*, **28**(5), 260–66.

Maternity Services Advisory Committee (1984) *Maternity care in action, Part II: care during childbirth (intrapartum care), a guide to good practice and a plan for action*. HMSO, London.

Meredith, S. (1983) Natural childbirth. *Midwife, Health Visitor and Community Nurse*, **20**, 228–30.

Moore, J. and Levy, V. (1982) Research into the management of controlled cord traction related to the incidence of postpartum haemorrhage. In A.M. Thomson (ed.) *Proceedings of the 1981 Research and the Midwife Conference*. Department of Nursing, University of Manchester.

Moore, J. and Levy, V. (1983) Further research into the management of the third stage of labour and the incidence of post partum haemorrhage. In A.M. Thomson and S. Robinson (eds) *Proceedings of the 1982 Research and the Midwife Conference*. Department of Nursing, University of Manchester.

National Childbirth Trust (1989) *Rupture of the membranes in labour, a survey*. NCT, London.

NM News (1981) *Nursing Mirror*, **153**(17), 5.

O'Driscoll, K., Foley, M. and MacDonald, D. (1984) Active management of labour as an alternative to caesarean section for dystocia. *Obstetrics and Gynecology*, **63**, 485–90.

O'Driscoll, K. and Meagher, D. (1980) *Active management of labour*. WB Saunders, Philadelphia.

Oakley, A. (1980) *Women confined: towards a sociology of childbirth*. Martin Robertson, Oxford.

Prendiville, W., Harding, J., Elbourne, D.R. and Stirrat, G.M. (1988) The Bristol third stage trial: active versus physiological management of third stage of labour. *British Medical Journal*, **297**, 1295–300.

Robinson, S., Golden, J. and Bradley, S. (1983) *A study of the role and responsibilities of the midwife*. Nursing Education Research Unit, Report No 1. Chelsea College, University of London.

Romney, M. (1984) Chair project. In A.M. Thomson and S. Robinson (eds) *Proceedings of the 1983 Research and the Midwife Conference*. Department of Nursing, University of Manchester.

Romney, M. (1987) The birthing chair, a random controlled trial. In S. Robinson and A.M. Thomson (eds) *Proceedings of the 1986 Research and the Midwife Conference*. Department of Nursing, University of Manchester.

Spencer, P. (1962) Controlled cord traction in management of the 3rd stage of labour. *British Medical Journal*, **1**, 1728–32.

Stewart, P. and Spiby, H. (1989) A randomized study of the sitting position for delivery using a newly designed obstetric chair. *British Journal of Obstetrics and Gynaecology*, **96**, 327–33.

Tasker, M., Verduijn, C.P., Bassett, C. and Murray, K. (1991) A randomized controlled trial of early amniotomy. *British Journal of Obstetrics and Gynaecology*, **98**, 1059–60.

Trowell, J. (1982) Possible effects of emergency caesarean section on the mother-child relationship. *Early Human Development*, **7**, 41–51.

Index

Page numbers appearing in **bold** refer to figures and page numbers appearing in *italic* refer to tables.